The four hemopoietic colony-stimulating factors (CSFs) are the major regulators in the body of the production and activity of two types of white blood cells - granulocytes and macrophages. Since these cells are primarily responsible for innate resistance to infections, the CSFs are now being used clinically in the treatment of patients with damaged blood-forming systems as a result of disease or cancer chemotherapy.

This book provides a detailed and up-to-date account of the discovery of the CSFs, their structure, molecular biology, and cellular receptors, the biology of the CSFs in vivo and in vitro, and their present and possible future clinical applications.

Written by two of the pioneers in the discovery of the CSFs, it is a clear and well-illustrated survey of the history, current knowledge, and future directions of this exciting field of investigation, and also serves as a guide to the more general areas of growth factor and cytokine research. It will prove an invaluable review for cell biologists interested in how growth factors act on the body, as well as for clinicians applying the fruits of modern biotechnology to improved patient care.

# THE HEMOPOIETIC COLONY-STIMULATING FACTORS

# THE HEMOPOIETIC COLONY-STIMULATING FACTORS

## From biology to clinical applications


DONALD METCALF

*The Walter and Eliza Hall Institute of Medical Research, Melbourne*

NICOS ANTHONY NICOLA

*The Walter and Eliza Hall Institute of Medical Research, Melbourne*


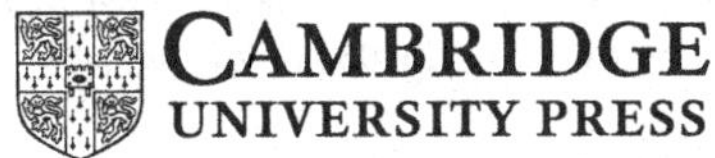

CAMBRIDGE UNIVERSITY PRESS
Cambridge, New York, Melbourne, Madrid, Cape Town, Singapore, São Paulo

Cambridge University Press
The Edinburgh Building, Cambridge CB2 2RU, UK

Published in the United States of America by Cambridge University Press, New York

www.cambridge.org
Information on this title: www.cambridge.org/9780521461580



First published 1995
This digitally printed first paperback version 2006

*A catalogue record for this publication is available from the British Library*

*Library of Congress Cataloguing in Publication data*
Metcalf, Donald.
The hemopoietic colony-stimulating factors : from biology to
clinical applications / Donald Metcalf, Nicos Anthony Nicola.
p. cm.
Includes bibliographical references and index.
ISBN 0-521-46158-8 (hc)
1. Colony-stimulating factors (Physiology) I. Nicola, Nicos,
1950– . II. Title.
[DNLM: 1. Colony-Stimulating Factors. 2. Hematopoiesis.
3. Receptors, Colony-Stimulating Factor. WH 140 M588c 1995]
QP92.M47 1995
612.1′12 – dc20
DNLM/DLC
for Library of Congress 94-23237
CIP

ISBN-13 978-0-521-46158-0 hardback
ISBN-10 0-521-46158-8 hardback

ISBN-13 978-0-521-03481-4 paperback
ISBN-10 0-521-03481-7 paperback

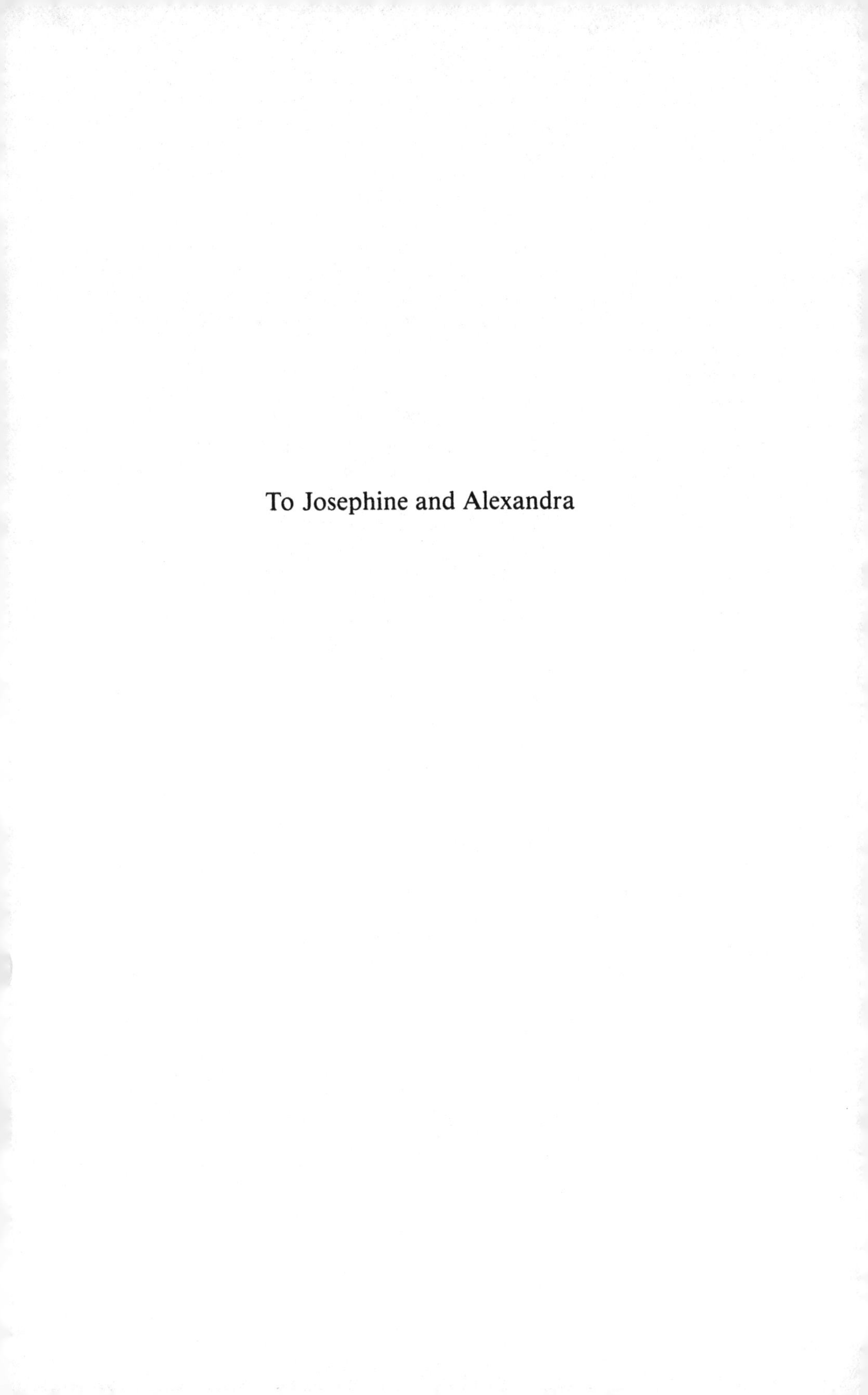

To Josephine and Alexandra

# Contents

# Preface

Our objective in writing this book was to prepare an up-to-date account of the colony-stimulating factors - hemopoietic regulators that have now entered clinical use. We assumed that this could be accomplished with sufficient documentation in a book of moderate length with perhaps some 600 references. However, we were discomfited to find that, in the past decade alone, there have been more than 12,000 publications on the colony-stimulating factors, and we were forced to exercise a higher level of selectivity than originally anticipated. We attempted to acknowledge the work of others by broad referencing, but inevitably we are probably guilty of overreferencing our own studies, which have lodged more firmly in our memories. For this we beg the indulgence of our colleagues.

On one matter we have exercised deliberate bias. It happens that most of what we know about the biochemistry and biology of the colony-stimulating factors was established first with murine systems and was only subsequently confirmed with human systems. We have noted a growing unawareness, particularly among our clinical colleagues, that this was so and have therefore written the account in a manner that makes the real sequence of discovery evident. The biology of mice and humans can differ significantly, but in most respects this is not the case for the colony-stimulating factors, and any pretensions to be dismissive of earlier mouse studies must be firmly checked. Progress has resulted from a fruitful interaction between both groups of investigators, and we are therefore happy to dedicate this account to all of our colleagues and competitors in acknowledgment of their achievements.

The authors are indebted to Richard Mahony and Peter Maltezos for preparing the text figures and to Elizabeth Hodgson for her meticulous preparation of the manuscript. We thank Louise Wardrop, Kerrie Ayberk, Josephine Marshall, and Helen Ried for their assistance in compiling the references.

# 1
# Historical introduction

Erythropoietin was the first humoral regulator of hemopoietic cells to be recognized and was discovered in the serum in 1906 as a consequence of some simple in vivo experiments on rabbits made anemic by bleeding (Carnot and Deflandre, 1906). While the purification of erythropoietin – from anemic human urine – was not completed until 70 years later (Miyake et al., 1977), extensive studies using impure preparations of erythropoietin were performed in animals during the 1950s and 1960s.

It was assumed that erythropoietin would be the prototype of comparable regulators for hemopoietic cells in other lineages. However, despite extensive in vivo studies using manipulated animals and tissue extracts, in the 60-year period until the mid-1960s, no convincing evidence was produced for the existence of comparable regulators.

The 30 years since that time have seen a major change in this situation, because at least 20 hemopoietic regulators have now been characterized. This has been achieved by the use of tissue-cultured hemopoietic cells to provide initial bioassay systems. For each of these regulators, only subsequently was it possible to undertake experiments in animals to verify the biological actions of the regulator. Initially during this period, the discovery process required the purification by separative biochemistry of the active factors from medium conditioned by tissues or cell lines. More recently, this method of discovery has been progressively supplanted by the initial detection of new regulators by direct expression screening of cDNA pools, using cell lines as bioassays. Furthermore, the biochemical characterization of the active molecules has been made from recombinant protein, which has then been used to establish the actions of the regulator on normal cells.

The colony-stimulating factors (CSFs) were the first regulators to be discovered after erythropoietin, and the history of their development (Table

1.1) bridges the transition between discovery by characterization of active native molecules and the subsequent discovery process using recombinant factors. For this reason, there was already extensive knowledge of the in vitro biological actions of the native CSFs before the first recombinant CSFs became available to permit in vivo studies in animals.

The CSFs were discovered as a consequence of the development of methods for growing granulocytic and/or macrophage colonies from bone marrow cells cultured in semisolid medium (Figure 1.1) (Bradley and Metcalf, 1966; Ichikawa et al., 1966). In such cultures, spontaneous proliferation of granulocytic and macrophage cells was not observed, and the formation of colonies required the addition of feeder cells, tissue fragments (Bradley and Metcalf, 1966), or medium conditioned by various tissues (Pluznik and Sachs, 1966). There was an obvious relationship between the amounts of such material added and the number and size of colonies developing, which offered a method for quantifying the stimulus being added.

The operational term "colony-stimulating factor" was applied to the active factor that it was necessary to introduce into the cultures by these maneuvers. It was felt to be a reasonable possibility that CSF might actually be a genuine regulator of granulocytic and macrophage cells, analogous to the known erythropoietic regulator erythropoietin.

Initial studies showed that a variety of organ tissues could stimulate granulocytic and macrophage colonies to develop when fragments of such tissues were co-cultured with marrow cells. Furthermore, comparable activity was demonstrable in medium (conditioned media) harvested from cultures of such organ fragments or from a variety of cell lines. Colony-stimulating activity, usually resulting in the formation mainly of macrophage colonies, was also observed when mouse or human sera or human urine was added to murine bone marrow cultures (Robinson et al., 1967; Foster et al., 1968b; Robinson et al., 1969).

Supporting the possibility that CSF might be a significant regulator of granulocyte and macrophage formation in vivo were observations that levels of colony-stimulating activity could be elevated in the serum or urine of mice or patients with infections and some types of leukemia – situations in which perturbations in these populations might be expected.

Beginning in the late 1960s, attempts were commenced in various laboratories to characterize the nature of CSF, also termed macrophage-granulocyte inducer (MGI). These indicated its likely protein nature, and initially the most extensively studied sources were human urine and medium conditioned by either mouse embryonic cells or mouse fibroblasts (Stanley and Metcalf, 1969; Landau and Sachs, 1971; Stanley et al., 1971).

Table 1.1. *Chronology of CSF publications*

| Event | Murine | | | | Human | | | |
|---|---|---|---|---|---|---|---|---|
| | GM-CSF | G-CSF | M-CSF | Multi-CSF (IL-3) | GM-CSF | G-CSF | M-CSF | Multi-CSF (IL-3) |
| First description of partially characterized native molecule | 1973 | 1980 | 1971 | 1974 | 1979 | 1979 | 1969 | — |
| Purification of native molecule | 1977 | 1983 | 1977 | 1982 | 1984 | 1985 | 1975 | — |
| Cloning of cDNA | 1984 | 1986 | 1987 | 1984 | 1985 | 1986 | 1985 | 1986 |
| First in vivo testing in mice | 1987 | 1986[a] | 1988[a] | 1986 | — | — | — | — |
| First clinical trials using recombinant CSF | — | — | — | — | 1987 | 1988 | 1992 | 1990 |

[a] In vivo testing in mice performed using cross-reactive human G-CSF or M-CSF.

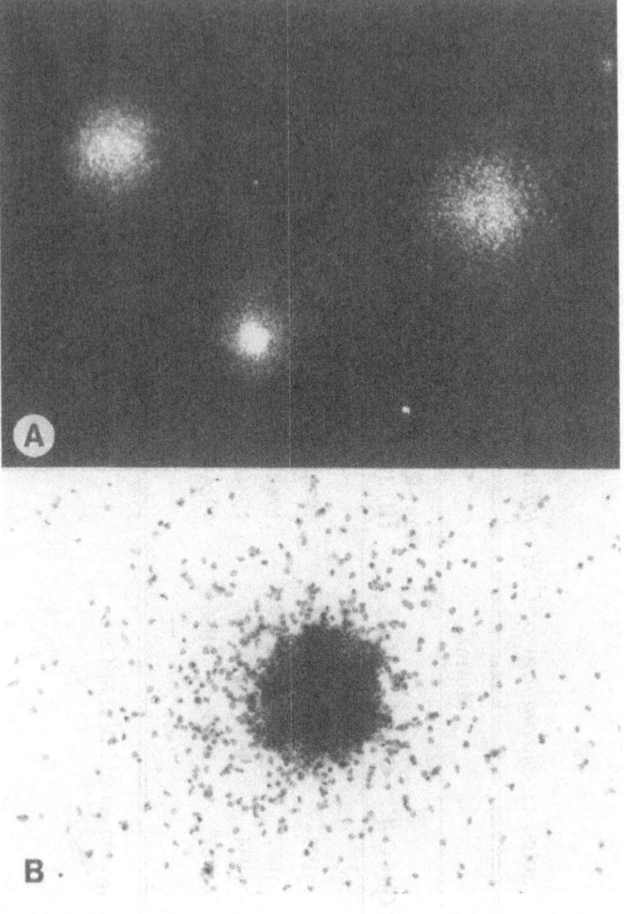


Figure 1.1. (A) Portion of an unstained culture of mouse bone marrow cells stimulated by a mixture of GM-CSF, G-CSF, and Multi-CSF showing the general appearance of the granulocyte-macrophage colonies developing after 7 days of incubation. (B) Granulocyte colony from such a culture after staining. Less mature cells are concentrated in the central region, and more mature cells migrate to form a corona around the colony.

This work led in 1975 to the purification of CSF from human urine, and this molecule appeared to be a glycoprotein of molecular weight (MW) 45,000 (Stanley et al., 1975). Oddly, this CSF appeared virtually unable to stimulate colony formation by human marrow cells in conventional agar cultures (Metcalf, 1974a) but was an effective stumulus for colony formation by mouse bone marrow cells. Unlike the original cultures that developed both granulocytic and macrophage colonies, the murine colony formation stimulated by human urinary CSF was predominantly macrophage in type, and this macrophage colony-stimulating factor was designated as M-CSF (alternatively, CSF-1).

While this work was in progress, it was observed that extracts of all mouse tissues contained detectable CSF (Sheridan and Stanley, 1971), as did medium conditioned by minced fragments of such tissues. Lung-conditioned medium appeared of special interest not only because its level of activity was higher than that from other tissues, but because the medium stimulated both granulocytic and macrophage colony formation, and the apparent molecular weight of the active factor was only 23,000 (Sheridan and Metcalf, 1973a). Because lung tissue from mice preinjected with endotoxin contained and produced higher levels of CSF than did control lung tissue (Sheridan and Metcalf, 1972), a program was commenced to purify the CSF in medium conditioned by lung tissue from mice preinjected with endotoxin.

Purification of this lung-produced form of CSF, given the name granulocyte-macrophage colony-stimulating factor (GM-CSF), was achieved in 1977 (Burgess et al., 1977) at the same time as parallel work achieved purification of murine M-CSF (CSF-1) from medium conditioned by mouse L-cells (Stanley and Heard, 1977). The murine M-CSF again appeared to be a markedly larger molecule (MW 70,000) than GM-CSF. Subsequent studies showed that M-CSF exists as a homodimer and that the monomeric polypeptide has a molecular weight of 26,000, more similar to that of native GM-CSF.

The period 1971–1978 saw the development of modified culture procedures that allowed the formation of erythroid, megakaryocytic, and multipotential hemopoietic colonies (Metcalf, 1984). Erythroid colony formation, as anticipated, required addition of erythropoietin (Stephenson et al., 1971), but erythroid colony formation from less mature precursors could be strongly enhanced by the addition of a variety of cell- or tissue-conditioned media, suggesting that other factors could stimulate the proliferation of earlier erythroid precursors. Eosinophil colony formation was recognized as occurring in cultures stimulated by many of the same types of crude conditioned media, including in particular mitogen-stimulated, lymphocyte-conditioned medium (Johnson and Metcalf, 1980). Part of this latter activity was subsequently shown to be due to the presence of a separate eosinophil regulator produced by T-lymphocytes – interleukin-5 (IL-5) (Sanderson, 1992). The formation of what were probably megakaryocytic colonies had been noted in cultures of mouse marrow cells stimulated by medium conditioned by the murine myelomonocytic leukemic cell line

WEHI-3B, and cells of the same tumor stimulated the formation in marrow cultures of curious dispersed colonies of novel morphology (Metcalf et al., 1969). However, the most efficient method for stimulating megakaryocytic colony formation was later found to be the use of mitogen-stimulated mouse lymphocyte-conditioned medium (Metcalf et al., 1975), an agent that also stimulated the formation of multipotential colonies (Metcalf et al., 1979).

These miscellaneous observations prompted attempts to establish the nature of CSF in both pokeweed mitogen–stimulated spleen lymphocyte-conditioned medium (SCM) and WEHI-3B-conditioned medium. In this laboratory, the assumption was made that distinct factors were likely to be responsible for stimulating these various colony types to develop, and initial results suggested that some separation of the biological activities seemed possible. However, other purification studies suggested that the various colony-stimulating activities in WEHI-3B-conditioned medium might be ascribed to a single-factor (Bazill et al., 1983), a conclusion eventually confirmed as purification studies were continued. The name "multipotential CSF" (Multi-CSF) was coined in this laboratory for the factor of MW 23,000–28,000 that stimulated colony formation by granulocytic, macrophage, eosinophil, megakaryocytic, blast, erythroid, mast, and multipotential cells (Cutler et al., 1985).

These conclusions were preempted by the successful completion of an apparently unrelated study investigating the active factor in WEHI-3B-conditioned medium that induced the enzyme 20$\alpha$-hydroxysteroid dehydrogenase in cultures of spleen cells or certain hemopoietic cell lines, thought at the time to be T-lymphoid in nature. This study, involving a rapid single bioassay, was completed promptly, and the name "interleukin-3" (IL-3) was coined for the active factor (Ihle et al., 1982). Subsequent analysis of the properties of this factor indicated that they were identical to those emerging for Multi-CSF (Ihle et al., 1983). A somewhat comparable analysis of the active factor in WEHI-3B-conditioned medium was based on a bioassay in which normal mast cells were stimulated to proliferate, and these studies identified an active factor, termed P-cell-stimulating factor. Subsequent amino acid analysis of this factor revealed it also to be IL-3 (Multi-CSF) (Clark-Lewis et al., 1984).

During an analysis of the CSF present in human placenta-conditioned medium, it was noted that a distinct form was present (termed CSF$\beta$) that was highly hydrophobic and selectively stimulated granulocytic colony formation (Nicola et al., 1979b). In parallel studies on the nature of the elevated levels of CSF in the serum of mice preinjected with endotoxin, the major form of CSF appeared to be M-CSF, but on chromatography, highly hydrophobic fractions were observed that again stimulated the formation almost exclusively of mature granulocytic colonies (Burgess and Metcalf, 1980). Both observations suggested the existence of a further type of CSF. Neither placenta-conditioned medium nor serum was a particularly suitable starting material for fractionation, but a survey of organ-conditioned media from mice preinjected with endotoxin revealed the presence of active material with the similar dual properties of high hydrophobicity and selective granulocytic colony-stimulating activity (Nicola and Metcalf, 1981). It was also noted that this candidate CSF had the capacity to induce differentiation in colonies of WEHI-3B leukemic cells. Using the twin bioassays of granulocytic colony formation and induction of differentiation in WEHI-3B colonies, this CSF was purified to homogeneity from mouse lung-conditioned medium as a glycoprotein of MW 25,000 and given the name "granulocyte colony–stimulating factor" (G-CSF) (Nicola et al., 1983).

Thus, by 1983, four distinct CSFs had been purified in small amounts from murine sources and had become available to the laboratories concerned for limited analyses of their in vitro biological actions on hemopoietic cells.

With the prototype example of human M-CSF, it was assumed that comparable human CSFs existed for the other three murine CSFs. In human placenta-conditioned medium, it was shown that two forms of CSF existed, termed initially CSF$\alpha$ and CSF$\beta$, which had biochemical and biological properties comparable with murine GM-CSF and G-CSF, respectively (Nicola et al., 1979b), and receptor competition studies confirmed that human CSF$\beta$ must be closely similar to murine G-CSF (Nicola et al., 1985).

The successful purification of human GM-CSF from medium conditioned by the Mo T-leukemic cell line was accomplished in 1984 (Gasson et al., 1984). In simultaneous studies, human G-CSF was purified from medium conditioned by a bladder cancer cell line 5637, initially under the name of "pluripoietin" (Welte et al., 1985), and by a squamous carcinoma cell line (Nomura et al., 1986). The successful purification of native human Multi-CSF (IL-3) (Zenke et al., 1991) was achieved only subsequent to the characterization of recombinant human Multi-CSF.

The period during which human GM-CSF and G-CSF were being purified overlapped the period during which cDNAs encoding the murine CSFs were being cloned. Two groups independently cloned cDNAs encoding murine IL-3 by direct expression screening of cDNA pools using continuous murine cell lines as the proliferation bioassay (Fung et al., 1984; Yokota et al., 1984). This was followed by the cloning of a cDNA for murine GM-CSF using amino acid sequence-based nucleotide probes and cDNA libraries from lung and a T-lymphocyte cell line (Gough et al., 1984). Cloning of cDNAs for human GM-CSF was accomplished by groups either using direct expression screening of cDNA pools from the human leukemic Mo cell line (Wong et al., 1985) or using murine cDNA probes on a human cDNA library (Cantrell et al., 1985). This was followed in 1986 by the cloning of cDNAs for human G-CSF using nucleotide probes based on amino acid sequence data from G-CSF (Nagata et al., 1986a; Souza et al., 1986).

A genomic clone encoding human M-CSF was isolated using a sequence-based cloning strategy (Kawasaki et al., 1985), and subsequently a cDNA encoding murine M-CSF was obtained (De Lamarter et al., 1987).

The successful cloning of a cDNA for human IL-3 was a more difficult feat, since murine-based probes were unsuccessful because of species divergence between the two molecules. It was eventually accomplished by direct expression screening of a primate cDNA library and the use of primate clones to probe a human cDNA library (Yang et al., 1986).

All four murine and human CSF cDNAs were expressed with various degrees of difficulty in bacterial, yeast, or mammalian expression systems, with the production of biologically active recombinant CSF. These studies indicated that the carbohydrate content of the native CSF glycoproteins was not necessary for biological activity in vitro.

Some early in vivo studies had been performed in mice using crude embryo-conditioned media containing high CSF levels (Bradley et al., 1969) or semipurified human urinary M-CSF (Metcalf and Stanley, 1971). These suggested that granulocytic and progenitor cell levels could be elevated by the injection of CSF. However, the ability to produce recombinant CSFs in relatively large amounts permitted the first effective studies to be performed on the action of fully purified CSFs on hemopoiesis in animals. The first such in vivo studies in mice were reported in 1986 for IL-3 (Multi-CSF) (Kindler et al., 1986; Metcalf et al., 1986a) and G-CSF (Fujisawa et al., 1986), and these were followed by comparable studies using GM-CSF and M-CSF. This work led to studies in primates of the actions of human GM-CSF, G-CSF, and Multi-CSF. The effectiveness of these CSFs in elevating white cell levels without obvious toxic effects in normal primates or primates with drug- or radiation-induced aplasia led to the commencement of human trials using purified recombinant CSF.

The first Phase I clinical study on injected CSFs analyzed the responses of AIDS patients to GM-CSF (Groopman et al., 1987), and this was followed by two Phase I studies on the responses of cancer patients to injected G-CSF (Gabrilove et al., 1988; Morstyn et al., 1988). The obvious capacity of these two CSFs to increase white cell levels with minimal adverse responses led rapidly to Phase II studies of both in marrow-transplanted patients and in cancer patients following chemotherapy. A general extension of such trials led to the first approval for clinical use of G-CSF and GM-CSF in 1992. Clinical trials of Multi-CSF and M-CSF were initiated during this same period, although to date neither has yet been licensed for medical use.

Since 1977 there has been a progressive recognition of the curiously pleiotropic actions of the CSFs on hemopoietic cells in vitro. However, the present clinical uses of CSFs are based largely on their actions as mandatory proliferative stimuli for granulocyte and monocyte-macrophage formation, and the present knowledge of the broader biological actions of CSFs on these populations has yet to be fully exploited in clinical applications.

During this same period, at least 15 other hemopoietic regulators were characterized, with increasing awareness of the existence and probable importance of regulator networks and the likelihood that these regulators were designed to function most effectively when acting in combination (Metcalf, 1993b). This knowledge has begun to reach the clinical trial stage with the first tentative use of regulator combinations. However, the critical assessment of the opportunities for therapy now available is a formidable problem. It cannot really be accomplished until laboratory studies provide a compelling case for the use of certain defined combinations for particular clinical problems. In short, the discovery and availability of recombinant hemopoietic growth factors have grossly outstripped the capacity for clinical assessment of these agents, and it is currently proving to be a logistical nightmare for pharmaceutical companies attempting their introduction into clinical medicine. This is not helped by the regulatory requirement that each first be demonstrated to be effective as a single agent when the biology of hemopoietic regulators indicates that they are most effective when used in combination.

# 2
# General introduction to hemopoiesis

To appreciate more clearly the roles played by the colony-stimulating factors in hemopoiesis, it is necessary to outline some aspects of the origin and organization of hemopoietic populations, the major cellular events occurring during hemopoiesis, and the general methods by which these events are regulated.

The first hemopoietic cells arise from nonhemopoietic precursors as a transient finite event in the blood islands of the yolk sac (Metcalf and Moore, 1971). Many of these cells then migrate to the fetal liver, where they build up to a large population (Figure 2.1) (Moore and Metcalf, 1970; Metcalf and Moore, 1971). The major recognizable cells in such populations are embryonic erythroid cells and macrophages, although populations of stem cells and progenitor cells are also present. At least in chickens, and presumably also in mammals, this yolk sac–derived hemopoietic population becomes replaced by a second population of hemopoietic cells arising de novo from nonhemopoietic precursors in the para-aortic region of the fetus (Dieterlen-Lievre and Martin, 1981). These fetus-derived hemopoietic populations replace the existing yolk sac–derived cells in the liver and then populate the developing spleen and bone marrow.

It is believed that no further de novo formation of hemopoietic cells occurs. As a consequence, throughout subsequent adult life, the hemopoietic populations are required to be self-sustaining as well as to generate continuously the large number of maturing cells in the eight major hemopoietic lineages that are needed to replace the relatively short-lived cells in the peripheral blood.

Soon after birth, hemopoietic populations decline in the liver, and the relative importance of splenic hemopoiesis also progressively declines so that, in the adult, most (>95%) hemopoietic tissue is located in the bone marrow in scattered locations throughout the body (Metcalf and Moore,

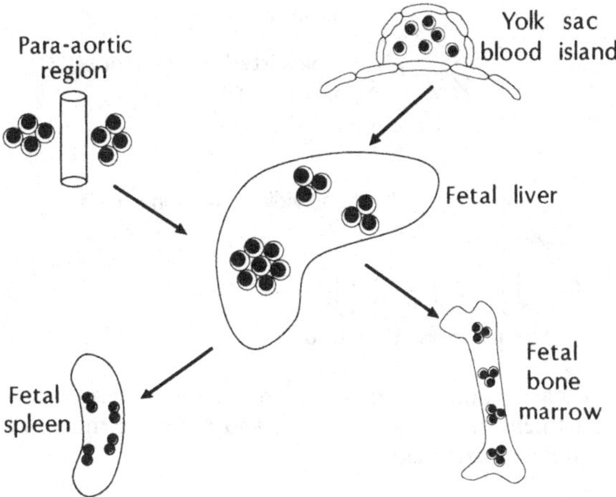


Figure 2.1. Schematic diagram of the early events in the development of the hemopoietic organs. Hemopoiesis begins in the yolk sac, from which cells migrate to the fetal liver. The fetal liver hemopoietic population is probably replaced during fetal development by a second wave of de novo hemopoiesis originating in the para-aortic region. The hemopoietic populations in the marrow and spleen are derived from migrants from the fetal liver.

1971). Particularly in the mouse, the spleen retains a capacity to expand rapidly its content of hemopoietic cells in situations requiring increased hemopoiesis, and if demand is extreme or the bone marrow is diseased the liver can also become reactivated as a hemopoietic organ.

While maturing cells in hemopoietic tissue are readily identifiable by their characteristic morphology and can be arranged into likely maturation sequences, these maturing populations are not organized in architecturally stratified layers, as is the situation in tissues such as the skin or gut. Instead, hemopoietic regions of the marrow and spleen appear to contain an almost random admixture of cells of different lineages and maturation stages. This is not true in all species, and in the chicken there is obvious segregation of granulocytic from erythroid populations in the marrow. Data from an analysis of the location of stem cells in mouse marrow have also suggested that there is some segregation of these cells, particularly to regions adjacent to the bone cortex (Lord and Wright, 1984). Despite these data, the overwhelming impression is that hemopoietic cells are mixed in a virtually random manner in marrow tissue.

Hemopoietic tissues also possess a network of specialized stromal cells. Although the precise identity and architectural arrangement of these cells

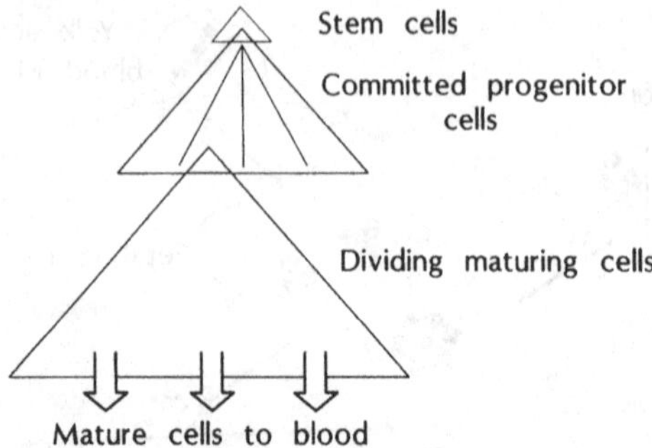


Figure 2.2. Three basic compartments in hemopoietic tissues. The cells in each succeeding compartment are the progeny of, and are more numerous than, the cells in the preceding compartment.

have yet to be characterized, they play a crucial role in permitting hemopoiesis and in regulating the cellular events that occur.

Identification of the nature and number of the more ancestral hemopoietic cells and their interrelationship has required the application of a number of clonal-analytical procedures. These analyses have indicated that hemopoietic cells in each lineage can be stratified into three major sequential cell populations, each of progressively larger size: stem cells, progenitor cells, and dividing maturing populations (Figure 2.2).

## Stem cells

Stem cells are a minor subpopulation of hemopoietic cells, numbering approximately 1 per $10^5$ marrow cells. When purified by complex cell-sorting protocols, stem cells have been shown to have the morphology of small to medium mononuclear (lymphocyte-like) cells. Most have a large nuclear to cytoplasmic ratio, and the nucleus often has prominent nucleoli. The cytoplasm is not basophilic and contains no granules. Under normal conditions, most of these cells are not in cell cycle, but the cells have an extensive potential capacity for self-generation and for the production of a large number of committed progenitor cells. It is now recognized that stem cells are a very heterogeneous group of cells, the heterogeneity probably being based on hierarchical parent–progeny relationships (Figure 2.3).

The most ancestral stem cells (termed repopulating cells) are capable of extensive self-renewal and are defined either by their capacity to repopulate hemopoietic and lymphoid organs on a long-term basis in irradiated animals or by their capacity to sustain long-term hemopoiesis in vitro.

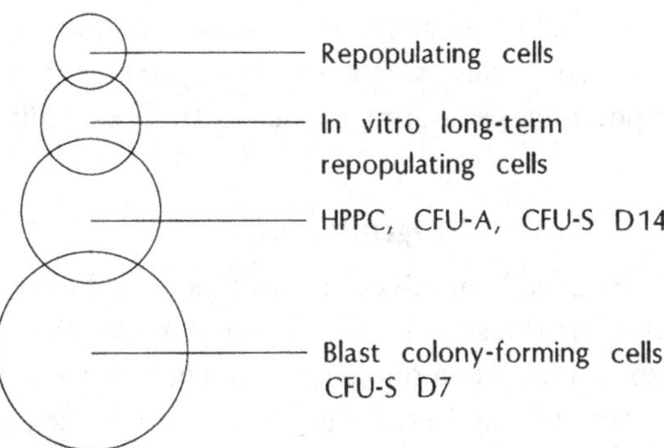


Figure 2.3. Hemopoietic stem cells are highly heterogeneous but are probably stratified in a hierarchical sequence of cells of increasing maturity with more restricted proliferative potential. HPPC denotes high proliferative potential cells.

In turn, their progeny stem cells (spleen colony–forming units, CFU-S) can be identified as being able (a) to form large hemopoietic colonies in the spleen of irradiated recipients (demonstrable at day 14 or, if more mature, persisting only until day 7) and (b) to form blast colonies or very large colonies of cells in multiple lineages in clonal in vitro cultures.

With highly enriched populations of murine stem cells ($Kit^+$ $Scal^+$ $Rh123^{lo}$ $Lin^-$ cells), 30 cells can permanently repopulate a lethally irradiated mouse, confirming the undoubted presence of repopulating cells in such preparations, yet all such cells can form blast colonies in appropriate agar cultures. As will be discussed later, the various stem cell assays must often detect the same stem cells, despite unequivocal evidence of hierarchical stratification within the stem cell population.

The least-mature subsets of stem cells certainly can form hemopoietic progeny in all eight major hemopoietic lineages, but the most mature of the hemopoietic stem cells may no longer generate T- or B-lymphocytes. This remains a somewhat unclear question, as does the possible existence of subsets of these mature stem cells committed exclusively to the formation of only T- and/or B-lymphocytes.

It is not possible to indicate how many progenitor cells an individual stem cell can generate. This depends on the stimuli applied to the stem cell and how much self-generation results. At one extreme, a stem cell might on occasion generate only two progenitor cells, while at the other extreme, a single stem cell can repopulate the hemopoietic tissues of an entire animal with evidence that such cells can then entirely repopulate secondary and tertiary recipients. Under in vitro culture conditions with appropriate stimuli and no evidence of self-renewal, individual stem cells can generate clones containing several thousand progenitor cells (Metcalf, 1991b), so their potential generating capacity can be exceedingly large.

## Progenitor cells

Progenitor cells are usually in cell cycle, have the morphology of medium to large mononuclear (blast) cells with agranular basophilic cytoplasm, and comprise up to 1% of hemopoietic cells. These are a transit population formed by stem cells and expending themselves in the production of maturing progeny. From analyses performed in vitro, these cells appear to have a minimal or no capacity for self-generation.

Progenitor cells are characterized by their capacity to form colonies of maturing progeny in semisolid cultures in response to stimulation by hemopoietic growth factors. The number of cells in such colonies can vary from five or ten thousand down to the lower limit for defining clones as colonies (usually 50 cells for most colony types). The variable size of these colonies is one of the parameters indicating the heterogeneity of progenitor cells even within one differentiation lineage. Cells forming colonies of small size are most likely to be the progeny of cells forming large colonies, a relationship most clearly evident in the erythroid lineage, where the progenitor cells are divided into two major classes - BFU-E, forming large, often multicentric (burst) colonies, and CFU-E, forming small colonies that are the equivalent of one of the subclones of a multicentric colony formed by BFU-E (Figure 2.4).

Progenitor cells appear to differ from stem cells in being committed, usually to a single lineage of differentiation. Bi- and trilineage-committed progenitor cells do exist but are less frequent than single-lineage progenitors and are likely to be the immediate ancestors of the latter cells. Bipotential granulocyte-macrophage progenitor cells are somewhat different, at least in the mouse, in being a major subset of progenitor cells in this closely related pair of lineages.

Most evidence indicates that differentiation commitment is irreversible, which means that progenitor cells cannot switch to another lineage or revert to multipotential stem cells.

## Dividing and maturing populations

These cells comprise the vast majority of cells present in hemopoietic tissues. They are the progeny of progenitor cells in a particular lineage and

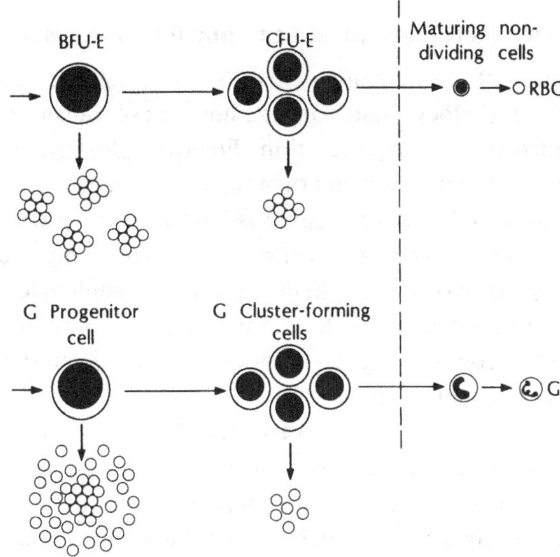


Figure 2.4. Progenitor cells in the erythroid lineage (BFU-E and CFU-E) can be identified by their ability to form colonies in semisolid cultures. Granulocyte progenitors (G) can be similarly detected. With increasing maturation, a progressive reduction occurs in the number of progeny generated by individual progenitor cells. RBC denotes red blood cell.

form a morphologically recognizable sequence of cells within each lineage – for example, myeloblasts → promyelocytes → myelocytes → metamyelocytes → polymorphonuclear neutrophils (the last cell type is often referred to throughout the text simply as "granulocytes").

The least mature of these cells have a considerable capacity for proliferation and can produce clones of subcolony size in semisolid cultures. Their capacity for proliferation is probably not strictly fixed, as proposed in earlier studies, but it is dependent on the level of stimulation exerted by relevant growth factors. Nevertheless, their proliferative capacity is limited in most lineages, although there are obvious exceptions in the T- and B-lymphoid lineages.

With progressive maturation, a progressive restriction is evident in the capacity of the cells for further proliferation, and typically the cells eventually mature to a postmitotic stage (e.g., metamyelocytes), after which no further cell division is possible. It is less clear whether macrophages are necessarily postmitotic cells, and under some circumstances apparently mature eosinophils may also exhibit a capacity for some cell division.

## Requirements for sustained hemopoietic cell formation

With the exception of at least some stem cells, the remaining cells that can form cells in the granulocyte-macrophage lineage are transit cells, which become expended by their proliferation. For example, myelocytes cannot self-renew and therefore expend themselves in generating metamyelocytes and polymorphs. Similarly, committed granulocytic progenitor cells cannot self-renew and will expend themselves by forming myeloblasts and myelocytes. Any capacity of the system to produce granulocytes and macrophages in a sustained manner therefore requires a continuous replenishment of lineage-committed progenitor cells by cells from the most ancestral, stem cell compartment.

The consequences of this arrangement are that when an agent like a CSF is used to stimulate granulocytic and/or macrophage formation by progenitor cells, the resulting increased cell production will terminate after a few days unless replacement progenitor cells are generated. The regulatory control of these different steps need not be identical; nevertheless, most regulatory factors do have actions at multiple levels. It becomes necessary, therefore, in the case of the CSFs to consider not only their actions on committed granulocyte-macrophage progenitor cells and their progeny, but also whether the CSFs have observable actions in stimulating progenitor cell formation by stem cells and possibly even stem cell self-renewal.

As will be seen, the CSFs do have proliferative actions on cells in all three of the major hemopoietic compartments, although the magnitude of this action varies at the different stages, as can the nature of other regulatory factors interacting with the CSFs to control cells in the different stages.

## General regulation of hemopoiesis

The events involved in the formation and function of blood cells are highly complex, since they include (as shown in Figure 2.5) precisely coordinated new cell formation occurring in the widely separate populations of hemopoietic cells scattered throughout the body, correct lineage commitment, the initiation and completion of maturation with fidelity, controlled release of mature cells, maintenance of circulating blood cell levels, selective exit of some but not all cell types to the tissues, functional activation of such cells when necessary, coupled finally with a system for detecting and eliminating effete cells.

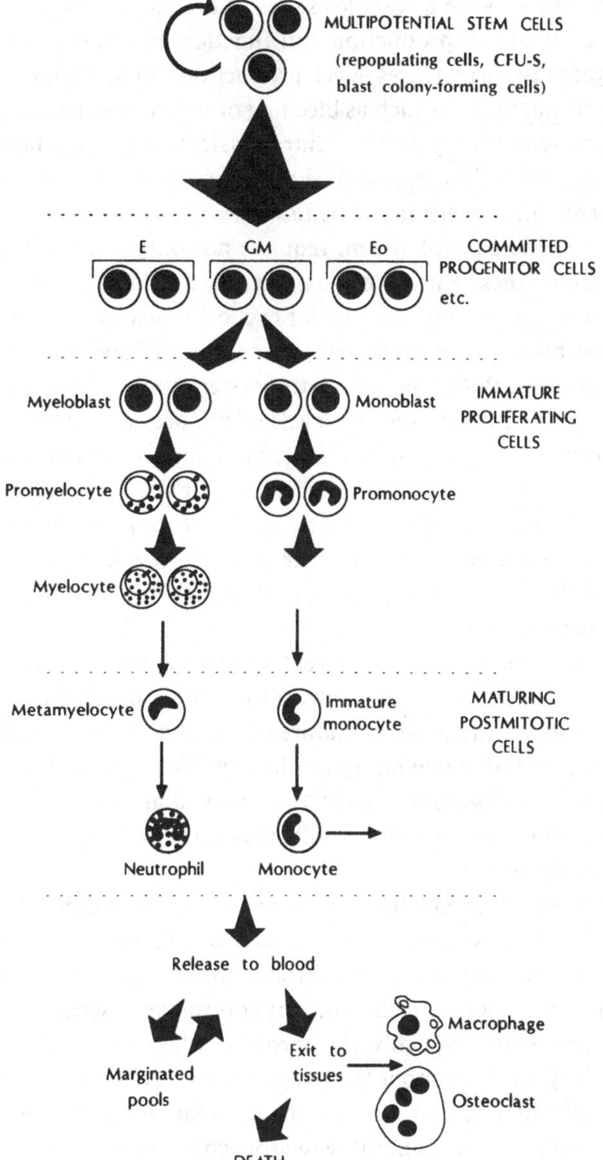


Figure 2.5. Schematic diagram of the major stages by which mature granulocytes and monocytes are generated. After release of mature cells from the bone marrow to the blood, the cells enter the tisues and, in the case of monocytes, undergo major changes in phenotype. E denotes erythroid progenitor cells; GM, granulocyte-macrophage progenitor cells; Eo, eosinophil progenitor cells.

The regulation of such a complex series of events must be arranged so that basal levels of cell production and function can be controlled with precision, yet massive increases in cell production can be achieved rapidly in response to emergencies such as bleeding or infections. The complexity and apparent redundancy of the control systems that have been documented by recent studies may well be necessary to accomplish these two quite different roles for hemopoietic tissues.

In principle, the control system requires not only a series of positive signals to initiate these various events, but also a balancing series of negative feedback signals to prevent major cyclic fluctuations in cell production and possibly to terminate amplified responses following restitution of normal conditions. Both types of control system could be activated by an inductive system based on sensing levels of mature cells, their products, or breakdown products or, alternatively, by an inductive system activated by tissue demands (e.g., oxygen deprivation or the presence of microorganisms). A feedback system based on monitoring of cell number or cell products would be elegant, but the weight of evidence suggests that the most likely induction systems that alter regulatory mechanisms are demand-generated (Metcalf, 1988a).

It was anticipated that quite different regulators would be necessary to control such different events as new cell production, release of mature cells, or functional activation of mature cells in the tissues. It may well be that there are exclusive regulatory mechanisms for some of these events; nevertheless, it has become evident that individual regulators can have actions on a wide range of these events, making the biology of such regulators extremely complex.

Regulation of cell production is achieved by what superficially appears to be a dual control system: (a) local control by microenvironmental cells located in the actual hemopoietic tissues, often involving intimate cell contact with hemopoietic cells, and (b) control by a series of humoral regulatory molecules, typically glycoproteins which can be produced by multiple cell types throughout the body. The two systems are not as separate as might first appear because the stromal cells have the capacity to produce many of the humoral regulators concerned and, under conditions of basal hemopoiesis, may be the major sources of these molecules. Furthermore, for at least some of the regulators, the stromal cells have an ability to produce them in a form held on the cell membrane, providing in part the molecular basis for the observed need for cell contact between stromal cells and responding hemopoietic cells if hemopoiesis is to be optimal. Although none have so far been discovered, it remains likely that stromal cells may produce unique regulatory molecules not produced elsewhere in the body. Alternatively, a regulator displayed on a stromal cell membrane might elicit responses in an adherent hemopoietic cell that are quite different from those elicited by the secreted form of the same regulator acting on nonadherent hemopoietic cells.

## Stromal control of hemopoiesis

The evidence supporting the role of stromal cells in hemopoiesis comes from two separate groups of observations. After discovery of the phenomenon of hemopoietic colony formation in the spleen or marrow of irradiated mice injected with bone marrow cells (Till and McCulloch, 1961), it was shown that such colonies were clones and that these colonies were generated by ancestral hemopoietic cells now regarded as more mature stem cells. Spleen colonies, when examined early (7 days), often appear to be composed of cells of only a single lineage, for example, erythroid, granulocytic, or megakaryocytic. Analysis of spleen colony populations indicated that the cell initiating such colonies, the CFU-S, was capable of self-renewal, and progeny CFU-S could form colonies of multiple types, indicating that at least some were multipotential. A consistent difference was noted between the relative frequency of erythroid versus myeloid colonies developing in the spleen or bone marrow - spleen colonies being mainly erythroid, whereas marrow colonies were granulocytic.

The conclusions from these and related observations were that hemopoietic stromal cells could somehow support, by what seemed to be a cell contact process, the self-generation of stem cells and the formation by them of maturing progeny. It was proposed that heterogeneity existed between such stromal cells, as evidenced by the differing cellular composition of the colonies formed, and that different stromal cells could commit stem cells to selective cell formation in a particular lineage (Trentin, 1989).

Subsequent observations on the progenitor cell content of spleen colonies have complicated the conclusions drawn from this phenomenon of spleen colony formation. All colonies, regardless of the morphological type of their dominant cell population, contain committed progenitor cells of multiple lineages, and there is no significant difference between the lineage commitment range of progenitors in erythroid versus granulocytic colonies (Johnson and Metcalf, 1979).

While it seems likely that stromal cells can support stem cell proliferation and progenitor cell formation in vivo, the morphological differences between colonies appear to be based more on a subsequent amplification and maturation of progeny formed by particular progenitor cells in any one colony. Thus, the difference between an erythroid stromal cell and a granulocytic stromal cell may relate more to their differing capacities to stimulate or permit the selective proliferation of maturing cells in the erythroid or granulocytic lineages.

The general conclusions reached from these in vivo studies have been strongly supported by studies on long-term survival and proliferation of hemopoietic cells in cultures of bone marrow cells (Dexter et al., 1984). In such cultures an adherent layer of mixed stromal cells develops. Not only are these adherent cells crucial for the sustained formation of stem and progenitor cells, but cell formation is clearly concentrated in islands of cells firmly bound to the adherent layers. The long-term cultures have not proved sufficient to define fully the mechanisms involved. However, some information is beginning to emerge. For example, recent studies have shown that expression by the stromal cells of membrane-bound stem cell factor (SCF), as distinct from secretion by the cells of SCF into the medium, is essential for the sustained production of a large number of stem and progenitor cells (Toksoz et al., 1992).

The role played by hemopoietic stromal cells is therefore crucial in hemopoiesis. While the precise mechanisms remain to be determined, at the very least the stromal cells provide a permissive microenvironment in which hemopoietic cells can be stimulated to proliferate and mature, and more likely the cells also provide a local source of many of the required specific regulatory molecules.

In contrast to these observations on the importance of stromal cell contact for the behavior of stem cells, the proliferation of progenitor cells can be readily stimulated in dispersed semisolid cultures to form colonies of maturing cells under conditions in which no cell contact is present. Based on these two sets of observations, it is often stated that cell contact with microenvironmental cells is more important in controlling stem cell behavior and their formation of progenitor cells, while humoral regulators are the major regulators of events from the progenitor stage onward. This may be so, but the data do not really allow such a broad distinction to be made, and it is probably better to regard both control systems as potentially influencing all stages of hemopoiesis.

## Hemopoietic regulators

To date, at least 20 hemopoietic regulators have been molecularly defined, and the implications raised by this large number require some discussion.

Table 2.1. *Hemopoietic growth factors grouped according to their known target cells*

| Target population | Hemopoietic growth factors |
|---|---|
| Stem cells | SCF, IL-1, IL-6, Multi-CSF (IL-3), GM-CSF, G-CSF, M-CSF, LIF, IL-12, flk-ligand |
| Granulocytes | G-CSF, GM-CSF, Multi-CSF, IL-6, SCF, IL-11 |
| Monocyte-macrophages | M-CSF, GM-CSF, Multi-CSF, O-CSF |
| Eosinophils | Multi-CSF, GM-CSF, IL-5 |
| Megakaryocytes | SCF, Multi-CSF, GM-CSF, IL-6, LIF, mpl-ligand |
| Mast cells | Multi-CSF, SCF |
| Erythroid cells | Early: SCF, Multi-CSF, GM-CSF; Late: Epo |
| T-Lymphocytes | IL-1, IL-2, IL-4, IL-10, IL-7 |
| B-Lymphocytes | SCF, IL-7, IL-4, IL-6, IL-2 |
| Dendritic cells | GM-CSF |

*Abbreviations:* SCF, stem cell factor; IL-1 through IL-12, interleukins-1 through -12; GM-CSF, granulocyte-macrophage colony-stimulating factor; G-CSF, granulocyte colony-stimulating factor; Multi-CSF, multipotential colony-stimulating factor; LIF, leukemia inhibitory factor; O-CSF, osteoclast colony-stimulating factor; Epo, erythropoietin.

The most relevant of these regulators for the present discussion are listed in Table 2.1 together with the hemopoietic cell types identified as responding to them in one manner or another. As evident from this table, multiple regulators have been identified as having actions on cells in any one lineage (Figure 2.6). Typically, at least five to six regulators are known to be active on cells in any one lineage. The quantitative importance of a particular regulator in controlling cell production in a lineage can vary according to the particular stage the cells are at in the lineage and the presence or absence of other regulators that interact with the regulator in question. Furthermore, it is evident from Table 2.1 and Figure 2.6 that all of the hemopoietic regulators are active on cells of more than one lineage, and there are no known examples of a regulator with actions restricted to cells of a single lineage.

### Regulator redundancy

This arrangement has resulted in a commonly expressed view that hemopoietic regulators exhibit extreme redundancy - that there are far more regulators with appropriate actions than are really required to achieve the production of any one hemopoietic cell type. If this is correct, it should follow that deletion of any one regulator would have no observable effect

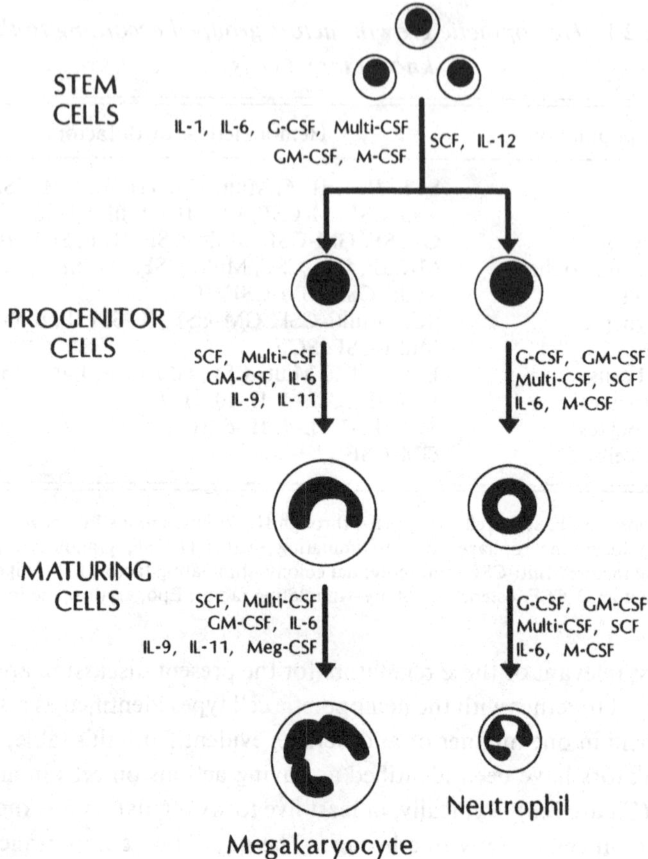


Figure 2.6. Schematic diagram showing the regulators involved in the formation of neutrophils and megakaryocytes. Note that, at each stage, multiple regulators can be shown to have proliferative actions. (Reproduced with permission from Metcalf, 1993b.)

on cell production, since its loss could readily be compensated for by the overlapping actions of other regulators.

However, there are alternatives to the redundancy hypothesis (Metcalf, 1993b). One possibility is that a hierarchy of regulators may exist - some with much greater importance or quantitative impact than others. Reasons will be given later why the CSFs are probably the most important regulators of granulocyte and macrophage formation even though, for example, SCF and IL-6 have some capacity to stimulate the formation of granulocytes.

A variant of this theme is that some regulators control basal levels of cell production, while others become important only in emergencies that require greatly increased cell production. This possibility is not fully resolved by existing data and has in particular led to the necessity for a careful examination of the effects of deleting CSFs, because CSF levels tend normally to be very low and become readily detectable only during emergencies. To preempt the discussion of these particular data, the conclusion to date is that there is no clear evidence for the existence of distinct "basal" versus "emergency" factors.

An important general concept to grasp is that hemopoietic regulatory factors are not exactly hormone-like in their biology. Unlike classical hormones, they do not have a single cell type as their source, and while they can often be detected in the circulation as would be expected of classical hormones, much of the production and action of hemopoietic regulators can occur locally. Thus, a particular regulator may be produced locally in the marrow at the site of responding immature hemopoietic populations while simultaneously, elsewhere in the body, a local inflammatory focus may be independently producing a high local concentration of the same regulator to achieve the local accumulation and activation of mature cells. Neither event will necessarily be detected by monitoring blood levels of that regulator. The general technical inability to assess local concentrations of regulators in these types of tissue continues to make it difficult to define the precise role played by a particular regulator in these various processes. Assessment of the situation is not helped by the capacity of some regulators to bind to the glycocalyx of some cells in a loose bonding that can potentially serve as a local, unmeasurable reservoir of a particular regulator (Gordon et al., 1987).

Given this biology of regulator production, it is somewhat naive to attempt to classify regulators as greater or lesser in importance either in basal or emergency circumstances by simple assessment of circulating regulator concentrations, although this is commonly implied in many publications. Because regulator production can occur at multiple local sites, including in particular hemopoietic tissues, circulating regulator concentrations can provide only a very incomplete view of actual regulator concentrations in various tissues.

A somewhat more sophisticated interpretation of the situation is to propose that certain regulators tend to act on early cells in a particular lineage, while others have their most important action on cells later in the sequence – the sequential notion of regulator control. This proposal has a certain elegance, and there are one or two cases where this interpretation may be reasonable. For example, in erythropoiesis it is evident that SCF and Multi-CSF have strong actions in stimulating the formation and initial cell divisions of the most ancestral committed erythroid progenitor cells (BFU-E), while, at least in a species like the mouse, erythropoietin has little or no action on such cells. Later in erythropoiesis, from the CFU-E stage onward, erythropoietin becomes the dominant regulator of erythroid cell proliferation. Unfortunately, this convincing example of sequential action is not typical of the situation in other lineages where individual regulators have readily demonstrable effects on cells at multiple stages in the lineage. On this basis, sequential action does not appear to be an adequate explanation for the existence of multiple regulators. Furthermore, whether or not a regulator appears to be active on cells of a particular lineage may be strongly influenced by what other regulators are acting on these cells. For example, in the megakaryocytic lineage, both SCF and IL-6, when acting alone, appear to be limited in their action to relatively mature precursors. Yet when either is combined with Multi-CSF, it becomes clear that each can exhibit significant proliferative actions on more ancestral cells in the sequence.

This introduces an important aspect of the biology of hemopoietic regulators, namely, the distinctive difference between the responsiveness of stem cells and most progenitor cells to stimulation by regulators. In vitro studies using purified populations of stem cells have consistently revealed that no single regulator can stimulate the proliferation of these cells (Li and Johnson, 1992). No combination of known regulators has yet been reported to stimulate stem cell self-renewal, but if the outcome of stimulation is assessed by production of progenitor cells and more mature progeny, stem cell proliferation requires combined stimulation by two or more regulators. This is in sharp contrast to the behavior of typical progenitor cells, whose proliferation can readily be stimulated by the action of single regulators.

From these facts, it becomes apparent that multiple regulators would be required if sustained cell production were to be achieved in any one lineage. Moreover, some progenitor cells have now been observed whose proliferation also appears to require multiple signaling by two or more regulators, extending the situations in which multiple regulators are necessary rather than redundant.

In vitro analysis has also revealed, as shall be discussed later for the CSFs, that the combination of two regulators can achieve greater levels of cell production by typical progenitor cells than can be achieved by the use of double the concentration of either regulator. Furthermore, where progenitors are bipotential or multipotential, the use of regulator combinations can achieve a broadening of the mature cell types being generated and, as in vivo studies have shown, a broadening of the distribution of the mature cells produced.

There is accumulating evidence, therefore, to support the view that the existence of a relatively large number of regulators with overlapping actions is not merely an example of biological redundancy; rather, the arrangement permits a subtlety and efficiency in cell production that can meet widely diverging requirements in health and emergencies (Metcalf, 1993b). Despite this conclusion, it should not be imagined that the injection of a single regulator in vivo would not achieve any observable effects on hemopoiesis. It is now common experimental and clinical experience that the injection of a single regulator can achieve remarkable biological responses. What the preceding discussion does make likely, however, is that the observed effects may not be due solely to the action of the injected regulator alone but may depend significantly on interactions with other regulators already present in the body.

The current controversies over the possible redundancy of hemopoietic regulators have made it of wide interest to determine the effects on hemopoietic populations of removing or suppressing each regulator. Two general approaches are possible: (a) the administration of neutralizing antibody to the regulator in question or (b) the identification or creation of animals in which the gene encoding the regulator has been inactivated in every cell. This is an active area of experimental investigation, particularly using the powerful approach in which the gene is inactivated in embryonic stem cells that are then used to generate chimeric animals. If chimerism involves either the sperms or ova, some of the progeny of such animals will have inactivation of one copy of the regulator gene, and by appropriate matings mice can be generated with homozygous inactivation of both genes.

Some of the regulators investigated by either approach are listed in Table 2.2. Certain comments can be made regarding the data obtained. In every case so far studied, suppression or deletion of a regulator has been observed to have some identifiable consequence, so no genuinely redundant regulators have been documented. In all cases, deletion of a single regulator has not resulted in a complete inability to produce cells in any one lineage. This result does indicate a degree of redundancy in hemopoietic regulators, but not complete redundancy. The effects of deletion can be quite subtle and appear to be compatible with a normal-enough life, at least for mice maintained under the protective conditions of pathogen-

Table 2.2. *Regulators examined by suppression or gene inactivation studies*

| Regulator | Consequences |
|---|---|
| Erythropoietin | Decreased erythropoiesis |
| GM-CSF | Defective resistance to lung infections |
| G-CSF | Neutropenia |
| M-CSF | Osteopetrosis, decreased macrophage populations |
| IL-2 | Elevated IgGl, IgE, and IgA reduced T-cell responses, autoantibody formation, inflammatory bowel disease |
| IL-4 | No IgE production, perturbed balance of Ig production, reduced TH2 cells |
| IL-6 | Increased rate of bone turnover, reduced T-cells, impaired resistance to infections |
| IL-10 | Elevated numbers of T- and B-lymphocytes and mast cells, inflammatory colitis |
| SCF | Decreased erythropoiesis |

free housing. While in each case distinctive deficiencies are identifiable, there is at least one instance (with M-CSF) where an eventual correction of the deficiency is achieved by the body.

Given the complexity of cellular processes required to activate hemopoiesis, it is not perhaps surprising that the control systems used should show evidence of both subtlety and fail-safe control systems.

## Regulator networks

The existence of, and interactions between, multiple hemopoietic regulators constitute a network of regulatory control, but this network is potentially far more complex.

Typically, each regulator can be produced by a wide variety of cell types – the most commonly involved being stromal cells, endothelial cells, fibroblasts, macrophages, mast cells, and lymphocytes. Curiously, individual cells, when induced, tend not to produce a single type of regulator but commonly to produce multiple types of regulators simultaneously. It is unclear why this should be a more efficient system, but it must be presumed that this arrangement has advantages. What is potentially possible with such an arrangement is that interactions between regulators, either competitive or enhancing, may also occur during the process of their production in addition to any interactions they may exhibit on responding cells.

There is also considerable potential complexity in the system controlling the production of hemopoietic regulators. For most regulators, the level of regulator production by cells under basal conditions is very low. The characteristic feature of regulator-producing cells is, however, that they can greatly amplify the transcription and production of a regulator when induced by appropriate signals and that this amplification can occur with great rapidity. The lability of the regulator-producing system is clearly of advantage in achieving rapid responses to emergencies but does require a system for producing appropriate inductive signals.

Figure 2.7 diagrams a very simple signaling network of the type that can be constructed by assembling data from individual in vitro experiments. In the diagram, an extrinsic signal (e.g., endotoxin) enters the body and either directly stimulates a cell (B) to increase transcription and production of a hemopoietic regulator or first stimulates another cell type (A) to produce an inducing signal for the regulator-producing cell. This

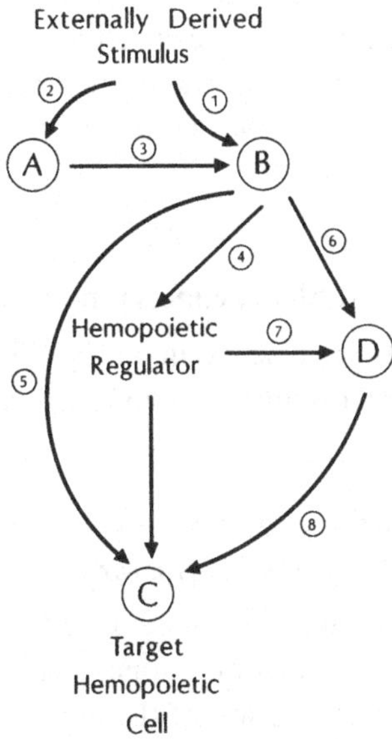


Figure 2.7. A simple regulator network showing some of the likely interactions among various cells. An externally derived stimulus such as endotoxin can initiate the production of a hemopoietic regulator (4) by cell (B) either by direct action (1) or by first stimulating (2) another cell (A) to produce an inducing signal (3) such as IL-1. The regulator-producing cell may simultaneously produce other factors (5) that have direct actions on the hemopoietic target cell or that influence (6) another cell (D) to produce factors with such actions (8). The hemopoietic regulator may also act directly (7) on such a cell to stimulate the production (8) of such factors.

regulator-producing cell will often simultaneously produce other factors that act directly on the hemopoietic target cell (C) to modulate the action of the hemopoietic regulator. Alternatively, these additional cell products may induce a further cell type (D) to produce factors influencing the response of the hemopoietic cell. The hemopoietic regulator itself may have a similar side action on such cells.

The scheme outlined is a relatively simple example of signal networking involving hemopoietic growth factors, and far more complex schemes can be devised, again based on observed actions of regulators on individual cell types in vitro. While all the individual events in such network diagrams may have been documented from isolated in vitro studies, they are necessarily theoretical models, and it is unknown whether the events actually occur in vivo and how important they are in the regulation of either basal hemopoiesis or enhanced hemopoiesis following emergencies.

The diagrams might again lead to the prediction that the injection of any single agent would be unlikely to override the dampening effects of the network or produce a measurable response in vivo. However, as noted earlier, the injection of a single agent can achieve reproducible responses, although networking may result in the occurrence of side effects of an injected agent on cells not themselves expressing receptors for the injected factor.

## Unresolved problems concerning hemopoiesis

It is relevant to the following discussion on the CSFs to comment briefly on certain unresolved general questions concerning hemopoiesis.

### *Is lineage commitment random or can it be influenced by extrinsic regulators?*

This is a central issue in hemopoiesis because it addresses the question of whether increased cell production in one lineage can be accomplished efficiently by the selective formation of the appropriate progenitor cells, or whether the process is an inherently wasteful one in which irrelevant progenitor cells are also formed that are not needed for the particular response.

When multipotential stem cells are stimulated to generate committed progenitor cells, analysis has shown that there is no fixed sequence in which committed progenitor cells are generated, because the initial daughter or granddaughter cells of multipotential cells can be a mixture of cells of virtually any lineage or lineage combination (Nakahata et al., 1982; Ogawa et al., 1983). This provides one answer to an old general question in cell biology, namely, whether cells generate like or unlike progeny at cell division. The same data have led to the conclusion that progenitor cell commitment is a stochastic event. However, the random nature of a process does not rule out the possibility that extrinsic regulators can influence the probability with which certain of these random events occur.

Four lines of evidence indicate that commitment can be influenced by extrinsic stimuli: (a) Apparently purified mouse hemopoietic stem cells can produce different types of progeny depending on whether they are injected intrathymically or intravenously or cultured in vitro. If injected intrathymically, T-lymphocytes are generated, whereas if they are injected intravenously, cells of all hemopoietic lineages are generated; if cultured in vitro, they generate progeny whose type depends on the growth factor combination used (Spangrude et al., 1988; Heimfield et al., 1991). (b) Various combinations of factors can induce the formation by stem cells of altered proportions of committed progenitor cells of various types (Metcalf, 1991b). (c) CSFs, when acting on bipotential granulocyte-macrophage progenitor cells, can bias subsequent cell formation into either the macrophage or granulocytic lineage (Metcalf and Burgess, 1982). (d) CSFs can induce specific differentiation commitment in certain multipotential cell lines (Heyworth et al., 1990). While, in total, the evidence makes a persuasive case, in each system it is difficult to account for every cell involved, leaving alternative possibilities that the effects may have been due to selection or amplification of a precommitted subpopulation.

It is evident in vivo that a puzzling wastefulness does occur in certain responses that might be expected to require changes in the cells of only a single lineage. For example, in response to bleeding, increases also occur in nonerythroid progenitor cells in the spleen (Metcalf, 1969), and as will be discussed later, in response to the injection of G-CSF, increases occur in progenitor cells in the blood that include lineages not stimulated by G-CSF – an apparently purposeless occurrence (Dührsen et al., 1988). This may indicate that a certain level of random commitment is inevitable during hemopoiesis, often meaning an unusable level of progenitor cell production.

### *Are an excessive number of progenitor cells formed?*

It is possible to use clonal cultures to estimate the total body progenitor cell number in an animal such as the mouse. The total number of progeny produced by such cells can also be established after the use of various types of stimuli in culture. The actual level of stimulation occurring in vivo can only be guessed at, so the actual number of progeny produced in vivo by these progenitor cells can only be approximated. However, conservative calculations indicate that, in the mouse, the number of progenitor cells available could produce approximately the required number of maturing progeny (Metcalf, 1984). These calculations appear to obviate the need to propose some radically different means of mature cell production in vivo. However, progenitor cells are a transitory population and estimates of the number of progenitor cells present at any one time cannot provide estimates of the rate of turnover of this population. While most progenitor cells appear to be in cell cycle in the adult, it cannot be ruled out that a significant number of them may die without producing maturing progeny. Animal models have recently been encountered in which puzzlingly high levels of mature cells are generated from what appear to be an unremarkable number of progenitor cells. It remains possible, therefore, that a certain level of abortive progenitor cell formation may normally occur, and if so, these cells may possibly be used to amplify hemopoiesis in emergency situations, reducing the need to generate additional progenitor cells.

### *What controls release of mature cells to the blood?*

In early studies on hemopoiesis, it was a popular notion that a leukocytosis was achieved simply by inducing the release of mature cells from the bone marrow, but a concerted effort to discover leukocyte-releasing factors was unsuccessful. Such factors with a simple releasing action may exist, but they have not yet been characterized. On the basis of present knowledge of the polyfunctional actions of most regulators, most researchers now feel that if an agent can accelerate the release of preexisting cells, it is also likely to stimulate new cell formation, and as will be discussed, CSFs have such dual actions.

The process of mature cell release is probably much more sophisticated than realized. Most researchers probably have a vague notion that mature cells may be relatively motile and actively penetrate a sinusoidal endothelial barrier during their exit from the marrow. This may be true for neutrophilic granulocytes but clearly not for enucleated red cells. Furthermore, the behavior of hemopoietic cells in culture indicates that certain cells such as immature erythroid or megakaryocytic precursors have a surprising capacity for extensive migration. This is the cellular basis for the formation of multicentric erythroid or granulocytic colonies and the typical widely dispersed nature of megakaryocytic colonies. Cell *retention* in the marrow may in fact be an active process. Selective expression of adhesion molecules may be a mechanism for retaining immature hemopoietic cells in the marrow, but this area of hemopoietic biology requires extensive investigation.

### What controls the levels of cells in the peripheral blood?

In normal health, the absolute numbers of various cells in the peripheral blood vary over only a relatively small range. Is there any regulatory system that monitors and maintains such levels, or do they simply passively reflect the level of new cell production in the bone marrow? The answer to this question probably varies from lineage to lineage. There is a strong presumption that red cell levels and/or their oxygen-carrying capacity are directly monitored by sensing cells that themselves produce, or signal the production of, erythropoietin. Such a surveillance system is not as easy to identify for cells of other lineages, and if animals are kept pathogen-free, abnormally low white cell levels do not appear to activate the transcription and production of relevant growth factors. Growth factor production increases promptly in a conventional animal subjected to a procedure that induces leukopenia. This leads to the conclusion that the response is triggered not by low leukocyte levels but by secondary infections and therefore represents a demand-generated response rather than one monitoring the number of cells. Conversely, there is no evidence so far for an overriding mechanism that responds to abnormally high white cell levels by inducing a reduction in progenitor cells or hemopoiesis.

The situation with platelets may be intermediate. Like excess red cell levels, the presence of excess platelets may well be life-threatening, and some mechanism may have developed to prevent such excess levels.

At present, therefore, outside the erythroid system there is no substantive evidence for the existence of regulatory mechanisms to monitor blood cell levels and to initiate corrections in hemopoiesis where necessary.

### Can mature hemopoietic cells exhibit any further capacity for proliferation in the tissues?

In the erythroid, granulocytic, and megakaryocytic lineages, the mature cells produced clearly enter an irreversible postmitotic state. Conversely, some T- and B-lymphocytes can exhibit both an extensive capacity for reactivation and mitotic activity in peripheral lymphoid tissues. Three mature cells remain in an ambiguous situation - mast cells, macrophages, and eosinophils. While these have a mature morphology, under certain circumstances some can be stimulated in vitro to exhibit continued proliferative activity. Does this ever occur in vivo when such cells seed in nonhemopoietic tissues? The answer in general seems to be no, except for a limited degree of macrophage proliferation that sustains the number of cells in peritoneal and pleural cavities. In abnormal situations such as inflammatory foci, some activation of local proliferative activity seems likely. However, the overall impression is that most of these cells behave as typical end cells, possibly because the environment in nonhemopoietic tissues lacks the special characteristics of the hemopoietic microenvironment.

The same general answer would appear to be the reason why circulating stem or progenitor cells do not initiate foci of hemopoiesis after lodging by accident in tissues such as the kidney or muscle. Such locations must be accessible to many of the necessary regulatory factors, but presumably what is again lacking is a conducive microenvironment. This conclusion is reinforced by the ready ability to graft hemopoietic tissue to almost any location in the body - but only if key stromal elements are also transferred.

# 3

# Key techniques in analyzing hemopoiesis

It is useful at this stage to comment on some of the major techniques used in analyzing cellular hemopoiesis, because an understanding of what each documents and what its limitations are is necessary to assess the importance or relevance of much that will follow in the discussion of the colony-stimulating factors.

## Identification and enumeration of stem cells

### *Repopulating cells*

The most ancestral stem cells can be identified and defined only by their capacity to repopulate for a sustained period all hemopoietic and lymphoid tissues of an irradiated recipient (Hodgson and Bradley, 1979; Harrison, 1980). To identify progeny of the injected repopulating cells, such assays require markers that, ideally, can detect cells in all major lineages, whether dividing or not. Thus, the use of markers such as Ly1.1 and Ly1.2 is ideal, permitting work with otherwise syngeneic donor and recipient mice. Sex markers and, to a lesser degree, marker chromosomes such as the T6 are also useful. With purified stem cells, as few as 30 cells can permanently repopulate an animal, often with evidence that the repopulating tissue is derived from a single cell. However, many such animals are chimeras because surviving host cells also contribute to hemopoiesis. The major disadvantage of this in vivo repopulation assay is that quantification is virtually impossible, and the assay cannot distinguish even two- to fivefold changes in the number of repopulating cells.

### *In vitro long-term culture-initiating cells*

These stem cells characteristically form cobblestone areas of primitive hemopoietic cells on appropriate supporting underlayers. Quantification of such cells is possible by limit dilution assay (Ploemacher et al., 1991), and the technique can be applied to both human and mouse cells. However, the cobblestone areas themselves cannot be assumed to be individual clones, since movement of cells outside the areas can result in the formation of secondary areas.

Some hierarchical stratification of the cells forming cobblestone areas is possible, based on how long such areas can be sustained and on their continuing capacity to generate stem and progenitor cell progeny (Ploemacher et al., 1991). This technique currently appears to be the most suitable method for identifying in vitro relatively ancestral stem cells, particularly when analyzing human populations.

### *Blast colony–forming cell assays*

Blast colony–forming cell assays are performed in semisolid cultures, and the blast colonies generated can therefore be enumerated as genuine clones (Suda et al, 1987; Metcalf, 1991b). All stem cells can form such colonies, and initially these are composed entirely of blast cells that on analysis prove to be progenitor cells. However, apparently similar colonies can be generated by some of the least-mature progenitor cells, so some overlap may exist between these two compartments. Such colonies lend themselves to further analysis of their content of progenitor cells by secondary reculture. At least with murine cells, blast colony–forming cells have never been detected in the common blast colonies grown from normal marrow, and it is possible that the stimuli used so far to initiate blast colony formation may suppress any capacity these cells might have had for self-generation.

### *Spleen colony formation*

The use of this technique has been largely restricted to murine populations (Till and McCulloch, 1961; Trentin, 1989). Two types of stem cell are detectable in irradiated recipient mice – one forming transient colonies enumerated after 7 days (CFU-S D7), the other forming colonies that persist for 14 days and are more often composed of multilineage populations (CFU-S D14). Both types of colony contain some cells that can form similar spleen colonies in secondary irradiated recipients. The CFU-S D14 cells are more ancestral than the CFU-S D7 cells, and both are relatively mature cells of the stem cell compartment.

### *High proliferative potential cells/colony-forming unit-agar assays*

According to the in vitro culture method used, stem cells or early progenitor cells can generate very large colonies (>2 mm in diameter) composed either of cells of multiple lineages or sometimes solely of macrophages (Bradley et al., 1980; Eckmann et al., 1988; Lorimore et al., 1990). Such assays are usually scored after at least 14 days of incubation, and the colonies concerned have almost certainly passed through an earlier phase of being composed wholly of blast cells. Thus, this assay probably detects the same types of stem cell detected in blast colony assays.

### *Comments*

There remains some confusion regarding the interrelationship between these various clonal assays with claims and counterclaims for the superiority of one over another for monitoring repopulating cells. It is possible that none of these assays satisfactorily monitors the small subset of genuine repopulating cells. Some of the apparent differences between the techniques probably originate from the fact that the technique itself commits the multipotential cells concerned into a restricted pattern of behavior with a differing end result (e.g., regarding self-generation or multipotentiality).

## Progenitor cell assays

Progenitor cell assays are based on the use of selective semisolid cultures using colony formation to identify the number, proliferative capacity, and lineage potential of the cells (Metcalf, 1984). The cultures, when performed properly, have a high detection efficiency, but each carries the risk of underestimating proliferative and lineage potentiality unless optimal culture conditions and combinations of appropriate stimuli are used.

Even with optimal stimulation, it is evident that wide heterogeneity exists between progenitor cells in any one lineage. In general, cells forming very large colonies are less numerous than those forming smaller clones and are presumably more ancestral to such cells. There is also clear heterogeneity in quantitative responsiveness to stimulation by any one growth factor, even between apparently similar progenitor cells.

It is usual to require clones to contain at least 40–50 cells before classifying them as colonies. Cells forming clones of smaller size (cluster-forming cells) are more numerous than colony-forming cells and presumably represent the early progeny of such cells. They are commonly not enumerated or described in publications. Nevertheless, they exist in all cultures and form part of the precursor pool in any one lineage. Many of these cluster-forming cells are already identifiable morphologically as cells such as myeloblasts or promyelocytes, which simply emphasizes the fact that the complete sequence of hemopoiesis can be reproduced in appropriate in vitro cultures. It is only in the erythroid lineage that such cluster-forming cells are separately identified and enumerated as the CFU-E. Thus, CFU-Es are the progeny of the erythroid progenitor cells, the BFU-E.

In the megakaryocytic lineage, a similar sequence occurs. The most ancestral progenitor cells form multipotential colonies containing a range of megakaryocytes and cells of other lineages. More mature progenitors form colonies of variable size but containing megakaryocytes at all stages of maturation, from small diploid precursors to polyploid mature cells. The most mature megakaryocytic progenitor cells form small clones of 2–32 cells, all of which are large polyploid cells.

## Liquid-/solid-state cultures

It is possible to culture stem cells in suspension in liquid culture and at subsequent times to monitor progenitor cell levels by clonal assays (Moore and Warren, 1987). This is in principle similar to a two-step solid-state culture in which blast colony cells are recultured. These two-step cultures are sometimes referred to as Delta assays.

## Long-term marrow cultures

Whole marrow suspensions are cultured in bottles for up to 6 months using special conditions and sera (Dexter et al., 1984). In principle, the successful establishment and maintenance of such cultures depends on the establishment of a satisfactory layer of adherent cells in the culture that serves as a hemopoietic stromal population. The hemopoietic cells commonly develop as foci of cells adherent to the underlayers, and such adherent cells can continuously generate stem and progenitor cells together with maturing cells in various lineages.

The disadvantage of the technique is that it is influenced by the variable quality of the adherent underlayer, and cell production at the clonal level cannot be monitored. In principle, the technique is equivalent to a cobblestone area assay, which offers a more feasible method for enumerating stem cells when used in a limit dilution format.

## Continuous cell lines

There are now available numerous murine and human continuous hemopoietic cell lines. The most useful of these are those retaining full dependency for survival and proliferation on stimulation by specific growth factors. Culture of such cells can be used in conventional suspension cultures, in clonal semisolid cultures, or in microwell suspension cultures. All of these systems have proved of value as convenient bioassays for growth factors. However, it should always be kept in mind that such cell lines may not respond exclusively to only one factor and cannot be used as specific bioassays for material potentially containing other growth factors, unless methods are used to rule out the possible activity of other factors. Most of these immortalized cell lines have retained little capacity for maturation, but some are clearly multipotential and can be induced to differentiate to cells of various hemopoietic lineages, offering valuable tools for analyzing the biology of this process (Heyworth et al., 1990).

There are corresponding continuous leukemic cell lines, some of which remain responsive to certain growth factors, and these are valuable both as bioassays for growth factors and for studies on the induction of differentiation, with or without maturation.

All conclusions drawn from the use of such immortalized cell lines must be regarded with caution until confirmed using normal cells.

## Serum-free versus serum-containing cultures

In principle, the regulators controlling cells could most precisely be analyzed if the cells were grown in adequate, fully characterized medium, thus avoiding the unwitting addition of potentially relevant factors in the fetal calf serum normally used in hemopoietic cell cultures. This has led to considerable use of serum-free hemopoietic cell cultures, with the consequent generation of data that seem elegant but often have little advantage over those obtained from conventional cultures.

Most current media for "serum-free" cultures contain a high concentration of "purified" bovine serum albumin. This is not a pure substance, and analysis has revealed the presence of a large number of other serum-derived proteins, many of which are delivered to the cultures in higher concentrations than by the addition of whole serum. Such "serum-free" cultures are as uncharacterized as serum-containing cultures. Furthermore, if such cultures contain a large number of cells, breakdown or secretion products of these cells potentially contribute further biologically active molecules available to the cells under study. Finally, important but irrelevant molecules can be omitted unwittingly from "serum-free" cultures with the production of misleading information.

With both serum-containing and "serum-free" cultures, it must always be acknowledged that important accessory factors may have been added inadvertently to the medium or have been generated in the cultures and that these accessory factors may have been needed to obtain the response observed. Anyone characterizing the apparent biological actions of a hemopoietic growth factor, whether performed in vivo or in vitro, must always accept this major caveat.

## Significance and limitations of bioassays for stem and progenitor cells

The assays discussed in the preceding section have been used for a variety of purposes, including an assessment of bone marrow reserve in various disease states or the repopulating potential of marrow collected for transplantation. Alternatively, such assays have been used to monitor responses to the injection of growth factors.

In principle, assays of stem cell numbers present no theoretical problems other than the difficulty of establishing which type of stem cell is being detected. Assays on progenitor cell numbers involve the special problem associated with any transit population. The number observed at any one instant cannot give any estimate of the rates of either formation or expenditure of such cells.

In an experimental animal such as the mouse, the entire marrow population can be collected from a whole femur and estimates made of the absolute cell number. This is not possible with human samples, where the only estimate possible is relative frequency – a measure potentially complicated by sampling variations and unknown levels of dilution of the sample by peripheral blood cells. For specimens of blood or cord blood cells, the latter problems do not arise and cell number can be expressed as absolute number per milliliter.

Estimates of lineage-committed progenitor cells in a marrow or peripheral blood sample have been shown to correlate in a general manner with repopulating capacity and are commonly used parameters for assessing the quality of such samples. They are likely to be inferior to estimates of multipotential progenitor cells [mixed CFC, colony-forming units – granulocytic, erythroid, macrophage, and megakaryocytic (CFU-GEMM), high proliferative potential cells (HPPC), or blast CFC] or estimates of $CD34^+$ cells, since these populations begin to include more mature members of the stem cell population.

Regardless of the monitoring system used, it is important to perform estimates on more than one lineage of cells by the use of replicate cultures with appropriate stimulating factors. It should also be kept in mind that combinations of factors are required to stimulate the proliferation of stem cells and some progenitor cells. Analyses using single stimulating factors inevitably underestimate the numbers of progenitor cells in any one lineage and, for many, their true potential for generating progeny in more than one lineage. It is also possible that optimal stimuli for fetal or cord blood populations may differ from those for adult hemopoietic cells.

As will be seen from the discussion to follow on the in vivo effects of CSFs, response patterns can vary widely in timing, the types of stem and progenitor cells appearing to respond, and the organ location of these responses. Studies in mice make it apparent that analysis of only a single tissue cannot reveal the full picture of responses occurring throughout the body and may even give misleading information. For example, greater responses can usually be observed in the spleen than the marrow, where levels of precursor cells may actually fall; this must be kept in mind in reading descriptions of responses in humans, where, of necessity, the observations are usually restricted to the marrow and peripheral blood. Because significant differences exist between response patterns to different growth factors in different organs, studies of mice will inevitably offer a more complete picture of the responses than is possible in humans.

## Assays for hemopoietic growth factors

### *Colony formation*

Most hemopoietic growth factors can stimulate colony formation of one type or another in semisolid cultures of normal hemopoietic cells. This colony formation has a characteristic sigmoid dose–response curve composed of three regions (Figure 3.1): (a) a subeffective concentration range where no or little colony formation occurs, (b) an ascending linear region

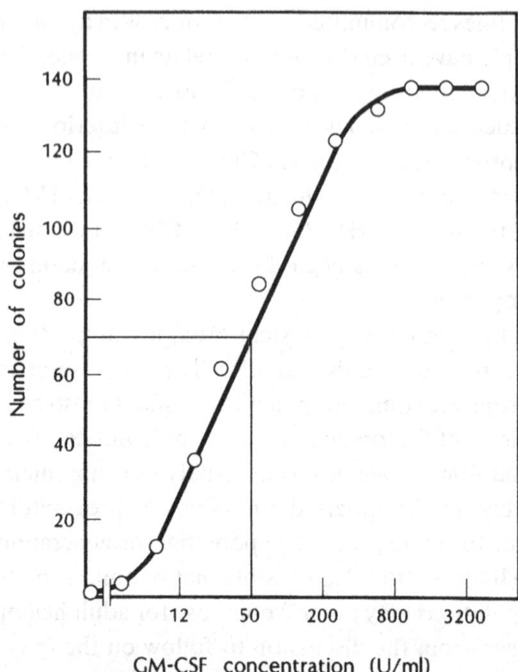


Figure 3.1. CSFs can be assayed in semisolid cultures of bone marrow cells. With increasing CSF concentrations, colony numbers increase until a plateau is reached, when all available progenitor cells have formed colonies. By convention, 50 U/ml is the CSF concentration in the culture stimulating the formation of the half-maximal number of colonies.

where an increasing number of colonies develop arithmetically as the concentration of growth factor rises logarithmically, the slope reflecting the heterogeneity in responsiveness of the clonogenic cells, and (c) a plateau region where the number of colonies does not increase because all available clonogenic cells have responded by forming colonies.

To establish a meaningful system of units for expressing biological activity in situations where the absolute number of target cells may vary widely with different growth factors and cell populations cultured, a colony-forming dose response can be converted to a percent maximal colony formation curve, and 50 U/ml is the number of units assigned to the concentration stimulating the formation of a half-maximal number of colonies (Figure 3.1).

For the granulocyte-macrophage CSFs, this unit system gives values of approximately $10^8$ U/mg purified protein, and throughout this book this approximation has been used for the specific activity of the CSFs.

An international unit system has recently been proposed, based on the assignment of an arbitrary number of units per milligram protein to an international standard preparation, but the value of such a standard remains to be determined.

### *Assays using factor-dependent cell lines*

Assays can be performed by using suspension cultures of CSF-dependent cell lines and either scoring cell proliferation by visual counting in microwell cultures or by tritiated thymidine uptake. Such assays can be converted to bone marrow units of activity by cross-assay of reference preparations of the factor in bone marrow cultures.

### *Receptor competition assays*

Useful assays can be developed in which the binding of a radiolabeled factor to an appropriate cell line can be competed for by pre- or co-incubation with a test sample. Such tests are highly specific and detect functional protein capable of receptor binding but tend to be relatively insensitive.

### *Immunoassays*

Immunoassays have become commercially available for many hemopoietic growth factors. They have the virtue of avoiding a common problem in bioassays, namely, that inhibitory material is often present in serum or tissue extracts that may prevent detection of active factors present in low concentrations. They are also highly specific and sensitive, outperforming most bioassays. However, they have one major disadvantage: They merely detect an intact antigenic epitope on the factor being measured and cannot distinguish between biologically active and biologically inactive molecules. Thus, they may well often overestimate concentrations of biologically active material in various situations.

Some regulatory factors are present in cells in unusually large amounts, and in this situation their presence can be detected by immunohistochemistry using suitable antibodies. However, the amounts of CSFs present in most cell types are usually too small to be detected by this approach.

### *Assays for mRNA*

Assays for mRNA measure levels of transcripts only, and there are many situations in which there is a major dissociation between transcription and the actual production of biologically active factors. The least-sensitive method is analysis by Northern gels or dot blots. RNase protection assays are more sensitive and polymerase chain reaction (PCR) analysis the most sensitive method. In situ hybridization is an elegant method for identifying cells exhibiting transcription, but the method is too insensitive to allow detection of the transcription of many growth factors in normal cells.

## Tests for direct action of a regulator

A hemopoietic regulator may act directly on a responding cell or indirectly by inducing the production by some adjacent cell of the true molecule responsible for eliciting the observed biological response. This problem applies both in vivo and in vitro but can at least be analyzed in vitro.

There are four procedures for certifying direct action. First and of paramount importance is the demonstration by autoradiography of cells incubated with radiolabeled factor that the responding cells actually express receptors for the regulator in question. The absence of detectable receptors does not rule out the possibility of a direct action, because receptors may be too few to detect or receptor expression may be induced during culture, but documentation of their presence provides some evidence.

Second, the most convincing functional documentation of direct action comes from the culture of a single cell - usually obtained by fluorescence-activated cell sorting but also by micromanipulation from developing clones. The use of single-cell deposition units is acceptable, but the cautious researcher will always verify the presence of a single cell by careful visual inspection.

Third, a somewhat less stringent test for direct action is to transfer day 2 or day 3 clones developing in cultures of hemopoietic cells in response to stimulation by the factor being tested to the surface of cultures containing the factor but no other cells. If the volume of agar surrounding the initial clone is kept small during transfer, then progressive growth of the transferred clone is evidence of direct action.

Fourth, a useful initial test is to determine in cultures of marrow or other cells whether the colony formation stimulated by addition of the factor increases linearly when an increasing number of cells are cultured. To be a valid index of direct action, this linearity must pass through zero. If linearity of colony formation occurs only when a threshold concentration of cultured cells is exceeded or if the response is nonlinear, then significant indirect actions in the culture are necessary for colony stimulation.

## Purification of factors

Most hemopoietic growth factors are produced in only minute concentrations by cells. The purification of these factors therefore requires a sequence of fractionation procedures in which the fractions containing the factor can be detected only by bioassay. It is not until purification is almost complete that the presence of the factor can become visible as an optical density peak. Useful separative procedures have been salting-out chromatography, affinity column separation based on carbohydrate content or binding characteristics of the factor to metal chelates, size separation by gel chromatography, charge separation by DEAE columns, and above all the eventual use of high-performance liquid chromatography fractionation often using at least two different systems.

The fold purifications required to purify CSFs have ranged up to 1 million-fold in difficult cases. The final criteria of purity are a single optical density peak coinciding exactly with the biological activity being measured, the presence of a single silver-staining band in native or reducing gels, and the presence of a single dominant sequence on amino acid sequencing. None of these criteria guarantees that the protein purified was the factor under study. This can be established only by cloning a cDNA using nucleotide probes synthesized on the basis of the amino acid sequence, then expressing the cDNA clone and showing that the resulting recombinant factor, when again purified, exhibits identical biological properties to those of the factor originally purified.

Opinions vary as to whether the concentration of a purified factor should be expressed in milligrams per milliliter or in biological units per milliliter. An essential criterion of purity is certainly that the biological activity per milligram protein should be known for the best preparations of that factor. Because recombinant factors can be expressed in an incorrectly folded, biologically inactive form, it is not sufficient to work with material using only a milligram per milliliter measurement. Similarly, biological activity can become lost in a previously active preparation, so all experiments must be performed using material that is repeatedly bioassayed to verify retention of full biological activity. Studies performed without such controls must be accepted with reservation.

# 4

# Biochemistry of the colony-stimulating factors

The colony-stimulating factors were originally described as biological activities in crude cell-conditioned media. Their intrinsic stability was a great advantage in their analysis and purification, but their heterogeneity, due primarily to differential glycosylation, and their extremely low concentration ensured that the purification of the CSFs would be extremely difficult and take up the better part of a decade. Even then, insufficient amounts of the CSFs were available from natural sources to allow detailed structural analysis and studies in vivo of their biological activities. With the advent of recombinant CSFs produced in *Escherichia coli,* it became apparent that glycosylation was not essential either for correct structure formation or for biological activity. This made it possible to perform detailed structural analyses of the CSFs as well as animal and clinical studies. The CSFs are all glycoproteins (Table 4.1), and despite having very little primary amino acid sequence homology, they have very similar folded structures; their stability and solubility are maintained by internal disulfide bonds (and intersubunit disulfide bonds in the case of M-CSF) and attached carbohydrate chains. In this chapter the purification, structural analysis, and structure–function studies of the CSFs will be described.

## GM-CSF

The major CSF activity in medium conditioned by lung tissue from endotoxin-injected mice was recognized to have distinctive biological and biochemical properties (Sheridan and Metcalf, 1973a). This CSF was termed GM-CSF and was purified to apparent homogeneity by Burgess et al. (1977) using a combination of ammonium sulfate precipitation, ion-exchange chromatography, binding to concanavalin A–Sepharose, and gel filtration. Subsequently, treatment of the preparation with neuraminidase and

Table 4.1. *Molecular properties of the CSFs*

| | GM-CSF | | Multi-CSF (IL-3) | | G-CSF | | M-CSF | |
|---|---|---|---|---|---|---|---|---|
| | Human | Mouse | Human | Mouse | Human | Mouse | Human | Mouse |
| Leader sequence (aa) | 17 | 17 | 19 | 26 | 30 | 30 | 32 | 32 |
| Mature sequence (aa) | 127 | 124 | 133 | 140 | 174, 177 | 178 | 338, 408, 523 | ND |
| Protein core (kDa) | 14.7 | 14.4 | 15.4 | 16.2 | 18.6 | 19.1 | 41, 49, 63 | ND |
| Glycosylated mass (kDa) | 18–33 | 18–30 | 23–35 | 22, 29, 34 | 22 | 25 | 45, 70, >200 | 70, >200 |
| Disulfides | Cys 54–96<br>Cys 88–121 | 51–93<br>85–118 | 16–84 | 17–80<br>79–140 | 36–42<br>64–74 | 42–48<br>70–80 | 7–90<br>48–139<br>102–146<br>157–159<br>31–31 | 7–90<br>48–139<br>102–146<br>157–159<br>31–31 |
| Glycosylation sites (N) | Asn 27, 37 | Asn 66, 75 | Asn 15, 70 | Asn 16, 86, (44, 51) | — | — | Asn 122, 140, 349, 383 | Asn 122, 140, 349 |
| Glycosylation sites (O) | Ser 9, Thr 10 | ND | ND | ND | Thr 133 | Thr 139 | Ser 277 GAG | Ser 277 GAG |
| Helical segments[a] | A: 13–28<br>B: 55–64<br>C: 74–87<br>D: 103–116 | | (19–27)<br>(56–68)<br>(71–85)<br>(103–121) | | 11–39<br>72–91<br>100–123<br>143–171 | | 13–24<br>46–64<br>71–87<br>110–130 | |
| Sequence identity (M/H) (%) | 52 | | 29 | | 80 | | 79 | |

*Note:* ND denotes "not determined."
[a] Predicted as opposed to experimentally observed helical segments are shown in parentheses.

reverse-phase high-performance liquid chromatography (HPLC) allowed the purification of larger amounts of homogeneous murine asialo GM-CSF (Sparrow et al., 1985) that provided amino acid sequence. Human GM-CSF was first described as a separate entity in human placenta-conditioned medium (Nicola et al., 1979b) and was subsequently purified to homogeneity from the HTLV-II-infected T-lymphoblast cell line Mo by Gasson et al. (1984) and Wong et al. (1985).

Human and murine GM-CSFs were of similar apparent molecular weight [24,000–33,000 by sodium dodecyl sulfate–polyacrylamide gel electrophoresis (SDS–PAGE)], and were clearly glycoprotein in nature since they bound to concanavalin A–Sepharose and showed reduced charge heterogeneity after neuraminidase treatment.

cDNA cloning revealed that both murine and human GM-CSFs (Gough et al., 1984; Lee et al., 1985; Wong et al., 1985) are synthesized with a 17-amino acid hydrophobic leader sequence that is proteolytically cleaved during secretion. The mature proteins consist of 127 amino acids for human GM-CSF and 124 amino acids for murine GM-CSF with core polypeptide molecular weights of 14,700 and 14,400. The two proteins share only 52% amino acid identity (Figure 4.1) and are species-specific in their biological actions. Nevertheless, they both contain two conserved intramolecular disulfide bonds (Cys 54–96 and Cys 88–121 in humans; Cys 51–93 and Cys 85–118 in mice), with only the first disulfide bond being required for biological activity (Shahafelt and Kastelein, 1989). The intramolecular disulfide bonds appear to result in a robust structure insensitive to most denaturing conditions (Nicola et al., 1979a).

Murine GM-CSF contains two potential *N*-glycosylation sites at Asn 66 and 75, while human GM-CSF contains two such sites at Asn 27 and 37. The confirmed sites of *N*-glycosylation in human GM-CSF are at positions Asn 27 and 37, which are of the complex acidic type (Schrimsher et al., 1987), but additional sites of *O*-glycosylation have also been inferred at the N-terminus, including Ser 9 and Thr 10. Nonglycosylated murine and human GM-CSFs produced in *E. coli* have the full spectrum of biological activities characteristic of glycosylated GM-CSF, but surprisingly the nonglycosylated forms have at least a 10-fold increased specific biological activity (DeLamarter et al., 1985; Moonen et al., 1987; Cebon et al., 1990b). Cebon et al. (1990b) purified the differentially glycosylated forms of human GM-CSF produced by phytohemagglutinin (PHA)-activated peripheral blood cells using a combination of antibody-affinity chromatography and reverse-phase HPLC. These molecules ranged in apparent molecular weight from 14,700 to 33,000, and with increasing

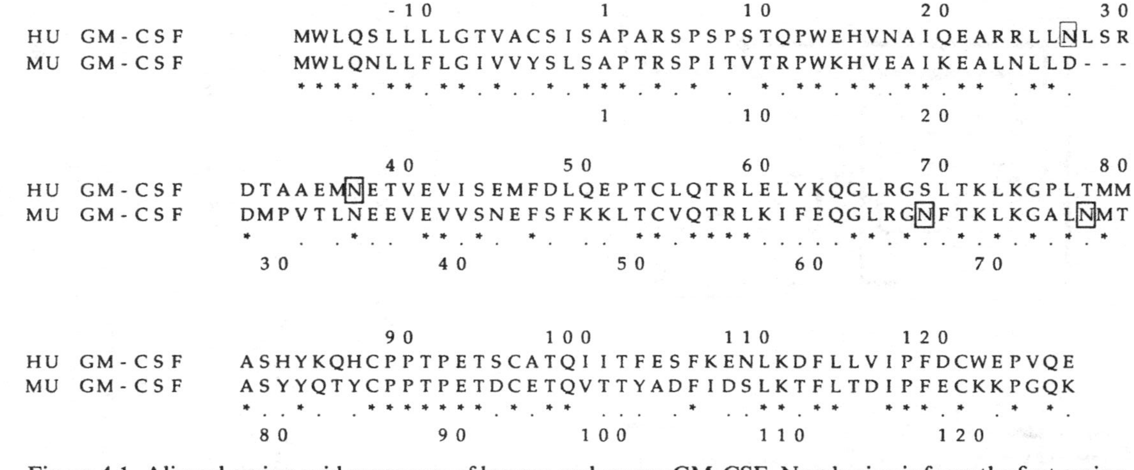


Figure 4.1. Aligned amino acid sequences of human and mouse GM-CSF. Numbering is from the first amino acid of the mature protein (+1). Identities are shown under the sequences with an asterisk and homologous substitutions with a dot. N-Linked carbohydrate attachment sites are shown by a box around the asparagine (N) residue.

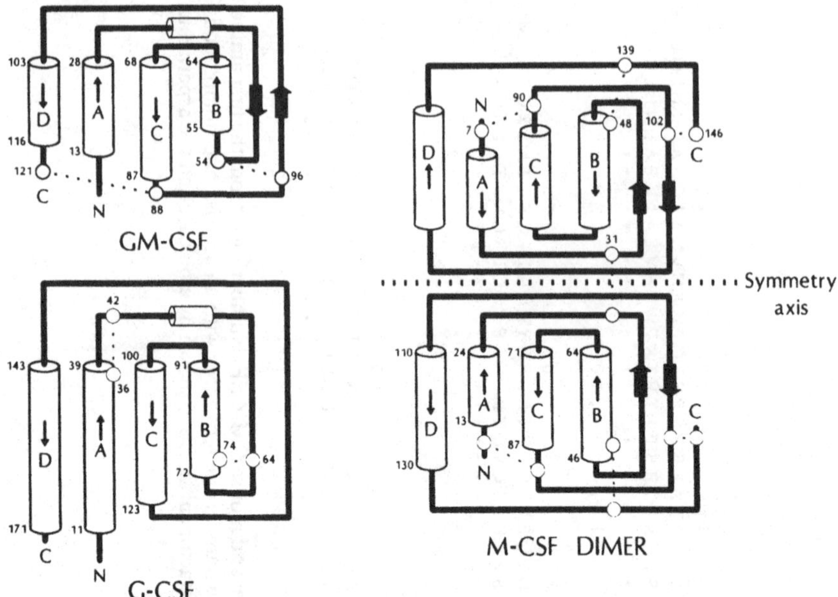


Figure 4.2. Helix topologies of the three known CSF structures. The four main helices (A–D) forming the antiparallel bundle are shown to scale as cylinders and the connecting loops as lines. $\beta$-Sheets are shown as arrows and short helical segments as cylinders. Disulfide bonds are shown as dots connected by dotted lines. The N- and C-terminal ends are indicated, as are the number of the first and last amino acids of each helix and the number of connected cysteine residues.

size and glycosylation, decreasing receptor-binding affinity and specific biological activity were observed.

Nonglycosylated GM-CSF has been crystallized and its three-dimensional structure determined by X-ray crystallography (Figures 4.2 and 4.3) (Diederichs et al., 1991; Walter et al., 1992). Like the other CSFs, it takes up the conformation of a four-$\alpha$-helical antiparallel bundle (A-/D-helices). The two long overhand loops connecting the A-/B- and the C-/D-helices each contribute a short antiparallel $\beta$-strand, and the A–B loop also contains another short $\alpha$-helical segment. The two disulfide bonds link the ends of C- and D-helices and the N-terminal end of B-helix to the C-D loop. The short chain length of the four major $\alpha$-helices and the large skew angle of the antiparallel helical pairs places GM-CSF in the short-chain four-$\alpha$-helical bundle subclass of this group of proteins, along with IL-4, interferon $\gamma$, IL-2, IL-5, and M-CSF.

The structural elements of GM-CSF responsible for binding to different receptor chains and biological activity have been established by a

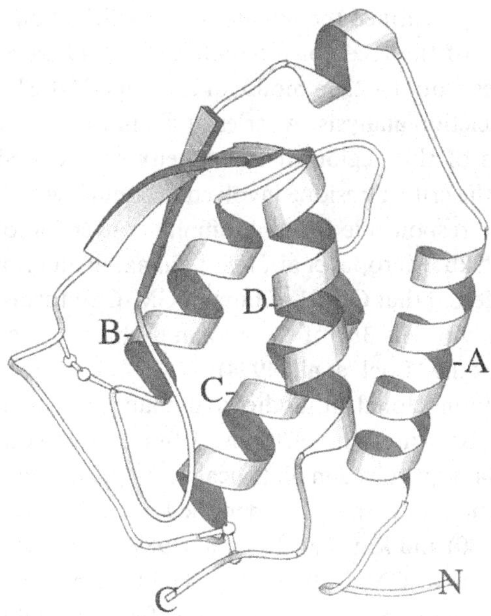


Figure 4.3. The structure of human GM-CSF determined by X-ray crystallography (Diederichs et al., 1991). Helices are shown as ribbons, $\beta$-sheets as arrows, and loops as strings. The N- and C-terminal ends and main helices are labeled. Disulfide bonds are indicated in ball-and-stick mode. The picture was created from the coordinates by the program MOLSCRIPT (Kraulis, 1991).

combination of scanning mutagenesis, interspecies chimeras, mapping of epitopes by neutralizing monoclonal antibodies, and peptide synthesis. Altmann et al. (1991) used a systematic substitution of proline for individual amino acids to show that the second predicted helix (B) of murine GM-CSF was not essential for biological activity. On the other hand, an analysis of human–mouse GM-CSF chimeric molecules (Kaushansky et al., 1989) showed that residues 21–31 and 78–94 (in the predicted A- and C-helices, respectively) were critical for high-affinity binding and biological activity, with a lesser contribution from the predicted D-helix. In vitro mutagenesis (Gough et al., 1987) and scanning deletion analysis (Shanafelt and Kastelein, 1989) of murine GM-CSF identified several regions in the molecule necessary for functional activity, including residues in the predicted A-, C-, and D-helices, but it was unclear whether these results identified a receptor-binding domain or critical structural elements. A more complete series of mouse–human GM-CSF chimeras, coupled with a series of selective binding and bioassays including mixed-species receptor subunits, identified the region of GM-CSF required for binding to the $\beta$-subunit of the receptor (Shanafelt et al., 1991a,b). This region included residues from 17–22 in mouse or human GM-CSF, in agreement with scanning deletion analysis. A series of alanine or specific amino acid point mutations of this region of the A-helix of GM-CSF have implicated Glu 21 as the critical residue involved in contact with the $\beta$-chain of the receptor and responsible for high-affinity conversion of the receptor (Lopez et al., 1992b; Meropol et al., 1992; Shanafelt and Kastelein, 1992). It has been suggested that Glu 21 of human GM-CSF forms a critical ion-pair interaction with His 367 of the human $\beta$-chain in the generation of high-affinity binding (Lock et al., 1994).

Neutralizing monoclonal antibodies to human GM-CSF have identified residues 77–94 (Brown et al., 1990) and 110–127 (Kanakura et al., 1991; Seelig et al., 1994) as involved in biological activity. Shanafelt et al. (1991a), using cross-species chimeras, also identified the region 77–82 (especially Thr 78 and Met 80) and Kaushansky et al. (1989) identified residues 78–94 as critical for human GM-CSF activity. The C-terminal contribution is not as well understood, however, since Shanafelt et al. (1991a,b) identified residues 122–126 as important, but this was not observed by peptide synthesis (Clark-Lewis et al., 1988b) or by the chimeric analysis of Kaushansky et al. (1989).

## G-CSF

The various names initially applied to G-CSF reflect the history of the purification of G-CSF from various cell sources and the use of different bioassays. Nicola et al. (1979b) showed that whereas most purification procedures could not clearly separate different CSF activities derived from human placenta-conditioned medium (HPCM), hydrophobic interaction chromatography on phenyl-Sepharose separated the CSF activities into two distinct peaks, termed CSF-$\alpha$ and CSF-$\beta$. A series of experiments showed that this was not an artifactual separation and, most important, that the biological activities of the two fractions were distinct. The more hydrophobic of these, CSF-$\beta$, stimulated the formation of predominantly neutrophilic granulocyte colonies, which were transient and peaked in number at day 7 – properties now characterized as those of G-CSF. CSF-$\alpha$, on the other hand, stimulated the formation of eosinophil, neutrophil, and macrophage colonies that peaked at day 14 – biological properties now recognized as those of GM-CSF.

Serum from endotoxin-injected mice induced terminal differentiation in the murine myeloid leukemia cell line WEHI-3BD$^{+}$, and this activity was initially termed granulocyte-macrophage differentiation factor (GM-DF) (Burgess and Metcalf, 1980). Neutralizing antisera to M-CSF inhibited most of the CSF activity in the serum but did not inhibit GM-DF. Moreover, GM-DF co-purified with a weak residual CSF activity that stimulated the formation of neutrophil colonies. In a survey of potential tissue sources of GM-DF activity it was noted that GM-DF in media conditioned by a variety of murine tissues had similar biochemical properties and could be distinguished from the majority of the CSF activity by several criteria including ammonium sulfate precipitation, binding to concanavalin A-Sepharose, and behavior on phenyl-Sepharose columns (Nicola and Metcalf, 1981). Again, GM-DF activity co-migrated with a neutrophilic G-CSF. Medium conditioned by lung tissue from endotoxin-injected mice was found to be the richest source of GM-DF, and a purification strategy was developed involving salting-out chromatography, phenyl-Sepharose and Biogel P-60 chromatography, and HPLC on a reverse-phase (phenyl-silica) and gel filtration (TSK G3000 SW) column (Nicola et al., 1983). Throughout the successive purification steps, GM-DF activity co-chromatographed exactly with CSF activity that selectively stimulated the formation of neutrophilic granulocytic colonies, and the active factor was named G-CSF. By these procedures, G-CSF was purified nearly 500,000-fold with a 30% yield and appeared as a homogeneous protein band of about MW 25,000 on silver-stained SDS–PAGE gels. Extraction of the gel showed that both WEHI-3BD$^+$ differentiation-inducing activity and G-CSF activity were associated with this homogeneous protein band.

Nicola et al. (1985) used the cross-species reactivity of G-CSF to show formally that partially purified GM-CSF$\beta$ from HPCM could also induce differentiation in mouse WEHI-3BD$^+$ cells and compete with purified mouse G-CSF for binding to murine receptor, thus identifying GM-CSF$\beta$ as human G-CSF. In parallel studies, Welte et al. (1985) purified a CSF activity from medium conditioned by the human bladder carcinoma cell line 5637, which induced differentiation in WEHI-3BD$^+$ cells and stimulated the formation of neutrophilic granulocytic colonies but also appeared to stimulate the formation of erythroid, megakaryocytic, and mixed colonies. This CSF was initially termed pluripoietin, but subsequent studies showed that the "pluripotent" effects of this molecule were spurious (Souza et al., 1986; Strife et al., 1987), and amino acid sequencing revealed it to be identical to human G-CSF (Nagata et al., 1986a). Using a human tumor cell line (CHU-2) that induces granulocytosis in nude mice, Nomura et al. (1986) also purified G-CSF and showed that it exclusively stimulated the formation of neutrophilic granulocytic colonies in cultures of human and mouse bone marrow cells.

Both human and murine G-CSFs were noted to be extremely stable molecules that were not irreversibly denatured by extremes of pH, temperature, or denaturants such as guanidine hydrochloride, urea, or SDS (Nicola, 1985). However, essential intramolecular disulfide bonds were inferred by the denaturation of G-CSF in the presence of reducing agents under the preceding conditions with no significant reduction in apparent molecular weight. The lack of binding of G-CSF to concanavalin A (Nicola and Metcalf, 1981) suggested that it did not contain typical mannose-containing carbohydrate. However, its charge heterogeneity in isoelectric focusing (isoelectric point 4.1–5.5) and the reduction of this heterogeneity after treatment with neuraminidase suggested that it did display sialic acid–containing O-glycosylation (Nicola and Metcalf, 1984). This has now been established by direct chemical analysis to result from attachment of *N*-acetylneuraminic acid $\alpha$-(2, 3)[galactase-$\beta$(1, 3)]-*N*-acetylgalactosamine to a single site at Thr 133, with or without a second *N*-acetylneuraminic acid residue linked $\alpha$-(2, 6) to the galactose residue (Oheda et al., 1988).

Both murine and human G-CSFs are synthesized with 30–amino acid leader sequences typical of secreted proteins (Nagata et al., 1986a; Souza et al., 1986; Tsuchiya et al., 1986).

The mature proteins contain 178 amino acids ($M_r$ 19,061) in mouse G-CSF and 174 amino acids ($M_r$ 18,627) in human G-CSF (Figure 4.4), and the larger apparent molecular weight on SDS–PAGE gels (22,000–25,000) is the result of the attached O-linked carbohydrate chain. Human and murine G-CSFs contain two homologous disulfide bonds (Cys 36–42 and Cys 64–74 in humans; Cys 42–48 and Cys 70–80 in mice) and a free cysteine each (Cys 17 in humans, Cys 89 in mice). The free cysteines are not accessible in the native folded structure and do not appear to be required for biological activity (Lu et al., 1989).

An additional form of human G-CSF has been described with the tripeptide Val-Ser-Glu inserted between residues 35 and 36 (Nagata et al., 1986a,b), but this molecule appears to have significantly lower biological activity than the shorter form of G-CSF. The most active forms of murine and human G-CSF have specific biological activities of $3 \times 10^8$ and $1 \times 10^8$ U/mg, respectively, with 50 U/ml being defined as that concentration stimulating 50% maximal colony formation in vitro (i.e., approximately 3 and 10 p*M*, respectively). Under appropriate conditions, the nonglycosylated forms of G-CSF are fully biologically active and are unaltered in their range of biological activities. However, G-CSF protein is a highly hydrophobic molecule, and the hydrophilic O-linked sugar chain dramatically

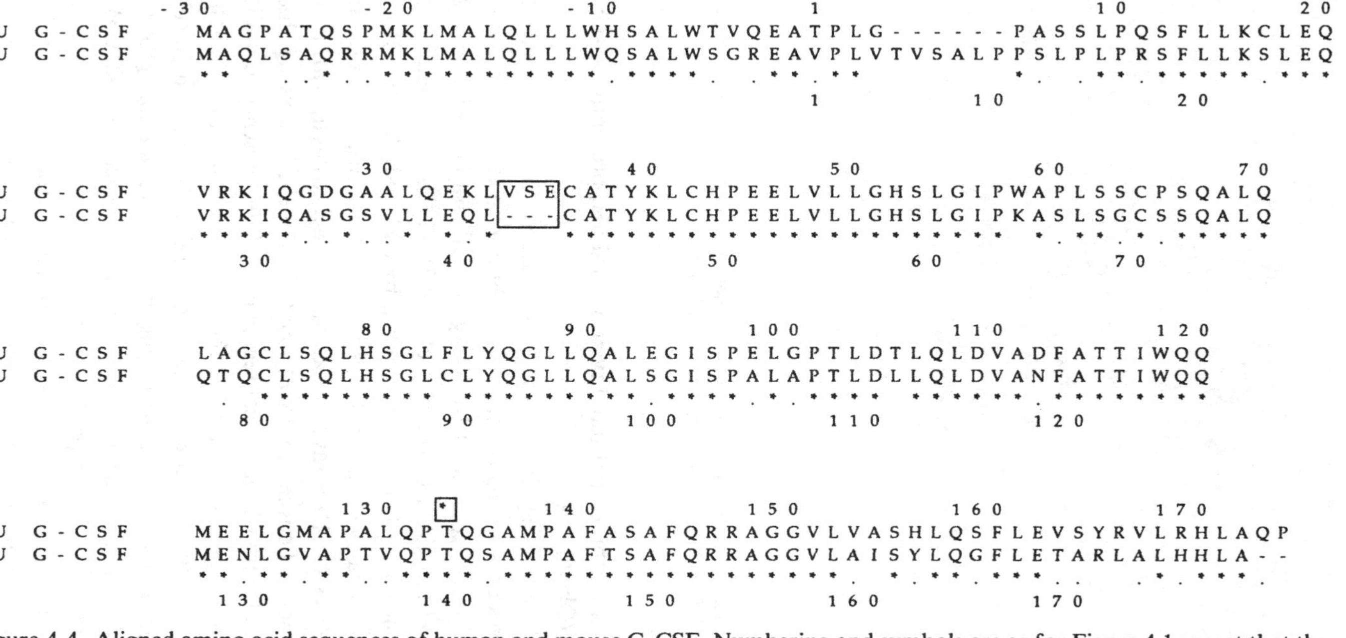


Figure 4.4. Aligned amino acid sequences of human and mouse G-CSF. Numbering and symbols are as for Figure 4.1 except that the boxed star indicates the single site of *O*-glycosylation and the boxed tripeptide is present in only one type of human G-CSF transcript.

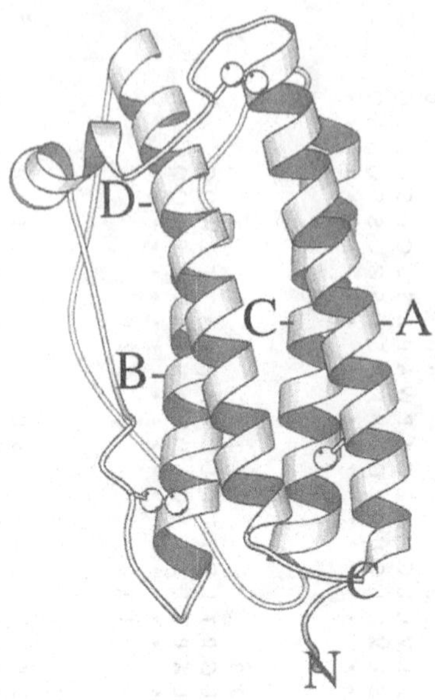


Figure 4.5. The structure of human G-CSF determined by X-ray crystallography (Hill et al., 1993). Representation is as for Figure 4.3.

increases its solubility and stability at neutral pH, preventing G-CSF aggregation (Oheda et al., 1990).

Early studies using circular dichroism (Lu et al., 1989; Oheda et al., 1990) suggested a strong $\alpha$-helical contribution to G-CSF structure, and this was directly confirmed by X-ray crystallography (Figures 4.2 and 4.5) (Hill et al., 1993; Lovejoy et al., 1993). G-CSF is a member of the four-$\alpha$-helical bundle cytokines typified by GM-CSF, M-CSF, IL-2, and interferon $\alpha$ (Parry et al., 1988, 1991; Bazan, 1990a,b). It consists of four long $\alpha$-helices (A–D) arrayed in an antiparallel fashion, with two long overhand loops between the A-/B- and C-/D-helices allowing chain reversal. The length of the helical segments and the presence of additional short $3_{10}$ and $\alpha$-helical segments in the A–B loop as well as the small skew angle between the helical pairs places G-CSF in the long-chain subclass four-$\alpha$-helical bundle structure (along with interferon $\alpha$ and growth hormone) and distinguishes it from the short-chain subclass [IL-2, GM-CSF, M-CSF, interferon $\gamma$, and predicted for IL-3 (Multi-CSF)]. In the G-CSF structure, the two essential disulfide bonds link opposite ends of the A–B loop to the C-terminal of the A-helix and the N-terminal of the B-helix.

Neutralizing monoclonal antibodies to human G-CSF recognize an epitope from residues 20–46, including the exposed A–B loop helical segments and the disulfide bond between Cys 36 and Cys 42 (Layton et al., 1991) (see Figures 4.2 and 4.5). Because this region includes residue 35, it is probable that the insertion of three amino acids on the longer form of human G-CSF would alter the receptor binding site. Non-neutralizing antibodies recognized various other regions, including the N-terminus (but not the C-terminus). Kuga et al. (1989) used site-directed mutagenesis to show that the N-terminal 11 amino acids were not required for biological activity but that substitution of residues Thr 1 Ala, Leu 3 Thr, Gly 4 Tyr, Pro 5 Arg, and Cys 17 Ser produced a mutant G-CSF (KW2228) that was about two-fold more potent in vivo and in vitro than wild-type human G-CSF. This mutant G-CSF was also more stable (Okabe et al., 1990) and had a higher binding affinity to the G-CSF receptor (Uzumaki et al., 1988). Single amino acid changes or deletion of Leu 35 or surrounding amino acids resulted in a loss of biological activity, confirming the importance of this site in receptor binding. Various other larger deletions or tandem repeats in different parts of the molecule also resulted in a loss of activity, but these may have resulted in dramatic structural alterations.

G-CSF shows significant similarity in its amino acid sequence and genomic organization to IL-6 (37% sequence identity) and to the chicken myelomonocytic growth factor (MGF) (32% sequence identity; Leutz et al., 1989). This presumably reflects their common origin from a primordial gene, which is reinforced by their similar predicted tertiary structures and binding to subunits of the same general receptor class. However, it is presently unclear whether chicken MGF is the precursor of murine IL-6, G-CSF, or both.

## M-CSF (CSF-1)

M-CSF was the first CSF to be purified. It was purified from human urine by Stanley et al. (1975) and subsequently purified to homogeneity by making use of absorption and elution from cells bearing M-CSF receptors (Stanley and Guilbert, 1981). In 1977, Stanley and Heard purified murine M-CSF from L-cell-conditioned medium by a combination of calcium phosphate gel, ion-exchange, and gel filtration chromatography, binding to the lectin concanavalin A, and a final step of gradient gel electrophoresis or calcium phosphate gel elution (Stanley and Heard, 1977; Stanley and Guilbert, 1981).

M-CSF differs from the other CSFs in several important respects. It is a homodimer with extremely variable levels and types of glycosylation. It contains intermolecular disulfide bonds, and the dimeric state is absolutely necessary for biological activity (Das and Stanley, 1982). It exists in both soluble and transmembrane cell-associated forms, both of which are biologically active (Stein et al., 1990). It is translated from multiple mRNA transcripts that produce proteins of different size and different levels of glycosylation (Cerretti et al., 1988; Baccarini and Stanley, 1990). Finally, it binds to a classical type III tyrosine kinase receptor, whereas the other CSFs bind to hemopoietin domain receptors (Nicola, 1991a,b). Mouse and human CSFs are 79% identical at the amino acid level (Figure 4.6), but although human M-CSF is fully active on mouse cells, mouse M-CSF is not active on human cells.

The longest human M-CSF transcript (encoded by a 4-kb mRNA) contains a 32-amino acid leader sequence, a 463-amino acid extracellular domain, a 24-amino acid transmembrane domain, and a 35-amino acid cytoplasmic tail. This transcript is transiently expressed at the cell surface as a disulfide-linked homodimer but is rapidly processed proteolytically by unknown enzymes to release a soluble 86-kDa homodimeric glycoprotein. Each 43-kDa subunit contains both N- and O-linked carbohydrate chains attached to a 26-kDa protein core (Manos, 1988; Rettenmier and Roussel, 1988).

A 1.6-kb mRNA codes for a form of M-CSF that has eliminated a coding region within exon 6 by alternative splicing (Figure 4.7). This form of M-CSF retains the transmembrane and cytoplasmic domains of full-length M-CSF and the initial N-terminal 149 amino acids but has lost most of the rest of the extracellular domain, including the putative proteolytic cleavage site. Consequently, it is expressed relatively stably at the cell surface as a 68-kDa homodimer, although it can be slowly released by proteolysis into the medium as a 44-kDa homodimer containing two sites of N-linked complex carbohydrate and no *O*-glycosylation (Rettenmier et al., 1987; Rettenmier and Roussel, 1988).

The 2.3-kb mRNA codes for a form of M-CSF that contains an additional 182 amino acids present in the longest transcript of human M-CSF. This segment contains two potential proteolytic sites (Gly-Gly-X), so, like the longer form of M-CSF, it is also rapidly proteolytically processed to release an 86-kDa homodimer.

Since soluble M-CSFs produced by each of the three transcripts are fully biologically active, it is clear that the receptor binding and activation sites of M-CSF are located in the first 149 amino acids, which has been confirmed by the production of an active 149-amino acid M-CSF in recombinant form in *E. coli* (Halenbeck et al., 1989). This observation also indicates that the many sites of glycosylation of M-CSF are not required for biological activity. Nevertheless, it has been observed in both mice and humans that the major form of M-CSF produced in vivo may be of very high apparent molecular weight (greater than 200,000) and has attached chondroitin sulfate (Price et al., 1992; Suzu et al., 1992b). M-CSFs produced by the 4- and 2.2-kb mRNAs, but not the 1.6-kb mRNA, contain a single glycosaminoglycan (GAG) attachment site (Ala-Ser-Gly) at Ser 277. These proteoglycan forms of M-CSF are fully biologically active and show a selective capacity to bind to type V collagen, but not to other types of collagen or fibronectin (Suzu et al., 1992a). Thus, the chondroitin sulfate chain may serve to localize these forms of secreted M-CSF to the extracellular matrix.

The disulfide bonding pattern of human M-CSF has been determined and shows that a single cysteine in each monomer (cys 31) forms an intermolecular disulfide bond, while the other six cysteine residues (all in the first 149 amino acids of each form of M-CSF) form three intramolecular disulfide bonds (Cys 7–90, 48–139, 102–146; Glocker et al., 1993; Yamanishi et al., 1993). In longer forms of M-CSF, additional intermolecular disulfide bonds may occur between Cys 157 and Cys 159 in each subunit (Glocker et al., 1993).

Despite its dimeric nature, the structure of M-CSF determined by X-ray crystallography (Figures 4.2 and 4.8) (Pandit et al., 1992) has revealed that each subunit in the M-CSF dimer takes up a three-dimensional conformation very similar to that of GM-CSF. Each subunit is a short-chain four-$\alpha$-helical bundle with two long overhand loops (A–B, C–D) that each contribute one strand to a short antiparallel $\beta$-sheet. However, unlike the related IL-5 and interferon $\gamma$ dimeric structures, where the opposite subunit contributes the D-helix to the four-$\alpha$-helical bundle, in M-CSF the subunits form independent four-$\alpha$-helical bundles with a head-to-head arrangement. The twofold symmetry axis runs perpendicular to the helix bundle axes with the A–B and C–D loops forming the major interface between the subunits. This arrangement results in a flat, elongated structure $80 \times 30 \times 20$ Å.

M-CSF shows distant sequence homology to SCF and the ligand for the flk-2 receptor (Lu et al., 1991; Lyman et al., 1993; Hannum et al., 1994). Although these do not form disulfide-bonded homodimers, they nevertheless do form noncovalent homodimers. This homology is reinforced by the conservation of some intramolecular disulfide bonds and the use in each case of type III tyrosine kinase receptors that contain five immunoglobulin-like loops in their extracellular domains. In addition, each of these growth factors is produced in both membrane-attached and soluble forms (Lu et al., 1991; Hannum et al., 1994). These observations

```
                  -30       -20       -10         1       10        20
HU M-CSF          MTAPGAAGRCPPTTWLGSLLLLVCLLASRSITEEVSEYCSHMIGSGHLQSLQ
MU M-CSF          MTARGRAGRCPSSTWLGSRLLLVCLLMSRSIAKEVSEHCSHMIGNGHLKVLQ
                  ***.* *****. ***** ******* ****. ****.******.***. **

                  30        40        50        60        70        80
HU M-CSF  RLIDSQMETSCQITFEFVDQEQLKDPVCYLKKAFLLVQDIMEDTMRFRDNTPNAIAIVQL
MU M-CSF  QLIDSQMETSCQIAFEFVDQEQLDDPVCYLKKAFFLVQDIIDETMRFKDNTPNANATERL
          .************.*********.**********.*****...****.****** *. .*

                  90       100       110       120       130       140
HU M-CSF  QELSLRLKSCFTKDYEEHDKACVRTFYETPLQLLEKVKNVFNETKNLLDKDWNIFSKNCN
MU M-CSF  QELSNNLNSCFTKDYEEQNKACVRTFHETPLQLLEKIKNFFNETKNLLEKDWNIFTKNCN
          **** .* *********..*******.*********.**.********.******.****

                      A
                 150       160       170       180       190       200
HU M-CSF  NSFAECSSQDVVTKPDCNCLYPKAIPSSDPASVSPHQPLAPSMAPVAGLTWEDSEGTEGS
MU M-CSF  NSFAKCSSRDVVTKPDCNCLYPKATPSSDPASASPHQPPAPSMAPLAGLAWDDSQRTEGS
          **** ***.***************.*******.***** ******.***.*.**. ****

                                                       ▼
                 210       220       230       240       250       260
HU M-CSF  SLLPGEQPLHTVDPGSAKQRPPRSTCQSFEPPETPVVKDSTIGGSPQPRPSVGAFNPGME
MU M-CSF  SLLPSELPLRIEDAGSAKQRPPRSTCQTLESTEQPNHGDR-LTEDSQPHPSAGGPVPGVE
          ****.* **..* .*************..*..* *   *. .....**.**.*.  **.*
```

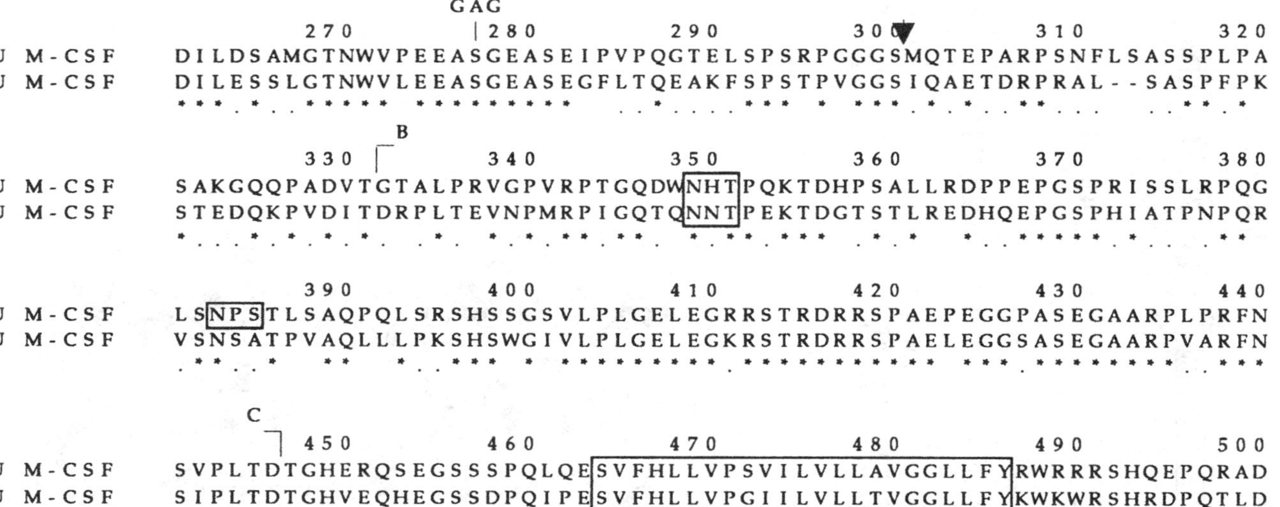


Figure 4.6. Aligned amino acid sequences of human and mouse M-CSF. Numbering and symbols are as for Figure 4.1 except that the transmembrane region is boxed, as are the tripeptide sequences that define N-linked glycosylation sites. Arrowheads define two potential proteolytic cleavage sites, and the serine at position 277 that defines the glycosaminoglycan attachment site is marked with the symbol GAG. The site labeled A at position 150 is the exon boundary for exon 5, and the two alternative splice sites at position 332 or 447 are labeled B and C.

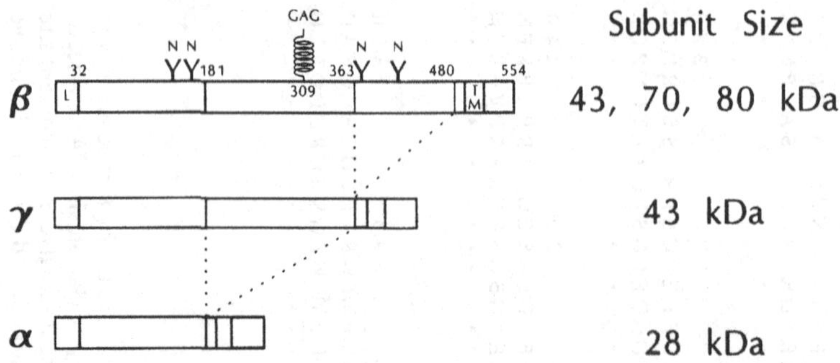


Figure 4.7. The protein structure of alternative M-CSF transcripts derived from the sequences of Figure 4.6. The leader sequence is labeled L, the transmembrane region as TM, glycosylation sites as Y, and the glycosaminoglycan (GAG) attachment site as a helix.

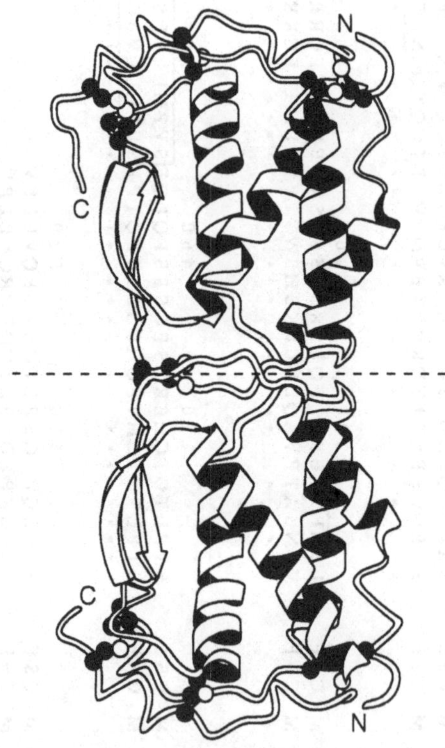


Figure 4.8. The structure of the human M-CSF dimer as determined by X-ray crystallography (Pandit et al., 1992). Representation is as for Figure 4.3, with the symmetry axis shown as a dashed line.

suggest that the structural organization of these growth factors may be similar (Bazan, 1991a).

## Multi-CSF (IL-3)

Murine IL-3 was first purified by Ihle et al. (1982) from conditioned medium of the myelomonocytic leukemic cell line WEHI-3B on the basis of its capacity to induce the enzyme 20α-hydroxysteroid dehydrogenase in cultures of spleen cells. Ihle et al. (1983) went on to show that this factor was the same as mast cell growth factor, P-cell-stimulating, and Multi-CSF, each of which was subsequently purified independently (Bazill et al., 1983; Clark-Lewis et al., 1984; Urdal et al., 1984; Cutler et al., 1985). In these studies, especially from the activated T-cell sources (Urdal et al., 1984; Cutler et al., 1985; Ziltener et al., 1988b), considerable size (16–45 kDa) and charge heterogeneity of Multi-CSF were noted due to extensive glycosylation differences. However, Multi-CSF (IL-3) could most readily be distinguished from other CSFs by its failure to bind to DEAE-Sepharose at neutral pH, indicating that it had a relatively high or neutral isoelectric point. Human Multi-CSF was not purified from natural sources until 1991 (Zenke et al., 1991), and its existence remained controversial until its expression cloning in 1986 (Yang et al., 1986). A cDNA for human Multi-CSF could not be isolated by cross-hybridization with murine Multi-CSF cDNA because Multi-CSF is among the least conserved of cytokines (29% sequence identity between mice and humans) (Figure 4.9) and does not act across these species.

Murine Multi-CSF is synthesized as a precursor with a 26–amino acid hydrophobic leader sequence that is proteolytically cleaved before secretion. The mature protein contains 140 amino acids (Fung et al., 1984), although the original form purified from WEHI-3B-conditioned medium was N-terminally truncated by 6 amino acids, presumably due to proteolytic degradation (Ihle et al., 1982). It contains four cysteine residues forming two intramolecular disulfide bonds (Cys 17–80, Cys 79–140) (Clark-Lewis et al., 1988b; Knepper et al., 1992). The predicted molecular weight of the protein is 16,200, and *N*-glycanase treatment of T-cell-derived murine Multi-CSF or tunicamycin treatment of T-cell cultures indeed produces Multi-CSF of this size (Ziltener et al., 1988b). Untreated murine Multi-CSF from this source showed discrete molecular weights of 22,000, 29,000, and 34,000 representing different *N*-glycosylated forms of Multi-CSF, and because murine Multi-CSF has four potential *N*-glycosylation sites at Asn 16, 44, 51, and 86, presumably three of these are used to

```
                             -10        1        10        20        30
HU  IL-3       M-------SRLPVLLLQLLVRPGLQAPMTQTTSLKTSWV-NCSNMIDEIITHLKQP
MU  IL-3       MVLASSTTSIHTMLLLLMLFHLGLQASISGRDTHRLTRTLNCSSIVKEIIGKLPEP
               *       *   .**** .*  ****.   . . .  .. ***..  *** .*  *
                                        1        10        20        30

                   40        50        60        70        80        90
HU  IL-3  PLPLLDFNNLNGEDQDILMENNLRRPNLEAFNRAVKSL--QNASAIESILKNLLPCLPLATA
MU  IL-3  ELK-------TDDEGPSLRNKSFRRVNLSKFVESQGEVDPEDRYVIKSNLQKLNCCLPTSAN
           *       ....    * ....** **. *  . .    ..   *.* *..*  *** ...
                         40        50        60        70        80

                100       110       120       130
HU  IL-3  APTRHPIHIKDGDWNEFRRKLTFYLKTLENAQAQQTTLSLAIF-------------
MU  IL-3  DSALPGVFIRD--LDDFRKKLRFYMVHLNDLETVLTSRPPQPASGSVSPNRGTVEC
          . .. . .* *.   .**.** **.  *.. ..  *
            90       100       110       120       130       140
```

Figure 4.9. Aligned amino acid sequences of human and mouse Multi-CSF (IL-3). Numbering and symbols are as for Figures 4.1 and 4.6.

account for the three observed molecular weights. In the baculovirus system, only Asn 16 and 86 were glycosylated (Knepper et al., 1992). In both systems there was no evidence for *O*-glycosylation of Multi-CSF. Recombinant murine Multi-CSF produced in *E. coli* is fully biologically active and has unaltered affinity for Multi-CSF receptors, suggesting that these glycosylation sites are not involved in the receptor-binding site.

During the analysis of murine Multi-CSF produced by WEHI-3B cells or in the baculovirus expression system, it was noted that proteolytically clipped forms of Multi-CSF were also fully active biologically. In the first case (Ihle et al., 1982), the first 6 amino acids were removed, and in the second, a proteolytic clip was introduced between Ala 127 and Ser 128 (Knepper et al., 1992), so these sites do not appear to be part of the active site of the molecule. Chemical synthesis of murine Multi-CSF has shown that the first 16 amino acids are not essential for activity and that a peptide corresponding to the first 79 amino acids of Multi-CSF has weak biological activity as long as the disulfide bond is intact (Clark-Lewis et al., 1986, 1988a). Monoclonal antibodies to the N-terminal 6 amino acids (Conlon et al., 1985; Ziltener et al., 1987) or the C-terminal end (Ser 130-Arg 135; Ziltener et al., 1988a) of murine IL-3 failed to neutralize biological activity. However, antibodies to amino acid residues 14–45 did neutralize the biological activity of murine IL-3 (Conlon et al., 1985; Ziltener et al., 1988a), suggesting that the predicted first $\alpha$-helix (A-helix) and the A–B loop are involved in receptor binding.

Human Multi-CSF is synthesized as a precursor with a 19–amino acid leader sequence and is secreted as a mature protein of 133 amino acids (protein core $M_r$ 15,400). It contains only two potential *N*-glycosylation sites (Asn 15 and Asn 70) and retains only one disulfide bond that is homologous to murine Multi-CSF (Cys 16–84) (Yang et al., 1986).

When neutralizing monoclonal antibodies to human Multi-CSF were used, two distinct epitopes at the N- and C-terminal ends of the molecule were recognized, namely, Val 14-Gln 45 and Phe 107-Glu 119 (Dorssers et al., 1991; Lokker et al., 1991; Kaushansky et al., 1992), and these fall within the predicted first (A) and fourth (D) helices (Parry et al., 1988, 1991). With both murine and human Multi-CSF, antibodies to the central region of the molecule (residues 56–74) were not inhibitory. Using gibbon–mouse chimeric IL-3 molecules, Kaushansky et al. (1992) showed that human receptor binding and biological activity were dependent on residues 15–22 and 107–119, consistent with the preceding data. Lopez et al. (1992a) have confirmed by site-directed mutagenesis the importance of the predicted A-helix in generating high-affinity binding and biological activity of human Multi-CSF, particularly in residues 21 and 22. Similarly, some mutations in the predicted D-helix (residues 104–108) resulted in reduced biological activity, while other mutations (at positions 101 and 116) actually resulted in higher receptor-binding affinity and biological activity. These authors suggested that the D-helix was involved primarily in interactions with the $\alpha$-chain of the Multi-CSF receptor, while the A-helix was involved in interactions with the $\beta$-chain to generate high-affinity binding. This may serve as a paradigm for the interactions of GM-CSF, Multi-CSF, and IL-5 with their respective $\alpha$-/$\beta$-chain heterodimeric receptors (Goodall et al., 1993; Kastelein and Shanafelt, 1993; Sprang and Bazan, 1993).

## Conclusions

Despite the lack of primary amino acid sequence homology of the CSFs, they each take up very similar folded structures based on the four-$\alpha$-helical bundle structure that is common to many cytokines. GM-CSF, Multi-CSF, and M-CSF belong to the short-chain submembers of this family, with M-CSF duplicating the basic design by the use of an intersubunit disulfide bond. On the other hand, G-CSF belongs to the long-chain group, along with IL-6 and LIF. These robust structures are further stabilized by intramolecular disulfide bonds and attached carbohydrate that allow the CSFs to function in the hostile environment of ongoing tissue reactions. Moreover, the common structures of the CSFs, and their relationship to almost all other cytokines that utilize hemopoietin domain receptors, reflects their common evolutionary origin from a molecule designed to bridge two receptor subunits. The structural elements in the CSFs that form two separate binding sites, either for common or for different receptor subunits, are beginning to be elucidated, and such studies promise to be extremely useful in the design of new-generation agonists and antagonists of CSF action.

# 5

# Biochemistry of the colony-stimulating factor receptors

The receptors for the colony-stimulating factors are responsible for detecting and responding to the presence of CSFs in the medium and initiating an appropriate biological response. Initially there appeared to be a great deal of complexity in the structure of CSF receptors. High- and low-affinity forms, cross-reactive and non-cross-reactive forms, and different molecular sizes for each type of CSF receptor have been described. With the molecular cloning of CSF receptor subunits (Figure 5.1), the situation has been considerably clarified, and a great deal of uniformity has emerged. The M-CSF receptor is a classical growth factor receptor of the tyrosine kinase type, while the other CSF receptors all belong to a superfamily of hemopoietin receptors (Table 5.1). They each function by forming homo- or heterodimeric receptor complexes that result in the activation of cytoplasmic tyrosine kinases and downstream signaling events. In this chapter the structure and function of CSF receptors will be reviewed with an emphasis on their common structural organization and signaling mechanisms.

## M-CSF receptor (c-*fms*)

The recognition that the feline retroviral oncogene (v-*fms*) encoded a cell-surface receptor that could bind M-CSF (Sherr et al., 1985) allowed the first molecular definition of a CSF receptor. The cellular homologue of the viral oncogene (c-*fms*) is a single-chain type III membrane glycoprotein with a single transmembrane domain of 25 amino acids, an N-terminal extracellular domain of 512 amino acids (including the leader sequence), and a C-terminal intracellular domain of 435 amino acids (Coussens et al., 1986; Rothwell and Rohrschneider, 1987).

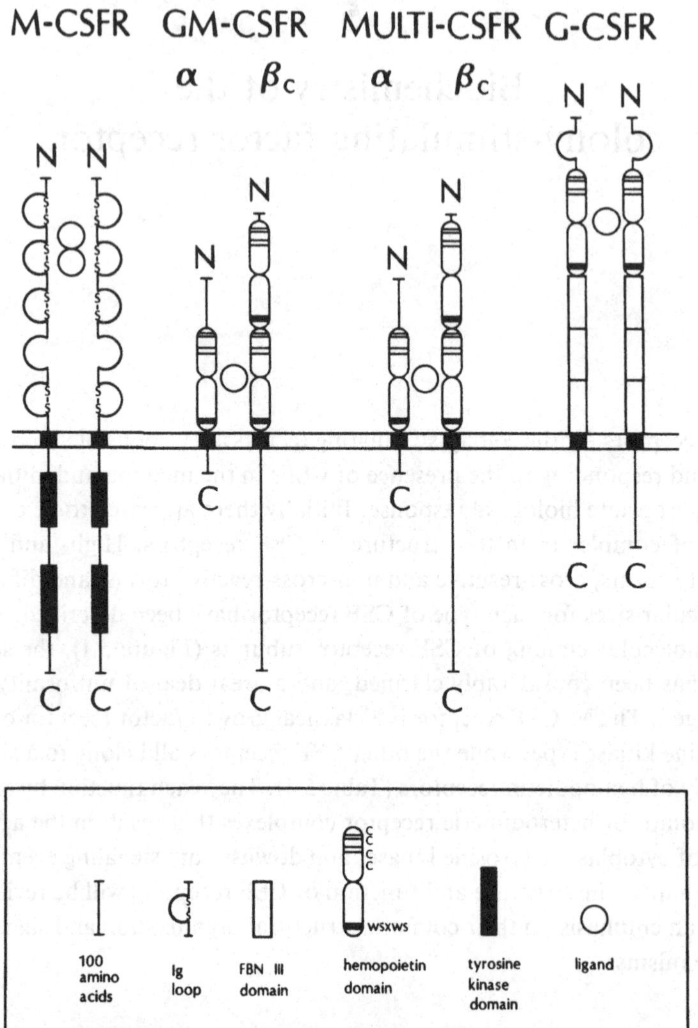


Figure 5.1. Subunit structures and structural elements of the CSF receptors. The M-CSF and G-CSF receptors are homodimers, while the Multi-CSF and GM-CSF receptors are heterodimers consisting of unique $\alpha$-chains and a common $\beta$-chain.

The extracellular domain contains the ligand binding site and presumably the site that leads to homodimerization of two M-CSF receptor molecules. It consists of five loop structures that appear to be homologous to immunoglobulin domains, and four of these contain the disulfide bonds characteristic of these structures. The M-CSF binding site has been localized

Table 5.1.. *Molecular properties of CSF receptors*

| Receptor | Structure | Molecular mass (kDa) | Intrinsic $K_D$ (n$M$) | Other subunits | High-affinity $K_D$ (p$M$) |
|---|---|---|---|---|---|
| hM-CSFR | $(Ig)_5TK$ | 150 | 1 | — | — |
| mM-CSFR | $(Ig)_5TK$ | 150 | 0.03 | — | — |
| hGM-CSFR$\alpha$ | (Ig)HD | 85 | 5 | $\beta_c$ | 20–30 |
| mGM-CSFR$\alpha$ | (Ig)HD | 55 | 5 | $\beta_c$ | 20–30 |
| hIL-3R$\alpha$ | (Ig)HD | 75 | 100 | $\beta_c$ | 100–300 |
| mIL-3R$\alpha$ | (Ig)HD | 75 | 45 | $\beta_{IL\text{-}3}$, $\beta_c$ | 100–300 |
| h$\beta_c$ | $(HD)_2$ | 120 | — | GM, IL-3, IL-5R$\alpha$ | — |
| m$\beta_c$ | $(HD)_2$ | 120 | — | GM, IL-3, IL-5R$\alpha$ | — |
| m$\beta_{IL\text{-}3}$ | $(HD)_2$ | 120 | 10 | IL-3R$\alpha$ | — |
| hG-CSFR | $(Ig)HD(FBNIII)_3$ | 150 | 0.5 | — | — |
| mG-CSFR | $(Ig)HD(FBNIII)_3$ | 150 | 0.5 | — | — |

to the ffrst three immunoglobulin-like domains, with an essential contribution from the third domain (Wang et al., 1993). There are 11 sites for potential *N*-glycosylation in the extracellular domain, and the mature protein has an electrophoretic mass of 150 kDa compared with the predicted 105 kDa of the unglycosylated molecule. The M-CSF receptor is co-translationally glycosylated in the rough endoplasmic reticulum by the addition of high-mannose oligosaccharides (130-kDa form), which are further processed to complex acidic-type sugars (150-kDa form) in the Golgi before presentation at the plasma membrane (Sherr, 1990).

The cytoplasmic domain contains sequences characteristic of tyrosine kinases, although this homology domain is split by a 72–amino acid kinase insert sequence that separates the ATP binding site ($GXGXXG_{594}$... $K_{616}$...) from the rest of the consensus catalytic site of tyrosine kinases. The kinase insert domain contains three potential tyrosine phosphorylation sites (Y699, Y708, Y723), with two further sites in the second tyrosine kinase homology domain (Y809) and near the C-terminus (Y969) (Figure 5.2).

The M-CSF receptor is structurally most closely related to the $\alpha$- and $\beta$-receptors for platelet-derived growth factor, the c-*kit* receptor for stem cell factor or Steel ligand, the flk-2 receptor whose ligand has recently been identified as homologous with M-CSF and SCF (Lyman et al., 1993; Hannum et al., 1994), and the KDR/flk-1 receptor for vascular endothelial cell growth factor (Quinn et al., 1993). Each of these receptors contains extracellular domains characterized by five immunoglobulin-like loops, contains an interrupted cytoplasmic tyrosine kinase domain, and recognizes homodimeric ligands. They each appear to require receptor homodimerization for activation of their tyrosine kinase domain and for signal transduction (Sherr, 1990).

The M-CSF receptor is expressed predominantly in macrophages (Byrne et al., 1981) and placental trophoblasts (Pampfer et al., 1992) but also in other tissues, including osteoclasts (Hofstetter et al., 1992) and their precursors, atherosclerotic intimal smooth muscle cells (Inaba et al., 1992b), and cells of the uterine endometrium (Pampfer et al., 1992). In the monocyte-macrophage cell series, receptor numbers increase with cellular maturation from a few hundred per cell on monocytes and their precursors to several thousand on activated peritoneal macrophages (Byrne et al., 1981) (Table 5.2). In all cases where they have been examined, the M-CSF receptors display a single class of binding affinity with an apparent equilibrium dissociation constant of about 30 p*M*. However, at 4°C, binding

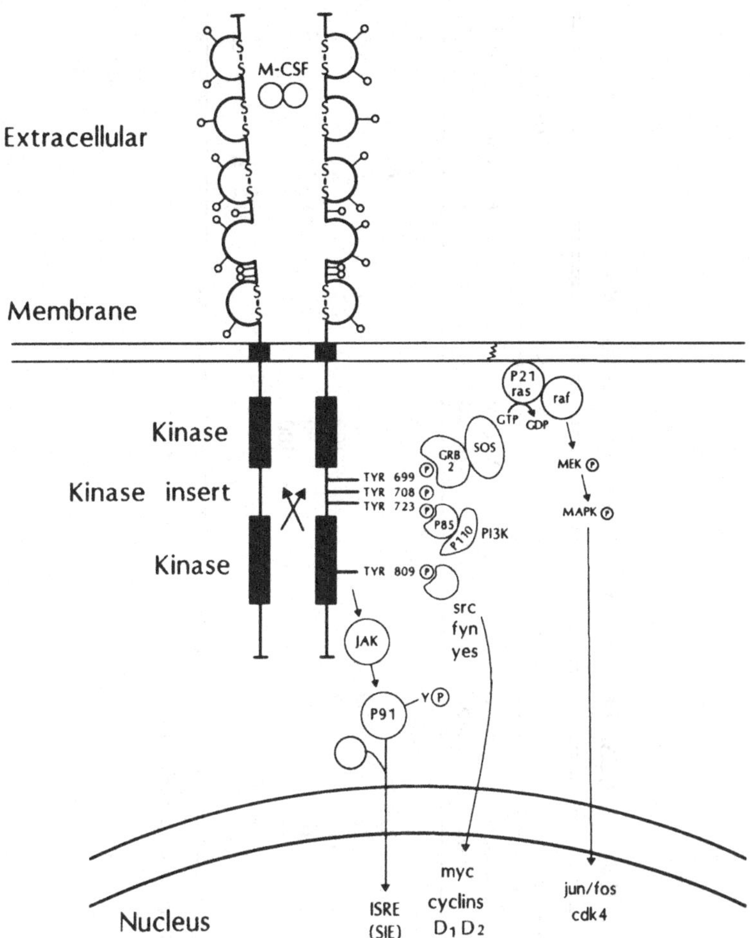


Figure 5.2. Signaling through the M-CSF receptor homodimer. Upon M-CSF binding, the cytoplasmic tyrosine kinase domains phosphorylate in trans a series of tyrosine residues (indicated) that serve as recognition elements for binding SH2-containing effector molecules such as GRB2, PI3 kinase, *src,* or JAK. These lead to the activation of nuclear transcription factors as shown.

of M-CSF to its receptor is essentially irreversible, so that a true equilibrium is not attained and the apparent equilibrium constant is better thought of as a steady-state constant with binding being accompanied by the loss of apparent binding sites (Stanley and Guilbert, 1981).

At 37°C, the binding of M-CSF is not irreversible, and measurement of the kinetic rate constants suggests an equilibrium dissociation constant

Table 5.2. *Distribution of CSF receptors on murine bone marrow cells*

| Cell | M-CSF | | GM-CSF | | Multi-CSF | | G-CSF | |
|---|---|---|---|---|---|---|---|---|
| | Percent labeled | Grain count | Percent labeled | Grain count | Percent labeled | Grain count | Percent labeled | Grain count |
| Blasts | 79 | 121 | 89 | 80 | 88 | 61 | 76 | 19 |
| Promyelocytes/myelocytes | 81 | 27 | 100 | 90 | 100 | 75 | 94 | 24 |
| Polymorphs | 75 | 22 | 100 | 65 | 100 | 26 | 100 | 44 |
| Promonocytes | 100 | 178 | 100 | 94 | 100 | 63 | 77 | 8 |
| Monocytes | 89 | 118 | 100 | 48 | 96 | 36 | 57 | 4 |
| Eosinophils | 0 | — | 93 | 29 | 100 | 61 | 0 | — |
| Lymphocytes | 23 | 78 | 0 | — | 0 | — | 0 | — |
| Nucleated erythroid | 0 | — | 0 | — | 0 | — | 0 | — |

*Note:* Data derived from autoradiography of adult marrow cells after incubation with $^{125}$I-labeled CSF.

of about 400 p*M*. After binding of M-CSF, rapid noncovalent homodimerization of the M-CSF receptor occurs followed by the formation of covalent disulfide bonds between the receptor chains. This, along with activation of the intrinsic tyrosine kinase activity of the receptor, leads to rapid internalization of receptor complexes through clathrin-coated pits and targeting to lysosomal degradation (Carlberg et al., 1991; Li and Stanley, 1991). This homologous downregulation of M-CSF receptors by M-CSF occurs more rapidly in mature macrophages than in monocytes and has been thought to form a feedback loop that limits the action of extracellular M-CSF (Guilbert and Stanley, 1986; Guilbert et al., 1986; Bartocci et al., 1987).

In addition to M-CSF-induced receptor internalization and degradation, which is dependent on receptor kinase activity, the M-CSF receptor can be downregulated by a variety of unrelated agents that do not bind directly to the M-CSF receptor. These include protein kinase C–activating agents such as phorbol esters (Downing et al., 1989) and bacterial lipopolysaccharide (LPS) (Chen et al., 1993), which downregulate the receptor by a mechanism distinct from that initiated by M-CSF. Activation of protein kinase C apparently activates, in turn, a protease that cleaves the M-CSF receptor in the extracellular domain near the transmembrane region. This releases the 100-kDa ligand binding domain into the extracellular space, where it may act as an M-CSF "scavenger" to achieve targeting of the remaining cell-associated 50-kDa domain for intracellular degradation. In this situation, the M-CSF receptor is not phosphorylated on serine or tyrosine, so it presumably remains in an inactive form (Downing et al., 1989). On the other hand, downregulation of M-CSF receptors by LPS involves activation of phospholipase C but is not inhibited by protein kinase C or protease inhibitors (Chen et al., 1993). Other cytokines such as interferon $\gamma$, GM-CSF, Multi-CSF, and interleukin-1 also result in acute downregulation of M-CSF receptors by an indirect, temperature-dependent mechanism (Walker et al., 1985; Chen, 1991), and in some cases (interferon $\gamma$) this form of downregulation mimics that of protein kinase C activators (Baccarini et al., 1992). The action of these proinflammatory agents in apparently downregulating the response to M-CSF is somewhat paradoxical, since the same agents induce M-CSF production and secretion. It may help to divert macrophages to activation rather than proliferation, prevent autostimulatory proliferative loops, or provide a self-limiting feedback loop to prevent overrecruitment of macrophages to inflammatory sites (Sherr, 1990).

### *M-CSF receptor signal transduction*

M-CSF binding results in homodimerization of the M-CSF receptor, and this extracellular event brings the cytoplasmic domains of the receptors together. The interaction of these two domains is thought to result in a conformational change that activates the tyrosine kinase domains so that they phosphorylate each other in trans on tyrosine residues. These residues include Tyr 697, 706, and 721 in the kinase insert domain, Tyr 807 in the kinase domain as well as other tyrosine residues (the equivalent human receptor residues are 699, 708, 723, and 809). Mutation analysis has shown that only phosphorylation of Tyr 721 is required for binding of phosphatidyl-inositol 3-kinase (PI3 kinase) to the activated receptor, and this residue occurs in the consensus sequence (Tyr-Val-Glu-Met) required for binding the P85 subunit of PI3 kinase to other tyrosine kinase receptors (Reedijk et al., 1992). The P85 subunit of PI3 kinase contains an *src* homology 2 (SH2) domain responsible for binding to the tyrosine phosphorylated site and for coupling it to the catalytic subunit p110. Tyr 697 has been identified as the binding site for GRB2, another SH2-containing adaptor molecule that couples receptor activation to the *ras* pathway (Van der Geer and Hunter, 1993). Other *src*-like kinases can also bind to the activated M-CSF receptor, but phospholipase C$\gamma$1 and the p21 *ras* guanine-nucleotide triphosphatase-activating protein (GAP), which also contain SH2 domains and bind to other activated tyrosine kinase receptors, do not (Figure 5.2). As a result, M-CSF does not stimulate phosphatidyl inositol turnover.

The kinase insert domains of the M-CSF receptor and v-*fms* could be deleted without affecting fibroblast transformation, suggesting that neither phosphorylation of the tyrosine residues in this region nor PI3 kinase binding is essential for this response (Taylor et al., 1989a). However, Van der Geer and Hunter (1993) found that both Tyr 697 and Tyr 721 in the kinase insert domain of the M-CSF receptor were required for rat-2 fibroblast proliferation in response to M-CSF. Similarly, substitution of Tyr 809 by phenylalanine significantly inhibited M-CSF-induced growth. Since this mutated receptor retained tyrosine kinase activity, PI3 kinase-binding activity, and the capacity to induce c-*fos*, c-*jun*, *jun B*, and c-*ets* 2, these events are not sufficient to signal cell proliferation (Roussel et al., 1990). The mutated receptor did not result in c-*myc* induction, and enforced expression of exogenous c-*myc* reinstated the M-CSF-dependent mitogenic response (Roussel et al., 1991). These data suggest that phosphorylation of Tyr 809 results in c-*myc* induction, which is required for the proliferative response. Since *src* itself, as well as the related kinases *fyn* and *fes*, also associate with this phosphorylated tyrosine (Courtneidge et al., 1993) and are activated in their kinase activity, they may play a role in *myc* activation. Recent data have also suggested that, like the other hemopoietic receptors, M-CSF receptor activation involves activation of JAK kinases and consequent phosphorylation of nuclear transcription factors related to those that interact with interferon response elements (Silvennoinen et al., 1993a,b).

Despite its failure to bind to or phosphorylate GAP, activation of the M-CSF receptor nevertheless does affect p21 *ras*. It increases GTP bound to p21 *ras*, perhaps by interacting with other proteins (such as GRB2) that lead to exchange of GDP for GTP on p21 *ras* (Smith et al., 1986). In other cell systems, GTP-activated p21 *ras* leads to activation of *raf* and hence the mitogen-activated protein kinase (MAP kinase) cascade that leads to transcriptional activation of *fos* and *jun* (Figure 5.2).

M-CSF is required continuously throughout the $G_1$ phase of the cell cycle in order for macrophages to enter the S phase of DNA synthesis. Activation of the M-CSF receptor induces mRNA and protein for a unique D1 cyclin within 2 hours and is required for its continued elevation during $G_1$. A more modest periodic increase in the mRNA for the related cyclin D2 is also induced after cyclin D1. Cyclin D1 forms a complex with a novel cyclin-dependent serine/threonine kinase p34 (cdK4), which is also coordinately expressed with cyclin D2. The transient expression of such complexes may be involved in cell cycle progression, possibly by phosphorylating the retinoblastoma gene product (Roussel and Sherr, 1993; Sherr, 1993).

### *Oncogenic transformation of the M-CSF receptor*

The transforming gene v-*fms* of the Susan McDonough strain of feline sarcoma virus induces the neoplastic transformation of fibroblasts and factor-dependent murine myeloid cell lines, as well as normal erythroid and B-lymphocyte progenitors (Heard et al., 1987; Wheeler et al., 1987). This indicates that proliferative signals generated by an activated M-CSF receptor are promiscuous; this has been confirmed by transfer of normal M-CSF receptors to factor-dependent myeloid and lymphoid cells, which allows the cells to proliferate in response to stimulation by exogenous M-CSF (Wheeler et al., 1987; Borzillo and Sherr, 1989).

The ligand-independent v-*fms* protein is a constitutively activated tyrosine kinase differing from the feline M-CSF receptor because of replacement of the C-terminal 50 amino acids by 11 novel amino acids and nine point mutations (Woolford et al., 1988). The C-terminal truncation disrupts a negative regulatory element of the receptor tyrosine kinase activity, but by itself, this is insufficient to create the transforming phenotype. Rather, mutations in the extracellular domain of the M-CSF receptor are required, and the single mutation, serine to leucine at position 301, was sufficient to create the transforming phenotype (Roussel et al., 1988). This does not alter M-CSF binding but may induce receptor dimerization and activation of kinase activity by trans-phosphorylation. The human M-CSF receptor can be mutated at several different extracellular sites to generate the transforming phenotype, including the region between the third and fourth immunoglobulin-like loops and within the fourth loop as well as codon 301 (Van Daalen Wetters et al., 1992). However, mutations in the M-CSF receptor in human leukemias are relatively rare, and the role of such mutations is not yet clear (Ridge et al., 1990; Tobal et al., 1990).

## GM-CSF receptors

GM-CSF receptors have been detected in low numbers (50–500) on cells of the monocyte-macrophage, neutrophil, and eosinophil cell lineages of both mice and humans with the number of receptors decreasing slightly with cellular maturation (Table 5.2) (Nicola, 1987a; Di Persio et al., 1988). Many primary human myeloid leukemic cells and even some lymphoid leukemic cells have been shown to retain GM-CSF receptors with similar binding characteristics to receptors on normal cells (Gasson et al., 1986; Kelleher et al., 1988; Budel et al., 1990). Although GM-CSF receptors have also been detected on several nonhemopoietic tumor cell lines (Dedhar et al., 1988; Baldwin et al., 1989), their significance is unclear. Nevertheless, GM-CSF receptors have also been detected, and may be functional, on normal human endothelial cells (Bussolino et al., 1989) and placental trophoblasts (Gearing et al., 1989b).

High-affinity ($K_D \approx 20$–$60\ \text{p}M$) and low-affinity ($K_D \approx 1$–$6\ \text{n}M$) receptors for GM-CSF have been described for both mice and humans (Walker and Burgess, 1985; Gasson et al., 1986; Park et al., 1986; Gearing et al., 1989b). However, low-affinity receptors have nearly always been detected with co-existing high-affinity receptors, while high-affinity receptors may represent the sole class of GM-CSF receptor on some cell types. Moreover, solubilization of high-affinity GM-CSF receptors in detergents results in their conversion to a low-affinity form with the same binding characteristics as the low-affinity receptor detected on intact cells (Nicola and Cary, 1992).

In the mouse, GM-CSF receptor binding is not competed for by other CSFs when competition experiments are performed at 4°C. However, at 37°C, GM-CSF receptors are indirectly downmodulated by Multi-CSF or high concentrations of M-CSF (Walker et al., 1985; Nicola, 1987a). In contrast, human GM-CSF receptors on a variety of cell lines are downmodulated at both 4° and 37°C by Multi-CSF and IL-5 (Elliott et al., 1989; Lopez et al., 1989; Budel et al., 1990). This apparent cross-reactivity is incomplete and is due in large part to a conversion of high-affinity receptors to a low-affinity form (Budel et al., 1990).

The basis for this phenomenon became clear with the molecular cloning of GM-CSF receptor subunits (Figures 5.1 and 5.3). The first receptor subunit to be cloned (subsequently termed the $\alpha$-subunit) was a low-affinity receptor from human placenta with a $K_D$ of about 5 n$M$ (Gearing et al., 1989b). It was recognized at the time that this receptor helped define an emerging receptor superfamily (the hemopoietin receptors) that included receptors for IL-6, erythropoietin, prolactin, and the $\beta$-chain of the IL-2 receptor characterized by homologies in the extracellular domain (conserved cysteine residues and the element Trp-Ser-X-Trp-Ser). Moreover, since this receptor subunit was specific for GM-CSF and was also expressed on hemopoietic cells, it was suggested that a second subunit must exist to generate high-affinity binding, and if this second subunit was shared with Multi-CSF receptors, it could explain indirect receptor downmodulation (Gearing et al., 1989b; Nicola, 1991a,b).

The second subunit (the $\beta$-subunit) of the human GM-CSF receptor was cloned by Hayashida et al. (1990) as KH97 and shown to reconstitute high-affinity binding of GM-CSF on simian fibroblasts. The $\beta$-subunit is also a member of the hemopoietin receptor superfamily, but unlike the $\alpha$-chain it contains a duplicated hemopoietin domain and a much longer cytoplasmic domain. Subsequently, it was shown that the $\beta$-subunit ($\beta_c$) is shared by the $\alpha$-chain receptors for Multi-CSF and IL-5 and is required in each case for the generation of high-affinity receptors and for biological signal transduction (Kitamura et al., 1991a,b; Tavernier et al., 1991).

The existence of high- and low-affinity GM-CSF receptors can now be explained by variable expression levels of $\alpha$- and $\beta_c$-receptor subunits. With an excess of $\beta_c$-chains, only high-affinity receptors are observed, but with an excess of $\alpha$-chains, both high- and low-affinity receptors are observed. Despite the fact that $\beta_c$-subunits can interact with complexes of $\alpha$-subunit and GM-CSF to generate high-affinity receptors, $\beta_c$-subunits demonstrate no detectable binding affinity for GM-CSF in the absence of $\alpha$-subunits. This arrangement also provides a ready explanation

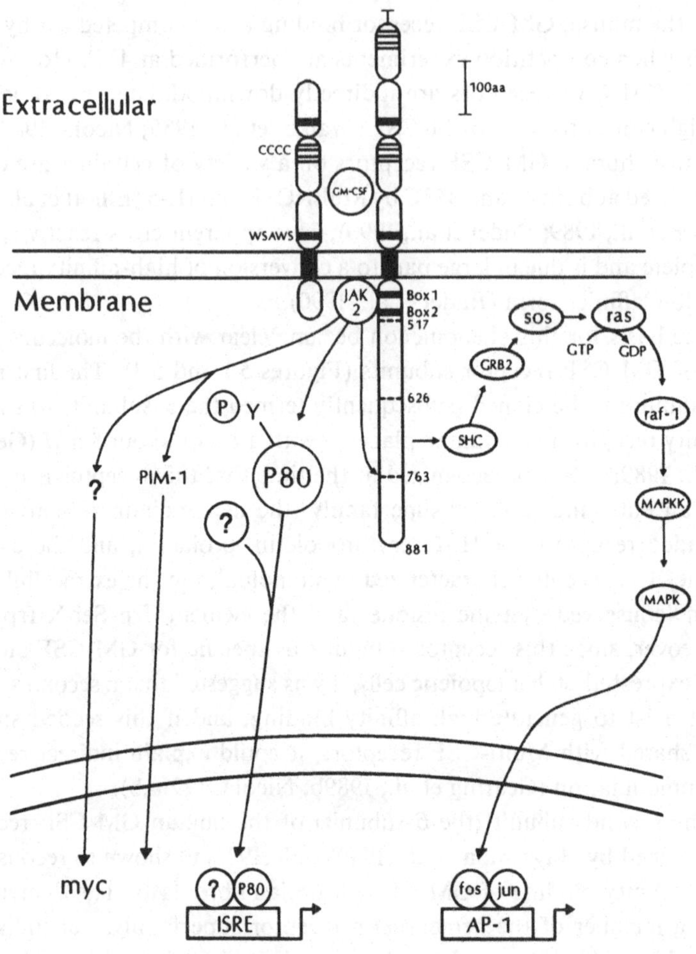


Figure 5.3. Signaling through the GM-CSF or Multi-CSF receptors. The conserved box 1 and box 2 elements in the juxtamembrane cytoplasmic domain of the $\beta$-chain are required for proliferative signaling and interact with JAK2, which in turn activates nuclear transcription factors directly. Other regions of the cytoplasmic domain activate tyrosine activity and signal transduction in a similar manner to the M-CSF receptor (see Figure 5.2).

for apparent cross-inhibition of the high-affinity binding of GM-CSF by Multi-CSF and IL-5, since these ligands compete for utilization of the common $\beta$-receptor subunit in forming their own high-affinity receptor complexes. The degree of cross-inhibition or downmodulation depends on the relative expression levels of the individual $\alpha$-receptor subunits and the common $\beta$-receptor subunit and would explain the variability of these phenomena with different cells (Figure 5.4). Finally, the use of a common $\beta$-receptor subunit by GM-CSF, Multi-CSF, and IL-5 also provides a rationale for their common biological activities since $\beta_c$ is required for biological signaling.

Analogues of the human GM-CSF receptor $\alpha$-subunits and $\beta_c$-subunit have also been described in the mouse (Gorman et al., 1990; Kitamura et al., 1991a; Part et al., 1992). However, with murine cells, receptor downmodulation is complicated by the existence of an alternative Multi-CSF-specific $\beta$-chain ($\beta$IL-3), and receptor cross-inhibition at 4°C has not been described.

In addition to CSF-induced GM-CSF receptor downmodulation, which has its explanation in the common usage of $\beta_c$, other agents (such as phorbol esters and the chemotactic peptide *f*-Met-Leu-Phe) can downmodulate GM-CSF receptors on neutrophils at 37°C (Walker and Burgess, 1985; Di Persio et al., 1988), but the mechanisms by which this occurs are not understood.

GM-CSF binding to high-affinity (but not low-affinity) receptors on a variety of cells results in their rapid internalization and the intracellular degradation of GM-CSF (Walker and Burgess, 1987; Nicola et al., 1988). The kinetic parameters associated with these events are cell type-specific and result in different patterns of internalization, but in all cases, they increase the apparent affinity of the binding interaction and lead to depletion of GM-CSF in biological reactions (Nicola et al., 1988).

## Multi-CSF receptors

Multi-CSF receptors are present in relatively low numbers (a few hundred to a few thousand) on blast cells, cells of the neutrophil and eosinophil series, monocytes and macrophages, and mast cells but are absent from mature lymphocytes and nucleated erythroid cells (Nicola and Metcalf, 1986) (Table 5.2). In general, receptor numbers decrease slightly as the cells mature, but a subpopulation of cells displays a very large number of receptors and includes cells with the morphology of neutrophil and eosinophil myelocytes as well as blast, monocytic, and lymphoid cells. This subpopulation of cells constitutes only a small fraction of bone marrow cells (~1%), and its relevance to overall biological responses to Multi-CSF remains unknown.

On most murine cell lines and normal hemopoietic cells, only a single class of binding affinity for Multi-CSF is detected by saturation binding and Scatchard analyses. Nevertheless, it is surprising that the apparent

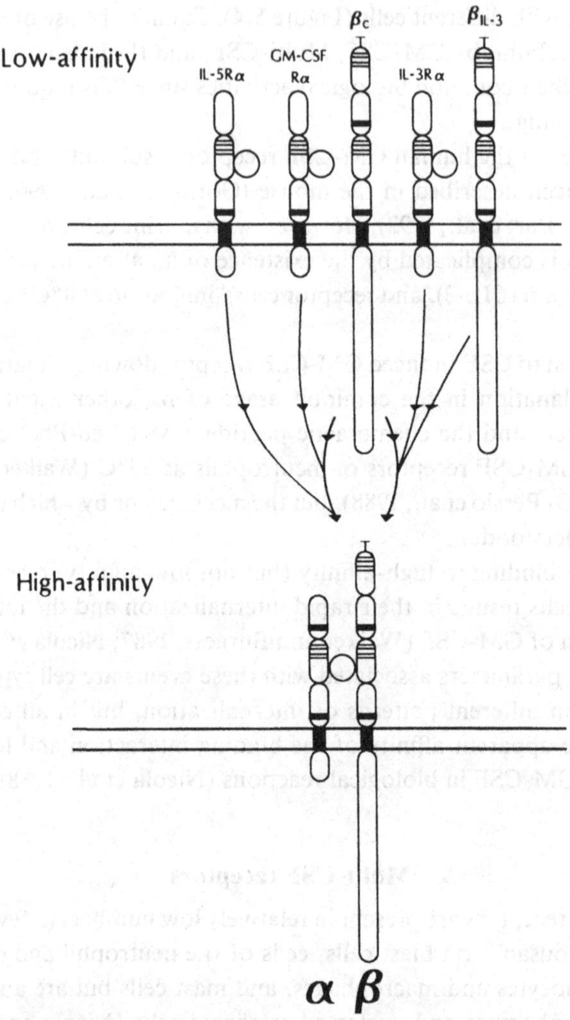


Figure 5.4. Receptor modulation and sharing of receptor $\beta$-subunits by the receptors for GM-CSF, Multi-CSF (IL-3), and IL-5. In the mouse, two alternate $\beta$-chains ($\beta_c$ and $\beta$IL-3) can be used by the IL-3 receptor $\alpha$-chain, while only $\beta_c$ can be used by the GM-CSF and IL-5 receptor $\alpha$-chains. In humans, only $\beta_c$ seems to be used by all three receptors. In all cases, ligand binding results in an $\alpha$-chain/$\beta$-chain heterodimer that has high-affinity binding characteristics and is signaling-competent. Competition for limiting numbers of $\beta_c$ by the different ligand-bound $\alpha$-chains results in apparent downmodulation of each other's high-affinity binding.

binding affinity at 4°C is significantly different on different cell types, varying from an equilibrium dissociation constant ($K_D$) of about 100 p*M* on murine bone marrow cells to about 1 n*M* on the factor-dependent cell line 32D (Nicola and Metcalf, 1986). In addition, very low-affinity Multi-CSF receptors have been detected on some cell lines (Schreurs et al., 1990). At 4°C, the binding of Multi-CSF to its receptor is fast, but the dissociation of bound Multi-CSF is very slow and barely detectable (Nicola, 1987b). The equilibrium dissociation constant calculated from these kinetic constants ($k_{off}/k_{on}$) is much lower (<1 p*M*) than the experimental value (100–1,000 p*M*) and indicates that the binding reaction cannot be considered to be a simple bimolecular equilibrium. This is now known to be the case and will be discussed later.

On human monocytes, both high-affinity ($K_D \approx 20$ p*M*) and low-affinity ($K_D \approx 700$ p*M*) receptors for Multi-CSF can be readily detected at 4°C (Elliott et al., 1989), while on human eosinophils and basophils only high-affinity receptors were observed (Lopez et al., 1989, 1990).

At 37°C, the binding of Multi-CSF to various cell lines is followed by rapid internalization ($k_e = 0.03$–$0.07$/minute) of the receptor–ligand complex and fairly rapid intracellular degradation ($k_h = 0.01$–$0.04$/minute). For bone marrow cells, the internalization process increases the apparent affinity of the interaction from a $K_D$ of about 250 p*M* to one of about 30 p*M*, a value that is close to the concentration of Multi-CSF required for half-maximal biological activity (~15 p*M*) at this temperature. On the other hand, receptor-mediated degradation of Multi-CSF implies that a steady supply of Multi-CSF is required to maintain the biological response at high cell concentrations (Nicola et al., 1988; Nicola and Metcalf, 1988).

On murine cells, Multi-CSF receptors are downregulated by Multi-CSF-induced internalization but are not transmodulated by other agents (Walker et al., 1985). In contrast, on human cells there is partial competition for high-affinity binding of Multi-CSF by GM-CSF and IL-5 at both 4° and 37°C (Lopez et al., 1989, 1990, 1991). This results from competition for a common $\beta$-chain for each receptor, as will be discussed later.

Chemical cross-linking of Multi-CSF to its cellular receptor(s) has revealed several species of receptor or receptor-associated subunits. Most commonly, one or two bands corresponding to proteins of 60–70 kDa have been observed, but sometimes bands of 120–140 kDa have also been observed (Nicola and Peterson, 1986; Park et al., 1986; Sorenson et al., 1986). Purification of the Multi-CSF receptor from B6SutA cells demonstrated tyrosine phosphorylation in a protein of about 130 kDa (Sorenson et al., 1989; Mui et al., 1992). These apparently disparate results can now be explained by the fact that the Multi-CSF receptor in the mouse exists in at least two different forms, each with multiple associated subunits.

The first mouse Multi-CSF binding subunit was cloned from a cDNA library from the mast cell line MC/9 after expression in COS7 cells and screening with an antibody (anti-AIC2) that had been shown to partially inhibit Multi-CSF binding. The cloned subunit was called AIC2, later AIC2A, and is now known as βIL-3 (Itoh et al., 1990).

βIL-3 contains a 22-amino acid hydrophobic leader sequence, a 417-amino acid extracellular domain, a single transmembrane region of 26 amino acids, and a long cytoplasmic domain of 413 amino acids. The cytoplasmic tail contains no tyrosine kinase consensus sequences or other recognizable signaling motifs despite the observation that Multi-CSF stimulates tyrosine kinase activity. On the other hand, the extracellular domain contains a duplication of a 200-amino acid domain that is homologous to domains in the erythropoietin, IL-4, IL-6, and IL-2 β-chain receptors (subsequently termed the hemopoietin domain).

βIL-3 is a glycoprotein of 120 kDa and binds Multi-CSF with a very low affinity ($K_D \approx 20$ n$M$ at 4°C) and with rapid dissociation kinetics ($k_{off} = 0.23$/minute) when expressed in simian fibroblasts or L-cells. It shows no intrinsic tyrosine kinase activity.

Because it was recognized that βIL-3 alone could not form a high-affinity Multi-CSF receptor, Hara and Miyajima (1992) used co-transfection of βIL-3 with a cDNA expression library from the B6SutA cell line and high-affinity binding conditions to detect additional subunits that conferred high-affinity binding to βIL-3. They obtained a clone SUT-1 that encoded a protein subsequently called mIL-3Rα. This protein consists of a 16-amino acid leader sequence, an extracellular domain of 315 amino acids, a transmembrane region of 24 amino acids, and a short cytoplasmic tail of 41 amino acids. The extracellular domain also contains a 200-amino acid hemopoietin domain as well as an N-terminal fibronectin III domain. mIL-3α expressed on simian fibroblasts cells is a 60- to 70-kDa glycoprotein with a very low affinity for Multi-CSF binding ($K_D =$ 45 n$M$). However, when co-expressed on simian fibroblasts or CTLL-2 cells with βIL-3, high-affinity ($K_D = 270$ p$M$) receptors with a very slow kinetic dissociation rate were generated. Moreover, although CTLL cells transfected with βIL-3 or mIL-3Rα alone could not proliferate in response to Multi-CSF, they did proliferate with a normal dose–response curve when both subunits were co-transfected.

The same authors showed that a second protein highly related to $\beta$IL-3 (91% identical), namely, $\beta_c$, could not bind Multi-CSF alone but could convert low-affinity binding to mIL-3R$\alpha$ to a high-affinity form ($K_D$ = 80–400 p$M$). When co-expressed with mIL-3R$\alpha$, $\beta_c$, like $\beta$IL-3, rendered CTLL cells responsive to Multi-CSF. When mIL-3R$\alpha$, $\beta$IL-3, and $\beta_c$ were all co-expressed together, there was no further increase in binding affinity or biological responsiveness to Multi-CSF, suggesting that $\beta$IL-3 and $\beta_c$ were functionally equivalent alternatives for the formation of high-affinity, signal-competent, Multi-CSF receptors (Figure 5.4).

Since $\beta$IL-3 is a unique affinity-converting subunit for Multi-CSF receptors, while $\beta_c$ is a common converting subunit for Multi-CSF, GM-CSF, and IL-5 receptors, it is apparent that Multi-CSF could compete for high-affinity binding of GM-CSF and IL-5 to their receptors (by sequestering $\beta_c$), while the reverse would not occur if there was sufficient $\beta$IL-3 on the cell surface. Such "hierarchical" one-way cross-competition has in fact been observed in bone marrow cells, but only at 37°C (Walker et al., 1985).

For human Multi-CSF receptors, clear equivalents of IL-3R$\alpha$ (Kitamura et al., 1991b) and $\beta_c$ (Hayashida et al., 1990) have been documented and cloned (the latter as KH97), but there appears to be no human equivalent of $\beta$IL-3. Presumably, $\beta_c$ represents the primordial gene, and gene duplication occurred in the mouse after separation of the species. If $\beta$IL-3 transduces special biological signals that are distinct from those transduced by $\beta_c$, such differences may be apparent in the response patterns to Multi-CSF by murine versus human cells. Alternatively, $\beta_c$ may have gained such functions through convergent evolution of human $\beta_c$ after the divergence of the species. In line with the poor conservation of Multi-CSF itself between mice and humans (29% identity), both IL-3R$\alpha$ (30% identity) and $\beta_c$ (56% identity) have diverged markedly, and no cross-species binding or biological activity of Multi-CSF has been observed.

As is the case with the murine receptor system, human $\beta_c$ does not have detectable binding affinity for Multi-CSF, GM-CSF, or IL-5 but can nevertheless convert each of their receptor $\alpha$-subunits to a high-affinity form (Nicola and Metcalf, 1991). For Multi-CSF binding, the hIL-3R$\alpha$ affinity ($K_D \approx 100$ n$M$) is converted to a $K_D$ of 100 p$M$. Since no alternative Multi-CSF-specific $\beta$-chain ($\beta$IL-3) exists in humans, it follows that, as long as $\beta_c$ is limiting in number, these growth factors will compete with each other for the formation of high-affinity receptors in a two-way cross-reactivity pattern. Such behavior has in fact been documented at both 4° and 37°C on a variety of cells, including monocytes, eosinophils, basophils, and leukemic cells (Elliott et al., 1989; Lopez et al., 1989, 1990, 1991). Moreover, this system has been experimentally reconstituted by co-transfecting hIL-3R$\alpha$, hGMR$\alpha$, and $\beta_c$ cDNA into NIH3T3 cells (Kitamura et al., 1991b).

## G-CSF receptor

The G-CSF receptor is relatively restricted in its distribution, being present at a few hundred copies per cell on all cells of the neutrophilic-granulocytic series and in even smaller numbers on a proportion of monocyte-macrophages (Table 5.2). The number of receptors increases with cellular maturation in mice (Nicola and Metcalf, 1985b), but for human myeloid cells, neutrophilic promyelocytes appear to have the highest number of receptors (Nicola et al., 1985). G-CSF receptors have also been reported on endothelial cells (Bussolino et al., 1989) and placental trophoblast cells (Uzumaki et al., 1989) but are not detected on other hemopoietic cells.

On all murine cells examined, a single class of high-affinity G-CSF receptor ($K_D \approx 100$ p$M$) has been observed. However, lower-affinity forms of the receptor ($K_D \approx 3$ n$M$) have been observed after detergent solubilization of murine NFS 60 cells (Fukunaga et al., 1990a), and it has been suggested that the low-affinity form of the receptor is a monomer, while the higher-affinity form is a dimer. If this is so, the G-CSF receptor must exist almost exclusively as a dimer on all intact cells studied. For human cells also, only a single affinity class of G-CSF receptor has been detected, but the apparent affinity has varied with investigator and cell type from 100 p$M$ to 1 n$M$. G-CSF receptors have been detected on some, but not all, human acute myeloid leukemia (AML) and chronic myeloid leukemia (CML) cells with characteristics similar to those of the receptor on human neutrophils (Nicola et al., 1985; Budel et al., 1989; Park et al., 1989). However, in some cases of Kostmann's syndrome (myeloproliferation with lack of neutrophil differentiation) and AML, it has been reported that an altered G-CSF receptor gene is present (see later).

With both mouse and human cells, chemical cross-linking of $^{125}$I-labeled G-CSF to its cellular receptor has revealed a binding protein of MW 150,000, although additional proteins of MW 110,000 and lower have also been detected with human cells. While some of these may represent degradation products of the receptor, it remains unclear whether other proteins form part of a functional G-CSF receptor (Nicola and Peterson, 1986; Hanazono et al., 1990).

Like the other CSF receptors, G-CSF receptors are downregulated by G-CSF-mediated receptor internalization and degradation at 37°C (Nicola et al., 1988) and are trans-downmodulated by a variety of agents. For mouse bone marrow cells, these agents include other CSFs (namely, Multi-CSF and GM-CSF), and for human neutrophils include GM-CSF, bacterial LPS, the chemotactic peptide *f*-Met-Leu-Phe (FMLP) (Nicola et al., 1986), tumor necrosis factor, and phorbol esters (Elbaz et al., 1991). The mechanism of trans-downmodulation of G-CSF receptors is still unknown, but it requires preincubation of the cells at 37°C, is relatively rapid, and, at least in the case of phorbol esters, involves the activation of protein kinase C (Elbaz et al., 1991).

Murine and human G-CSF receptor cDNAs were obtained by expression cloning from NFS 60 and human placenta, respectively (Fukunaga et al., 1990b,c; Larsen et al., 1990). The receptors are homologous (63% sequence identity), and the largest transcripts of each are 812 amino acids in length, including relatively long cytoplasmic tails of 187 amino acids. The extracellular domains of these receptors represent structural mosaics including an N-terminal immunoglobulin-like loop (~90 amino acids) and a membrane-proximal set of three repeats of a fibronectin type III-like module (~300 amino acids in total). Between these elements is an approximately 200-amino acid domain (hemopoietic) that is conserved in many hemopoietic receptors, including GM-CSF receptor $\alpha$-chains, Multi-CSF receptor $\alpha$-chains, and the common $\beta$-chain(s), and contains the landmark four cysteine residues and WSXWS motif (Figure 5.5). The G-CSF receptor extracellular domain is most closely related to the receptor for LIF and the common $\beta$-chain (gp 130) for the IL-6, LIF, ciliary neurotropic factor, oncostatin-M, and IL-11 receptors (Bazan, 1991b).

Site-directed mutagenesis of the receptor for G-CSF has revealed that only the N-terminal half of the hemopoietin domain is required for G-CSF binding, so the roles of the other structures in the extracellular domain, if any, remain to be elucidated (Fukunaga et al., 1991).

The cytoplasmic domain of the G-CSF receptor is also related to those of other hemopoietic receptors and, in particular, is 50% identical to that of the IL-4 receptor. It contains the box 1 and box 2 elements described for the common $\beta$-chain and for gp 130, and mutagenesis of these elements suggests that they are required for the proliferative effect of the G-CSF receptor. However, using FDC-P1 cells transfected with intact G-CSF receptor or site-directed mutants (a cell line that responds to G-CSF by induction of the myeloid differentiation marker myeloperoxidase), Fukunaga

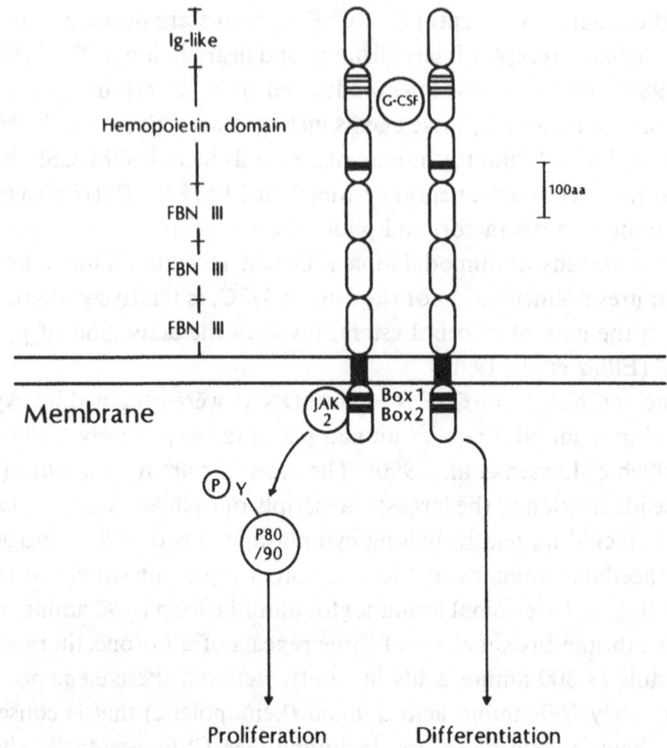


Figure 5.5. Signaling through the G-CSF receptor homodimer. As for the GM-CSF and Multi-CSF receptor β-chains, the box 1 and box 2 cytoplasmic elements mediate proliferative signaling via ligand-dependent activation of JAK1 kinase activity. The C-terminal end of the cytoplasmic domain appears to be required for the induction of cellular differentiation.

et al. (1993) showed that a quite different cytoplasmic element near the C-terminus was required for the differentiation-inducing effects of the G-CSF receptor, which was confirmed in another cell line (Dong et al., 1993).

Dong et al. (1994) have detected G-CSF receptors that are mutated in this same cytoplasmic region in some patients with Kostmann's syndrome or AML, both being disease states in which granulocytic cells proliferate but are unable to differentiate into mature cells. However, this does not seem to be a common defect in these diseases (Sandoval et al., 1993).

Proliferative signaling by activated G-CSF receptors is associated with activation of the kinase activity of bound JAK1 kinase (Nicholson et al., 1994), and by analogy with $\beta_c$, this probably results in activation of transcription factors that bind to G-CSF-responsive genes (see later).

## Binding sites in the extracellular domains of the GM-CSF and Multi-CSF receptors

There are at least three important points of interaction between the ligands, GM-CSF and Multi-CSF, and the two components of each receptor ($\alpha$- and $\beta$-chains).

The first is between the growth factor and the $\alpha$-chain. With both ligands this occurs in the absence of the $\beta$-chain, appears to be absolutely specific for each $\alpha$-chain–ligand pair, and is of low affinity ($K_D = 5$–100 n$M$) with a relatively fast on-rate ($10^8$–$10^9$ $M^{-1}$ minute$^{-1}$) and fast off-rate ($t_{1/2} = 3$–5 minutes) (Gearing et al., 1989b; Kitamura et al., 1991a). Although, in both cases, the binding site on the growth factor has been mapped to some extent (involving primarily the D-helix and a small part of the A-helix), the binding site on the receptor $\alpha$-chains has not been determined.

The second interaction site is between the growth factor and the $\beta$-chain of the receptor. For $\beta_c$, no interaction is detectable unless the $\alpha$-chain is also present, but for the murine $\beta$IL-3 receptor, a low-affinity interaction with Multi-CSF is observable. A mutagenesis study of the $\beta$IL-3 receptor showed that both hemopoietin domains were necessary for Multi-CSF binding, but domain swapping between $\beta$IL-3 and $\beta_c$ (which does not itself bind Multi-CSF) suggested that the membrane-proximal hemopoietin domain of $\beta$IL-3 contained the Multi-CSF binding site and bound Multi-CSF with the same affinity as $\beta$IL-3, while the N-terminal domain presumably played only a structural role. Swapping individual amino acids in this domain of $\beta$IL-3 with the residues present in $\beta_c$ revealed that a number of amino acids had minor effects on Multi-CSF binding affinity, but alteration of the sequence Ile-Pro-Lys-Tyr beginning at position 367 completely eliminated Multi-CSF binding (Wang et al., 1992). In the model of hemopoietin domains represented by the X-ray structure of the growth hormone–growth hormone receptor complex (Figure 5.6) (de Vos et al., 1992), this corresponds in sequence alignment to the loop between the B′ and C′ strands of the C-domain $\beta$-barrel. This same loop forms several site II contacts with the growth hormone A-helix, and a similar region of the human IL-2 receptor $\beta$-chain is also involved in contacting IL-2.

The strong sequence homology of $\beta_c$ with $\beta$IL-3 suggests that a similar site may be involved in contacting Multi-CSF, GM-CSF, and IL-5. However, because $\beta_c$ affects the binding of these ligands only in the presence of the respective receptor $\alpha$-chains, it is possible that binding of the ligand

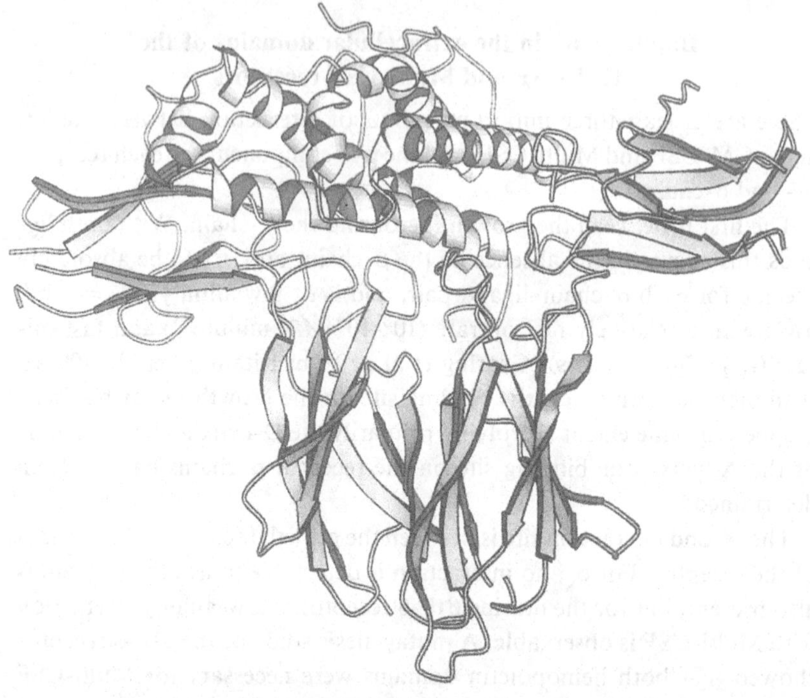

Figure 5.6. The X-ray structure of the growth hormone–receptor complex (de Vos et al., 1992). Growth hormone, like the CSFs, is a four-$\alpha$-helical bundle structure and results in homodimerization of the receptor. The receptor subunits are structurally related to the $\alpha$- and $\beta$-subunits of the GM-CSF, IL-3, and G-CSF receptors and contain two $\beta$-barrel structures consisting of seven antiparallel $\beta$-strands. The site I and site II contacts on each receptor subunit are formally equivalent to interactions with the $\alpha$-subunit or the $\beta$-subunit, respectively, for the CSFs.

to the $\alpha$-chain alters its conformation so that it can be recognized by $\beta_c$ or that contacts with both the ligand and the $\alpha$-chain are required for a stable high-affinity complex to form. In this context, there is a formal analogy with growth hormone binding to its receptor, since site II interactions with the second receptor subunit occur only after site I interactions with the first receptor subunit have occurred. This analogy suggests a two-step binding mechanism for Multi-CSF and GM-CSF:

$$L + \alpha \rightarrow L\alpha$$
$$L\alpha + \beta \rightarrow L\alpha\beta$$

Indeed, only this type of mechanism would result in apparent high-affinity receptor binding competition between GM-CSF, Multi-CSF, and

IL-5, since preexisting complexes of $\alpha$- and $\beta$-subunits would not allow for competition. Moreover, antibodies that recognize only the human GM-CSF receptor $\alpha$-chain binding site inhibit high-affinity binding and biological action of GM-CSF at the same concentration as they inhibit the interaction between GM-CSF and isolated receptor $\alpha$-chains (Nicola et al., 1993).

The site on human $\beta_c$ that contacts GM-CSF to effect high-affinity conversion has been mapped by site-directed mutagenesis to the same site as that on murine $\beta$IL-3, and a single amino acid residue, His 367, has been shown to be essential (Lock et al., 1994). This residue presumably forms a salt bridge with the A-helix residue Glu 21 on human GM-CSF, since mutation of either residue on the growth factor or on $\beta_c$ eliminates high-affinity binding.

The third interaction site is a ligand-induced association between the $\alpha$- and $\beta$-subunits of each receptor. This is quite independent of the high-affinity receptor formation that results from contact of the $\beta$-subunit with the ligand itself and seems to be the crucial interaction that leads to biological signaling. For example, the human GM-CSF and human Multi-CSF receptor $\alpha$-chains can be co-expressed with murine $\beta_c$ in murine CTLL or FDC-P1 cells without any detectable contribution of $\beta_c$ to high-affinity binding of the respective human ligands (Metcalf et al., 1990; Kitamura et al., 1991a). Nevertheless, at high CSF concentrations, commensurate with their low-affinity binding, these human ligands are fully capable of signaling cell proliferation in the murine cells. In fact, when the low affinity of their binding interaction is taken into account, each ligand-bound complex is just as efficient as a high-affinity receptor in delivering a proliferative stimulus. Similarly, mutations in GM-CSF or in human $\beta_c$ that abrogate high-affinity binding still result in proliferation-competent receptor complexes (Lopez et al., 1992b; Shanafelt and Kastelein, 1992; Lock et al., 1994). It must be concluded that GM-CSF or Multi-CSF binding to the respective receptor $\alpha$-chains induces a conformational change in the $\alpha$-chain that allows recognition by the $\beta$-chain at a site distinct from the contact point of the ligand with the $\beta$-chain. This association is then the critical event for biological signaling.

## Biological signaling by Multi-CSF and GM-CSF receptors

Because isolated receptor $\alpha$- or $\beta$-chains are incapable of biological signaling, it is clear that the ligand-induced physical association of $\alpha$- and $\beta$-chains is a critical event in biological signaling. As a minimum event, this extracellular noncovalent "cross-linking" of receptor subunits translates the binding event to a physical association of the receptor subunit cytoplasmic domains, although the further association of other transmembrane molecules cannot be ruled out and is indeed probable.

For both Multi-CSF and GM-CSF receptors, both the cytoplasmic tails of the $\alpha$- and $\beta$-receptor subunits are required for signaling (Sakamaki et al., 1992), and in this respect, they differ from IL-6 receptors, where the cytoplasmic domain of the $\alpha$-chain is dispensable for biological activity (Kishimoto et al., 1992). However, this does not imply that the basic mechanism of IL-6-mediated signaling is different from that of Multi-CSF and GM-CSF, since IL-6 binding to its $\alpha$-chain leads to physical association of two $\beta$-subunits (known as gp130; Kishimoto et al., 1992).

Despite the lack of any intrinsic tyrosine kinase activity of the various subunits of the Multi-CSF and GM-CSF receptors, it is well documented that both of these growth factors stimulate tyrosine phosphorylation of a substantially overlapping set of cellular substrates in responsive cells (Isfort and Ihle, 1990; Kanakura et al., 1990; Linnekin and Farrar, 1990). One substrate is $\beta_c$ itself, but not the $\alpha$-chain of the receptor. The most likely site of phosphorylation is Tyr 750, but this site does not contain any consensus sequences for interaction with SH2 domain–containing proteins, and deletion analysis suggests that it is not required for inducing cellular proliferation (Sakamaki et al., 1992). Other tyrosine phosphorylated substrates include *vav, fps/fes*, *raf*, *shc*, and MAP kinase (Carrol et al., 1990; Okuda et al., 1992; Welham et al., 1992; Mui et al., 1992; Hanazono et al., 1993; Sato et al., 1993). These proteins have been implicated in other cell signaling pathways, either because they contain SH2 or SH3 domains that can interact with tyrosine phosphate residues in activated receptors (*vav*, *shc*), interact with p21 *ras* (*raf*), have intrinsic tyrosine kinase activity (*fes*), or are involved in the induction of specific genes (MAP kinase). More recently, both GM-CSF and Multi-CSF have been shown to phosphorylate the cytoplasmic tyrosine kinase JAK2 on tyrosine and activate its kinase activity (Silvennoinen et al., 1993a,b; Ihle et al., 1994). Because JAK2 and closely related members of this family (JAK1 and TYK2) play an essential role in signaling by interferons $\alpha$, $\beta$, and $\gamma$ (Ihle et al., 1994) and are associated with activation of several different but related cytokine receptors (erythropoietin, growth hormone, prolactin, IL-6, LIF, and ciliary neurotropic factor), this may represent a critical signaling event (Stahl and Yancopoulos 1993; Ihle et al., 1994).

JAK2 has been shown to associate with $\beta_c$ in either a ligand-dependent or -independent manner, but not to the $\alpha$-chains of the receptor. Nevertheless, the cytoplasmic domain of the GM-CSF receptor $\alpha$-chain is required to activate the tyrosine kinase activity of JAK2, which results in phosphorylation of $\beta_c$ and other cellular substrates. Among these substrates is probably the 91-kDa component and possibly other components of the ISGF3 (or similar) transcription complex that is involved in interferon signal transduction (Larner et al., 1993).

Deletion analysis of the $\beta_c$ cytoplasmic domain has shown that the membrane-proximal region of about 60 amino acids is sufficient for stimulating cell proliferation in factor-dependent cell lines, at least in the presence of serum (Sakamaki et al., 1992; Sato et al., 1993). This region shows some sequence similarities with other cytokine receptors including the IL-2 receptor $\beta$-subunit, the IL-4 receptor, erythropoietin receptor, G-CSF receptor, and the common $\beta$-subunit (gp130) of IL-6, LIF, ciliary neurotropic growth factor, oncostatin-M, and IL-11, and in these receptors also this region is essential for cellular proliferation. Mutant $\beta_c$ receptor chains that contain only these 60 cytoplasmic residues retain the capacity to bind and activate JAK2 as well as to induce the expression of *myc* and the serine/threonine kinase PIM-1 (Sato et al., 1993; Ihle et al., 1994). Proliferation by these transfected cells is sensitive to inhibition by the tyrosine kinase inhibitor herbimycin, as is the induction of *myc*, suggesting that a kinase, possibly JAK2, is critical for proliferative signaling by GM-CSF and Multi-CSF. On the other hand, PIM-1 appears to enhance the proliferative response but is not essential.

Other deletion mutants of $\beta_c$ have revealed another cytoplasmic domain between residues 626 and 763 that is not essential for cell proliferation in serum but is responsible for the majority of the tyrosine phosphorylated proteins, including *shc*, *raf*-1, and MAP kinase, as well as the activation of *raf*-1 and MAP kinase activity, activation of GTP-bound p21 *ras*, p70S6 kinase activity, PI3K activity, and the induction of the immediate early response genes c-*fos* and c-*jun* (Sato et al., 1993). These elements are part of the signal pathways induced by classical tyrosine kinase receptors such as those for epidermal growth factor and platelet-derived growth factor (Schlessinger and Ullrich, 1992). In these pathways, cross-phosphorylation of consensus receptor tyrosine residues provides recognition sites for docking proteins that contain *src*-homology domains (SH2 and SH3) (such as *shc*, *grb*2, PI3K p80 subunit, GAP) and act as adaptors to couple the receptors to enzymic activities. Such activities include PI3K, which may activate protein kinase C, as well as SOS and *vav*, which activate *ras* by exchanging GDP for GTP. This in turn leads to activation of *raf* kinase, which leads to activation of MAP kinase and the induction of specific genes. Although these events do not appear necessary for GM-CSF- or Multi-CSF-induced cell proliferation in serum, it is possible that other serum growth factors perform these functions in cells expressing the truncated $\beta_c$ mutants.

## Conclusions

All of the CSF receptors require receptor dimerization for high-affinity binding and for biological signal transduction. In two cases (M-CSF and G-CSF) this is achieved by dimerization of identical receptor subunits, while in the other two cases (GM-CSF and Multi-CSF) unique $\alpha$-receptor subunits dimerize with a common $\beta$-receptor subunit. The M-CSF receptor is a classical type III receptor tyrosine kinase, but all of the other CSF receptor subunits belong to the hemopoietin receptor superfamily for which the growth hormone–receptor dimer complex provides a good model of the structure and mechanism of complex formation. Although the hemopoietin receptor subunits have no demonstrated intrinsic enzyme activity, it is becoming clear that they also utilize tyrosine kinases in biological signaling. Indeed, it appears that there are many common events in signaling by tyrosine kinase receptors and hemopoietin receptors, including the use of JAK kinases and other SH2-containing signaling molecules to activate common pathways.

There are still many problems to solve. Almost nothing is known about nonproliferative signaling by CSF receptors. There is some suggestion that the regions of the $\beta$-receptor subunits and, by implication, the signaling pathways used for differentiation induction will be different from those used for cell proliferation. Different model systems will be required to address this issue properly. Can single $\alpha$-chain receptors utilize multiple $\beta$-chains to achieve different types of signaling events in different cells? Do $\alpha$-chains have any unique signaling capacities? Which other growth factors will be united into receptor families by the use of common $\beta$-chains? How are responses to multiple growth factors that use $\beta$-chains coordinated at the cell surfaces? These questions may soon be answered if progress to date is any indication.

# 6

# Molecular genetics of the colony-stimulating factors and their receptors

A new era in the study of the structure and biological activities of the colony-stimulating factors was ushered in by the molecular cloning of cDNAs encoding the CSFs and their cellular receptors, as well as the production of recombinant proteins. New insights into the physiology of CSF action have also been gained from the structures of the genes and promoter elements of the CSFs and their receptors. In some cases, the results have been unexpected, as was the case with multiple transcripts, all of which encode membrane-anchored forms of M-CSF. In other cases, such as alternative transcripts of CSF receptors that encode soluble forms, the results suggest novel mechanisms of biological regulation of CSF action. It is already clear that the control of CSF gene expression is extremely complex, with some mechanisms controlling RNA stability, others the constitutive transcription rate in different cells, and yet others the transcription rate inducible by biological regulators in a cell-specific manner. In this chapter, the chromosomal localization and structure of the CSF and receptor genes will be described along with the occurrence of alternative transcripts and the regulation of gene expression.

## GM-CSF

The gene encoding human GM-CSF is on chromosome 5q21–31 (Huebner et al., 1985; Yang et al., 1988), and the corresponding mouse gene is on chromosome 11A5–B1 (Barlow et al., 1987) (Table 6.1). Both genes contain four exons and produce a single transcript of 780 bp (Miyatake et al., 1985; Stanley et al., 1985) (Figure 6.1). In both cases, control of GM-CSF expression occurs both transcriptionally and post-transcriptionally as a result of conserved AT-rich sequences in the 3′ untranslated region of the gene.

Table 6.1. *Molecular genetic characteristics of the CSFs*

| Factor | Chromosomal location of the gene | Size of the gene (kbp) | Size of transcripts (kb) | Number of exons |
|---|---|---|---|---|
| hGM-CSF | 5q21–31 | 2.5 | 0.78 | 4 |
| mGM-CSF | 11A5–B1 | 2.5 | 0.78 | 4 |
| hMulti-CSF | 5q21–31 | 2.2 | 0.9 | 5 |
| mMulti-CSF | 11A5–B1 | 2.7 | 0.9 | 5 |
| hG-CSF | 17q11–22 | 2.5 | 1.5 | 5 |
| mG-CSF | 11D–E2 | 2.5 | 1.5 | 5 |
| hM-CSF | 1p13–21 | 20 | 4, 2.3, 2.0, 1.6 | 10 |
| mM-CSF | 3F3 | 20 | 4, 2.6, 1.4 | 10 |

Shaw and Kamen (1986) and Caput et al. (1986) noted that there was a conserved sequence (AUUUA or TTATTTAT) at the 3′ untranslated region of mRNAs for GM-CSF, several inflammatory cytokines (IL-1, tumor necrosis factor, and interferons) and proto-oncogenes. A 62-bp AT-rich sequence from the human GM-CSF gene was shown to destabilize globin mRNA in recombinant constructs (Shaw and Kamen, 1986), and the demonstration of cytoplasmic proteins that recognize the AUUUA element (Malter et al., 1990; Hamilton et al., 1993) suggests that specific recognition events are involved. Recent data suggest that selective degradation of such RNAs is coupled to ribosome binding or translation of the mRNA (Aharon and Schneider, 1993). Since activation of GM-CSF production by monocytes, endothelial cells, and fibroblasts involves mRNA stabilization as well as increased transcription (Seelentag et al., 1987; Kaushansky, 1989), production signals may also serve to inhibit the AUUUA-binding proteins.

Transcriptional regulation of GM-CSF expression involves multiple promoter and enhancer elements in the gene that have been identified by nucleotide sequence homology, transcription factor binding and footprinting, and functional analysis using reporter genes. Upstream of the TATA box are a GC-rich region (GC box), and NF-KB binding site (on the noncoding DNA strand), and two conserved sequence elements known as cytokine consensus elements (CK-1 and CK-2) or conserved lymphokine elements (CLE-1 and CLE-2) (Figure 6.2). CK-1 sequences are conserved in the genes for GM-CSF, IL-3, IL-2, and G-CSF, while CK-2 sequences are conserved in the genes for GM-CSF and IL-3.

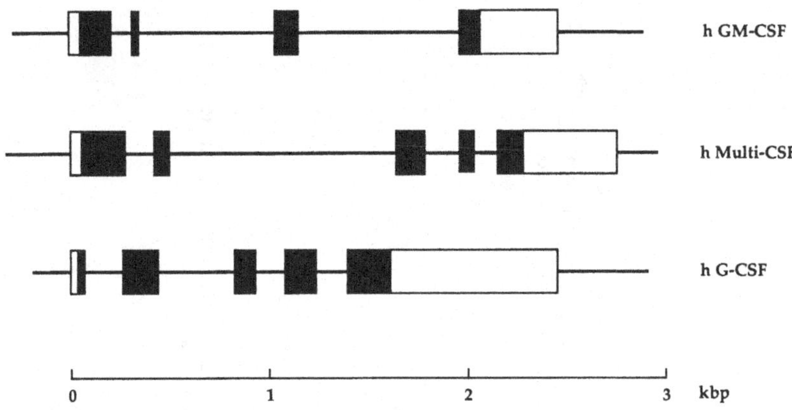


Figure 6.1. Genomic organization of the human GM-CSF, Multi-CSF, and G-CSF genes. Exons are shown in boxes with coding segments in black and noncoding segments in white.

The GC box appears to be responsible for constitutive expression of GM-CSF, and three proteins that can bind to this element and activate transcription in vitro have been identified, one of which is closely related to the transcription factor SP-2 (Arai et al., 1992).

The CK-1 box forms a binding site for a ubiquitous nuclear protein, NF-GMa, which can be induced by tumor necrosis factor treatment of fibroblasts, so it may represent a control element for stromal cell production of GM-CSF (Shannon et al., 1988, 1990; Nimer et al., 1989). The CK-2 box forms a binding site for the nuclear protein NF-GMb, which is induced in T-cells after activation with phorbol esters (Shannon et al., 1988), and this construct along with the GC box results in highly inducible expression in T-cells stimulated with phorbol ester and calcium ionophore (Miyatake et al., 1988). The relationship of NF-GMb to NF-KB, which has a similar binding specificity, is not clear (Arai et al., 1992).

Closer to the TATA box is another sequence element called the CATTA/T box or CLEO box, which is homologous to sequences in the genes for IL-4, IL-5, and G-CSF (Nimer et al., 1988b, 1990; Arai et al., 1992). Nuclear factors (NF-CLEOa and NF-CLEOb) bind to the 3′ and 5′ halves, respectively, of this element and may provide phorbol ester/$Ca^{2+}$-inducible (NF-CLEOa) or -inhibitory (NF-CLEOb) signals for transcription (Miyatake et al., 1991). It has been shown that one of the protein complexes binding to CLEO contains both NF-AT and AP-1 proteins (c-Jun/c-Fos), which are inducible by phorbol ester/$Ca^{2+}$ (Tokumitsu et al., 1993).

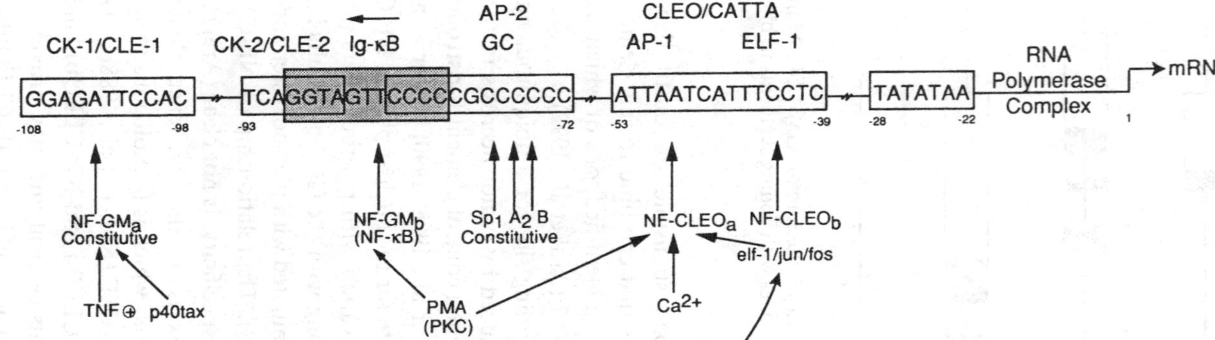


Figure 6.2. Promoter and enhancer elements in the human GM-CSF gene 5′ of exon 1. Nucleotides are labeled relative to the transcriptional initiation site. Recognized sequence elements are boxed and labeled.

Cockerill et al., (1993) found only one DNase I–hypersensitive site (reflecting an active chromatin structure), within the GM-CSF/IL-3 locus that was inducible by treatment of T-cells with phorbol ester and calcium ionophore. The site was also blocked by cyclosporin A, a powerful immunosuppressant that blocks GM-CSF and IL-3 transcription as well. This site was 3 kb upstream of the GM-CSF gene, and the enhancer contained four copies of a functional binding site (TGAGTCA) for the nuclear transcription factor AP-1. The fourth of these is embedded in a longer sequence that is also homologous to the NF-AT site of the IL-2 promoter, and this segment conferred strongly inducible, cyclosporin-inhibitable expression of a chloramphenicol transferase marker gene. The mechanism of action of NF-AT (Schumacher and Nordheim, 1992) is shown in Figure 6.3. Activation of protein kinase C and $Ca^{2+}$ release by activation of the T-cell receptor results in the induction of a nuclear AP-1-like protein (NF-ATn) and the translocation of a cytoplasmic factor NF-ATp to the nucleus. These form a transcription complex that binds to NF-AT nucleotide sequences and activates gene transcription.

## Multi-CSF (IL-3)

Like the GM-CSF gene, IL-3 is encoded by a unique gene on chromosome 5q23–31 in humans (Le Beau et al., 1986; Yang et al., 1988) and on chromosome 11 band A5–B1 in mice (Barlow et al., 1987; Ihle et al., 1987) (Table 6.1). In both mice and humans, the IL-3 gene contains five exons and produces a single mRNA of 850–900 bp (Campbell et al., 1985; Todokoro et al., 1985; Yang et al., 1986) (Figure 6.1).

It is tightly linked to the GM-CSF gene, being separated by only 9 kbp in humans and 14 kbp in mice, and in both species it is in the same transcriptional orientation and 5′ to the GM-CSF gene.

The $5q^-$ syndrome involves an interstitial deletion of chromosome 5 between breakpoints at 5q11–21 and 5q22–34 and is associated with myelodysplasia and leukemia development after treatment with chemotherapy (van den Berghe et al., 1985). Although the extent of deletion in cases of $5q^-$ is variable, a common region involving 5q22–23 is involved, but although this is close to the GM-CSF and IL-3 genes, these genes are not always deleted in the $5q^-$ syndrome. More recent data suggest that the interferon regulatory factor-1 gene (IRF-1) may be the element involved in this syndrome (Willman et al., 1993).

In one case of acute B-lymphocytic leukemia associated with eosinophilia and with a t(5; 14) (q31; q32) translocation breakpoint, it has been

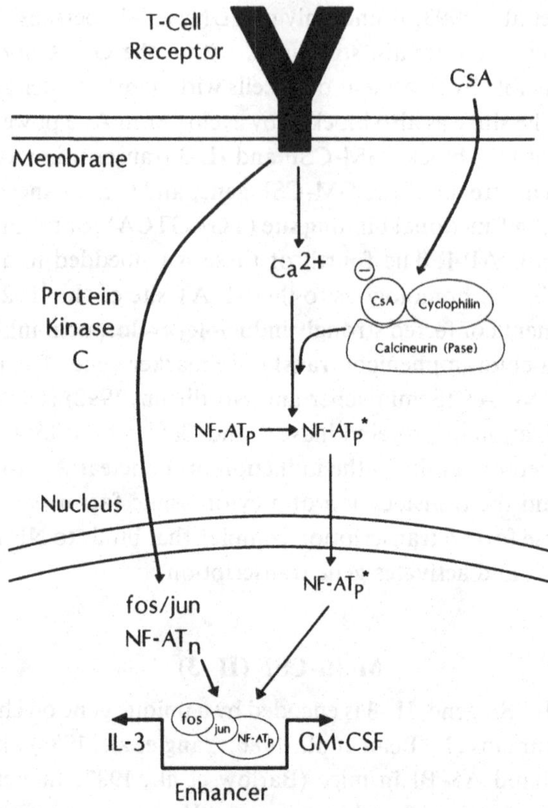


Figure 6.3. Mechanism of action of NF-AT transcription factor during T-cell activation. AP-1 elements (*fos/jun*) are induced by protein kinase C and $Ca^{2+}$, while NF-ATp is a cytoplasmic factor activated by the $Ca^{2+}$-dependent phosphatase calcineurin. NF-ATp then moves to the nucleus and with *jun/fos* forms a transcriptional complex that binds to the NF-AT enhancer that regulates GM-CSF and Multi-CSF (IL-3) transcription. Cyclosporin A is thought to mediate its immunosuppressive effects by binding to cyclophilin and inactivating calcineurin.

shown that the IL-3 gene is juxtaposed next to the IgH genes and that this may result in overexpression of the IL-3 gene (Meeker et al., 1990).

In normal T-cells, expression of the IL-3 gene appears to be tightly linked to, and dependent on, expression of the GM-CSF gene (Gough and Kelso, 1989). In part, this may be due to the cyclosporin-inhibitable enhancer between these two genes discussed earlier and to the use by the IL-3 gene of an enhanced element in the (CLE-2/GC box) promoter region of the GM-CSF gene (Nishida et al., 1991). However, unlike the GM-CSF gene, which is widely expressed, the IL-3 gene appears to be expressed mainly by activated T-cells and mast cells (see Arai et al., 1990).

Like the GM-CSF gene, the IL-3 gene contains the 5′ promoter sequences CLE-1 (CK-1), CLE-2 (CK-2), and the GC box at positions −127 to −49 from the transcription start site (Figure 6.4). However, CLE-1 and CLE-2 do not appear to be necessary for transcription stimulation by retroviral $p40^{tax}$ or by phorbol ester/$Ca^{2+}$ signals. Additional upstream control elements have been recently described. An AP-1 site at position −301 is required for maximal transcriptional activation, and immediately downstream of it is a strong repressor element (NIP). The AP-1 site is essential for inducible transcription in T-cells (via c-*jun*/c-*fos*), and an Elf-1 binding site (an Ets-like nuclear factor) 6 bp upstream of the AP-1 site is also required for maximal activity (Gottschalk et al., 1993).

At position −157 is a sequence termed ACT-1 or NF-IL-3A (Mathey-Prevot et al., 1990; Shoemaker et al., 1990). The 5′ end of this sequence (GATGAATAAT) binds an inducible T-cell-specific DNA-binding protein (NF-IL-3A) similar to the octamer-1-nuclear factor, and the 3′ end (TACGTCT) is homologous to the cAMP-responsive element (CRE). These elements appear to be required for inducible expression of the IL-3 gene by T-cell activators (Davies et al., 1993; Gottschalk et al., 1993; Park et al., 1993).

As with the GM-CSF gene, expression levels of IL-3 mRNA are also controlled post-transcriptionally by mRNA stabilization involving AU-rich sequences (Ryan et al., 1991).

## G-CSF

The human G-CSF gene is located at chromosome 17q11–22 (Kanda et al., 1987; Le Beau et al., 1987; Simmers et al., 1987), and the mouse gene is located on a syntenic region of chromosome 11D–E2 (Table 6.1) (Tsuchiya et al., 1987; Buchberg et al., 1988). Both genes contain five exons, span about 2.3 kbp of DNA, and encode mRNAs of about 1,500 nucleotides (Figure 6.1). The human G-CSF gene lies proximal to a common breakpoint in the t(15; 17) translocation present in acute promyelocytic leukemia but is not rearranged in malignant clones (Le Beau et al., 1987; Simmers et al., 1987). The human and mouse genes are highly homologous, with 69% nucleic acid identity in both coding and noncoding regions. However, two transcripts have been described for the human gene and only one for the mouse. The two human mRNAs are produced with the use of two alternative donor splice sequences (9 bp apart) at the 5′ terminus of the second intron with a common splice acceptor site within intron 2. This results in the presence or absence of nine nucleotides (three amino acids) at the 3′ end of exon 2, whose addition encodes a G-CSF of lower

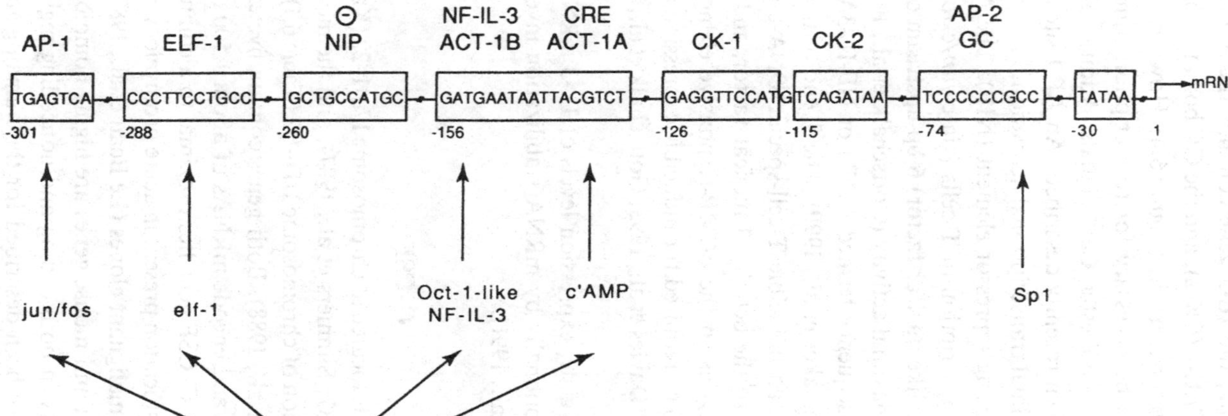


Figure 6.4. Promoter and enhancer elements in the human Multi-CSF (IL-3) gene 5′ of exon 1. Nucleotides are labeled relative to the transcriptional initiation site. Recognized sequence elements that correspond to nuclear factor binding sites are boxed and labeled.

specific activity (Nagata et al., 1986b). However, the transcript with the extra nucleotides appears to be a minor one in normal human cells and is not present in mouse cells even though both splice donor sites exist.

As for the other CSFs, both transcriptional and post-transcriptional mechanisms have been implicated in the control of expression of G-CSF. G-CSF mRNA contains repeated AU-rich sequences (in the 3′ untranslated region) that confer message instability ($t_{1/2} < 15$ minutes). Upon induction by agents such as bacterial LPS, IL-1, tumor necrosis factor, phorbol esters, or cycloheximide, the mRNA is transiently stabilized, possibly by interference with RNA-binding proteins or RNase activity (Koeffler et al., 1988; Ernst et al., 1989; Demetri et al., 1990). In some tumor cell lines, constitutive G-CSF expression is thought to result from message stabilization possibly through a *ras*-dependent pathway (Demetri et al., 1990).

The human and mouse G-CSF genes are highly homologous for about 300 bp upstream of the transcription initiation site, and this region is sufficient for constitutive and inducible (by LPS, tumor necrosis factor, and IL-1) expression of G-CSF by macrophages (Nishizawa and Nagata, 1990; Nishizawa et al., 1990) (Figure 6.5). Within this region are several potential regulatory elements. At positions −189 to −170 there are sequences with homology to the CK-1 and NF-IL-6 elements (GPE1-G-CSF promoter element), and at position −69 there is a CK-2 homologous element. At position −115 there is an octamer element (ATTTGCAT) (GPE2) thought to be important in the transcriptional control of immunoglobulin genes. Using reporter constructs in embryonic fibroblasts, Shannon et al. (1992) found that the CK-1, NF-IL-6, and octamer sequences (but not the CK-2 or upstream PU-1 site) were required for induction by tumor necrosis factor $\alpha$ (TNF $\alpha$) and IL-1$\beta$, with the octamer sequence contributing the differential response to IL-1$\beta$ compared with TNF$\alpha$. In macrophages, the CK-1 element was necessary for LPS inducibility but did not by itself confer LPS inducibility (Nishizawa and Nagata, 1990), suggesting the involvement of other proximal nuclear binding proteins, possibly NF-IL-6, which binds adjacent to this sequence. Similarly, the octamer sequence did not confer inducibility on the G-CSF gene in macrophages (Nishizawa et al., 1990) or cell types other than embryonic fibroblasts (Shannon et al., 1992), suggesting that its action is cell-specific. Another sequence element of 19 nucleotides (GPE3), beginning at position −98, is unrelated to known regulatory elements but, along with GPE1 and GPE2, is required both for constitutive gene expression in the tumor cell line CHU-2 and for LPS-inducible expression in macrophages (Nishizawa and Nagata, 1990; Asano and Nagata, 1992).

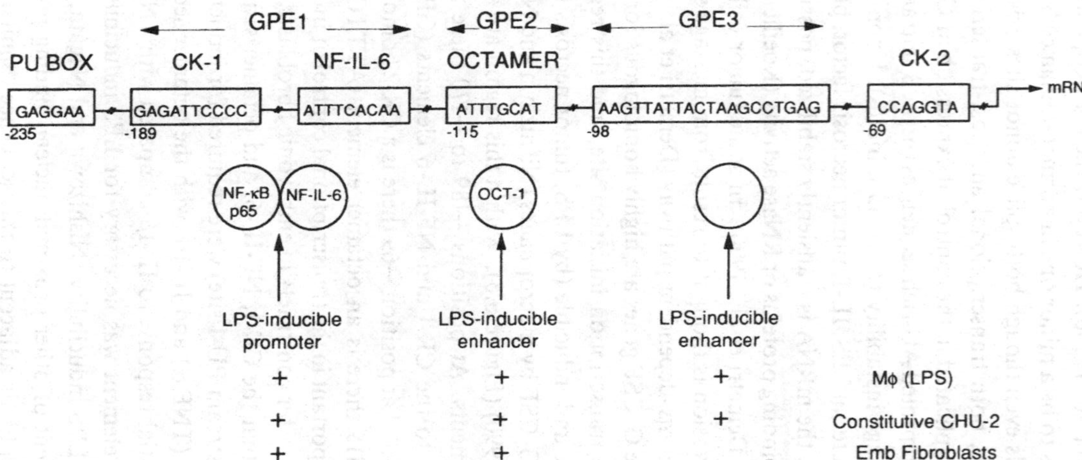


Figure 6.5. Promoter and enhancer elements in the human G-CSF gene 5′ of exon 1. Nucleotides are labeled relative to the transcriptional initiation site. Recognized sequence elements that correspond to nuclear factor binding sites are boxed and labeled. Plus signs indicate the elements that are active in LPS-activated macrophages $M\phi$(LPS) and embryonic fibroblasts stimulated with tumor necrosis factor (TNF) or IL-1, and that are constitutively active in CHU-2 cells.

## M-CSF

The human M-CSF gene is located on chromosome 1p13–21 (Morris et al., 1991), although it had originally been assigned to chromosome 5q33, and the mouse gene is located on chromosome 3F3, in an identical location to the *op* (osteopetrosis) locus (Table 6.1). In osteopetrotic (op/op) mice, a single base insertion leads to a frameshift in the M-CSF coding sequence (Yoshida et al., 1990; Wiktor-Jedrzejczak et al., 1991).

Both human and mouse M-CSF genes span about 20 kbp of DNA and consist of 10 exons (Ladner et al., 1987; Harrington et al., 1991) (Figure 6.6). Unlike the situation with the other CSFs, there are multiple transcripts of the M-CSF gene involving the alternative use of the 10 exons by differential splicing. The largest transcript is approximately 4 kb in length and utilizes all of the coding sequences in all exons except exon 9. Exon 10, which encodes the 3′ untranslated region of this mRNA, contains three copies of AU-rich sequences that confer message instability in human monocytes (Horiguchi et al., 1988). An approximately 2.3-kb mRNA is identical to the 4-kb mRNA, except that the smaller exon 9 is used to encode the 3′ untranslated region. The protein products of these

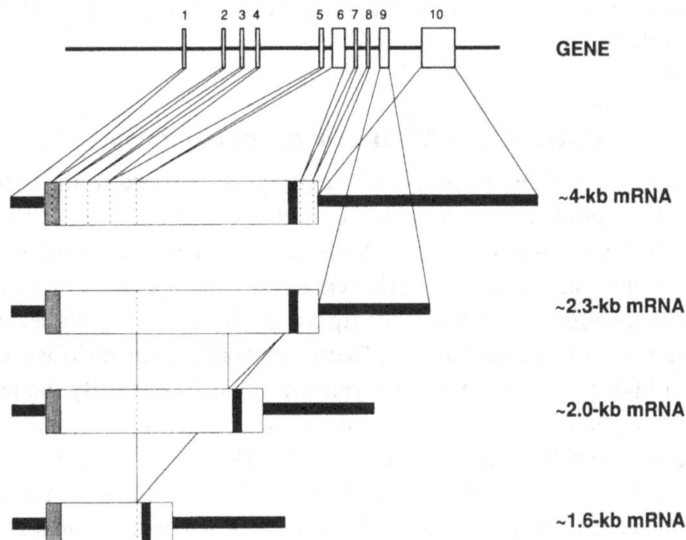


Figure 6.6. Structure of the human M-CSF gene and its alternative mRNA transcripts. Exons 1–10 are shown as boxes and untranslated 5′ and 3′ ends of the mRNAs are shown as black bars. The leader sequence codons are lightly stippled, and the transmembrane codons are heavily stippled in the mRNAs.

mRNAs are identical 522-amino acid transmembrane precursors. Two other differential splicing events involving exon 6 have also been observed. The first, which generates a 2.0-kb mRNA, is a splice event between exon 5 and the 5′ end of exon 6 so that 348 bases of exon 6 are deleted. The second, which generates a 1.6-kb mRNA, is a splice event between exon 5 and the 5′ end of exon 6 so that 894 bases of exon 6 are deleted. The latter event eliminates the proteolytic cleavage site encoded in exon 6 and produces a form of M-CSF that is relatively stably expressed at the cell surface (Kawasaki et al., 1985; Ladner et al., 1987, 1988; Wong et al., 1987; Cerretti et al., 1988).

The 5′ region of the M-CSF gene is highly conserved between mice and humans and displays a number of sequence elements homologous to known promoter and enhancer elements, including SP-1, AP-1, AP-2, NF-1, NF-IL-6, CK-1, and CK-2 sites (Harrington et al., 1991). As mentioned earlier, the CK-1 site may represent an NF-KB site, and DNA footprinting analysis has demonstrated an NF-KB binding site at position −377 to −368 of the M-CSF promoter in TNF$\alpha$-stimulated HL-60 cells (Yamada et al., 1991). IL-2 is known to activate NF-KB, and IL-2 stimulation of human monocytes activates NF-KB binding to the M-CSF promoter and activates M-CSF gene transcription (Brach et al., 1993). However, the role of the other promoter elements in M-CSF gene transcription is currently unknown.

## GM-CSF and Multi-CSF receptor $\alpha$-chains

The human GM-CSF receptor $\alpha$-chain gene was mapped to the pseudoautosomal regions of the X and Y chromosomes by a combination of analysis of human–mouse cell hybrids, in situ hybridization of human chromosomes, and human genetic pedigrees (Gough et al., 1990) (Table 6.2). This region is localized at the tip of the short arms of the sex chromosomes and recombines at high frequency during male meiosis, resulting in a high degree of genetic polymorphism at this site. By the use of pulsed gel electrophoresis, the human GM-CSF receptor $\alpha$-chain gene has been shown to span at least 45 kbp of DNA and is located within 1,180–1,300 kbp of the telomere in close proximity to the CpG island B5 (Rappold et al., 1992). The human IL-3 receptor $\alpha$-chain also maps to the pseudoautosomal region of the sex chromosomes (Yp13.3 and Xp22.3) within 190 kbp of the GM-CSF receptor $\alpha$-chain gene (Kremer et al., 1993; Milatovich et al., 1993). In contrast, the murine GM-CSF receptor $\alpha$-chain gene maps to the telomeric band $D_2$ of the mouse autosomal chromosome 19 (Disteche et al., 1992).

Table 6.2. *Molecular genetic characteristics of CSF receptors*

| Receptor | Chromosomal location of the gene | Size of the gene (kbp) | Alternative transcripts | Number of exons |
|---|---|---|---|---|
| hGM-CSFR$\alpha$ | X,Y PAR | — | 3 | — |
| mGM-CSFR$\alpha$ | 19D2 | — | — | — |
| hIL-3R$\alpha$ | X,Y PAR | — | — | — |
| mIL-3R$\alpha$ | — | — | — | — |
| h$\beta_c$ | 22q12.2–13.1 | — | — | — |
| m$\beta_c$ | 15 | 28 | 3 | 14 |
| m$\beta_{IL\text{-}3}$ | 15 | 28 | 2 | 14 |
| hG-CSFR | 1p35–34.3 | 16.5 | 3 | 17 |
| mG-CSFR | 4, 19 | — | — | — |
| hM-CSFR | 5q33.3 | 60 | 2 | 22 |
| mM-CSFR | 18D | — | — | — |

The frequent loss of sex chromosomes in some human myeloid leukemias suggested that either the GM-CSF or IL-3 receptor $\alpha$-chain genes might be involved as recessive oncogenes (Gough et al., 1990), but gross structural lesions of the GM-CSF receptor gene have not so far been observed in human leukemias (Brown et al., 1993).

A number of transcripts of the human GM-CSF receptor $\alpha$-chain gene have been observed. The major transcript is an mRNA of 2.8 kb coding for the originally cloned receptor (Gearing et al., 1989b). A second transcript (approximately 10-fold less abundant in human bone marrow and placenta) arises from alternative splicing of the gene and replaces the C-terminal cytoplasmic 25 amino acids with 35 new amino acids. This form of the receptor is functional (Crosier et al., 1991). A third transcript represents approximately 20% of the GM-CSF receptor $\alpha$-chain transcripts in placental tissue and encodes a soluble receptor in which the transmembrane and cytoplasmic domains have been deleted and replaced with 16 new amino acids (Ashworth and Kraft, 1990; Raines et al., 1991).

## GM-CSF and Multi-CSF receptor $\beta$-chains

The common $\beta$-subunit of the human GM-CSF, Multi-CSF, and IL-5 receptors appears to be encoded by a single gene located on chromosome 22q12.2–13.1 (Table 6.2) (Shen et al., 1992). In the mouse, however, two closely related genes, AIC2A and AIC2B, are homologous to the human

$\beta$-subunit, with the AIC2A molecule being an IL-3-specific $\beta$-subunit and the AIC2B molecule being a shared $\beta$-subunit for the GM-CSF, IL-3, and IL-5 receptors. Both genes are closely linked on mouse chromosome 15 near the *sis* proto-oncogene, a region that is syntenic with human chromosome 22q12.3–13.1 (Gorman et al., 1992). The two genes arose by duplication and retain identical structures (14 exons spanning 28 kbp of DNA) with highly homologous intron sequences (90% identity) and 5′ upstream sequences (95% identity). Exon 1 and part of exon 2 encode 5′ untranslated sequences, and the signal sequence is encoded in exon 2. Exons 3–10 encode the duplicated hemopoietin domain, exon 11 encodes the transmembrane domain, and exons 12–14 encode the cytoplasmic domain along with 3′ untranslated sequences and a polyadenylation signal on exon 14 (Figure 6.7). The transcription initiation sites for both genes are 30 nucleotides downstream of the TATA box. The 5′ region upstream of the gene contains several consensus sequences including three PU-1 recognition sequences (at −51, −71, and −257), a GATA sequence (at −138), an AP-3 binding site (at −242), an octamer sequence (at −375), and two interferon $\gamma$-responsive elements (at −384 and −444). Little is known about the control of transcription of these genes, but it is interesting that interferon $\gamma$ upregulates human $\beta$-chain expression in monocytes at both the transcriptional and post-transcriptional levels (Hallek et al., 1992). Alternative transcripts of AIC2A and AIC2B have also been described involving deletion of exons 6 and 7, or exons 5, 7, and 8, but the functional consequences of these deletions are unknown (Gorman et al., 1992).

## G-CSF receptors

The human G-CSF receptor is encoded by a single gene on chromosome 1p35–34.3 (Inazawa et al., 1991) and contains 17 exons spanning approximately 16.5 kbp of DNA (Seto et al., 1992) (Table 6.2). However, in the murine genome two unlinked G-CSF receptor genes have been localized on chromosomes 4 and 19 (N. Gough and S. Rakar, unpublished data). The gene on the distal portion of chromosome 4 is syntenic with the human gene on chromosome 1, but it is unclear whether both murine genes are functional or whether one represents a pseudogene.

The exonic organization of the human G-CSF receptor gene is similar to that for AIC2A and AIC2B, as well as for other hemopoietic receptors, with separate exons encoding the various functional elements of the receptor (Figure 6.7). Exons 1 and 2 encode the 5′ untranslated region of

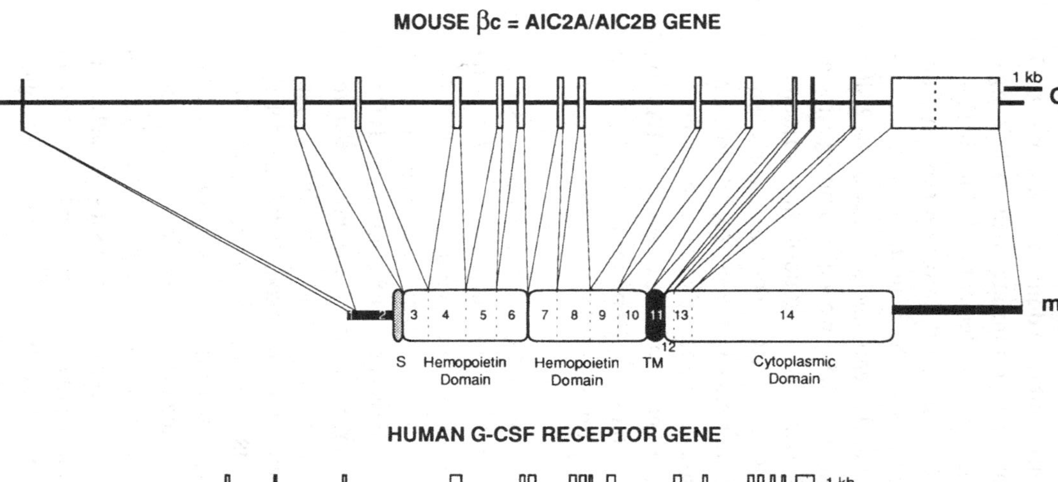


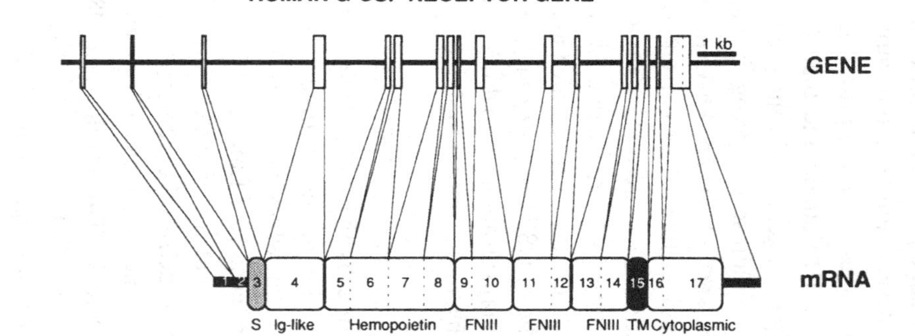


Figure 6.7. Structure of the murine AIC2A/AIC2B ($\beta$IL-3/$\beta$c) and human G-CSF receptor genes, as well as the major transcripts. Exons are shown as boxes and untranslated regions of the mRNA as black bars. The structural domains of the receptor codons are labeled (S, signal sequence; TM, transmembrane domain).

the mRNA, exon 3 the signal sequence, exon 4 the immunoglobulin-like domain, exons 5–8 the hemopoietin domain, exons 9–14 the three fibronectin III domains, exon 15 the transmembrane domain, and exons 16–17 the cytoplasmic domain along with the 3′ untranslated region. This organization suggests that the primordial genetic element coded for half of a fibronectin III domain and that the hemopoietin domain evolved from the bringing together of four such exons. The 5′ upstream genomic sequences contain several recognizable elements, including two AP-2 sites (at −305 and −185), an AP-1 site at −815, two GF-1 binding sites at −1,025 and −1,100, and several GC-rich regions. At position −120 is an 18-nucleotide sequence CCTGGGAGGAAGGGGCTG that is complementary to conserved sequences at similar sites in the myeloperoxidase and neutrophil elastase genes, which are also selectively expressed in neutrophils. The G-CSF receptor gene does not contain a classical TATA box, but the major transcriptional initiation site is 20 bp upstream of the cap site, with a minor initiation site 10 bp upstream of the cap site (Seto et al., 1992).

A single major G-CSF receptor transcript (3.7 kb) has been observed in human cells that are receptor-positive (Fukunaga et al., 1990c; Larsen et al., 1990), but multiple transcripts have been identified by cDNA cloning, all of which can arise by alternative splicing of the gene. The first transcript encodes a functional G-CSF receptor of 831 amino acids (form 1). The second transcript contains an 88-nucleotide deletion relative to form 1 that deletes the transmembrane domain and alters the translation reading frame so that 150 new amino acids are encoded after the deletion point (form 2). This results in a 748-amino acid-secreted soluble form of the human G-CSF receptor that retains the capacity to bind G-CSF. The third transcript has an 81-nucleotide insertion within the cytoplasmic domain resulting in a functional receptor of 863 amino acids (form 3) (Fukunaga et al., 1990c). The fourth transcript contains a 419-nucleotide deletion in the cytoplasmic domain relative to form 1 that generates an altered shorter cytoplasmic domain and an altered 3′ untranslated region (Larsen et al., 1990). All forms of the receptor retain G-CSF binding activity, and while form 1 appears to be the major transcript in most cells, the other forms have also been detected at lower levels (Fukunaga et al., 1990c). The functional significance of the different transcripts is unknown, but it is interesting that some C-terminal deletions of the G-CSF receptor may result in altered capacities to induce terminal differentiation (Dong et al., 1993, 1994; Fukunaga et al., 1993).

## M-CSF receptor (c-*fms*)

The M-CSF receptor is encoded by the cellular homologue (c-*fms*) of the feline oncogene v-*fms* (Sherr et al., 1985). The human M-CSF receptor gene is on chromosome 5q33.3 (Le Beau et al., 1986), while the mouse gene is on chromosome 18D (Sola et al., 1988) (Table 6.2). The mouse gene maps to a common proviral integration site (FIM-2) involved in Friend virus-induced myeloid leukemias. This site spans one of the gene promoters and leads to overexpression of apparently normal M-CSF receptor mRNA (Gisselbrecht et al., 1987). Although the human gene maps to chromosome 5q, it is distant from the interstitial deletion that occurs in the $5q^-$ syndrome.

The c-*fms* gene encompasses approximately 60 kbp of DNA and consists of 21 or 22 exons depending on which promoter is used (Roberts et al., 1988). Exon 1 is the 5′ noncoding exon and is separated by 26 kbp from exon 2, which encodes the signal peptide for the receptor. The exon 1–containing transcript is driven from a promoter that is only 359 bp downstream of the 3′ end of the B-type platelet-derived growth factor receptor and is active only in placental trophoblast cells. In monocytes and macrophages, a separate promoter leads to initiation of transcription at exon 2 (Visvader and Verma, 1989). A 775-bp fragment of DNA, immediately upstream of exon 1, mediates gene transcription in placental and fibroblast cells but not macrophages, while a 550-bp gene fragment immediately upstream of exon 2 mediates transcription in macrophages, but not other cells, at multiple initiation sites (Roberts et al., 1992). Neither of these promoters contains classical promoter elements (TATA or CAAT boxes or SP-1 sites), although the upstream promoter (placental) contains consensus sequences for helix–loop–helix nuclear proteins and PU-1 sites, while the downstream promoter (macrophage) contains consensus sequences for CK-1, helix–loop–helix transcription factors, Myb, and PU-1 (Roberts et al., 1992). On the other hand, Yue et al. (1993) found that the murine M-CSF receptor in macrophages was controlled primarily at the level of transcriptional elongation through DNA sequences encoded in intron 2 and that these were also responsive to downregulation by phorbol esters, LPS, and M-CSF.

A final level of control has been described by Weber et al. (1989), who suggested that a labile protein induced by macrophage differentiation and downregulated by phorbol esters stabilizes M-CSF receptor mRNA. On the other hand, Gliniak et al. (1992) showed that when a M-CSF receptor retroviral construct was transfected into myeloid FDC-P1 cells, GM-CSF and Multi-CSF transcriptionally activated an RNase activity that caused selective degradation of M-CSF receptor mRNA and consequent loss of M-CSF receptor and responsiveness (Gliniak and Rohrschneider, 1990; Metcalf et al., 1992b). The relative contributions of these different mechanisms of control and the involvement of specific transcription factors remain to be definitively resolved.

## Conclusions

The genetic control of CSF action is mediated at several different levels. The use of different transcripts, by alternative splicing, of M-CSF and several of the CSF receptors may produce molecules with distinct biological activities, although in many cases this has not yet been formally established. The mRNAs for the CSFs have intrinsic instability that can be modulated by exogenous agents, which could allow for very rapid control of CSF expression in response to a changing extracellular environment. The promoter and enhancer elements of the CSF and receptor genes are complex and generally highly conserved among species. They contain multiple, overlapping, consensus binding sequences for nuclear transcription factors, and the subtle interplay of these factors in controlling transcription rates is only beginning to be elucidated. There is little doubt that these elements represent a versatile and highly coordinated means by which the producing cell can respond to multiple extracellular signals impinging on any given cell.

Several of the CSF and receptor genes are clustered on human chromosomes (particularly the 5q and sex chromosomes), and while none have yet been definitely associated with chromosomal aberrations in human disease, it is possible that more subtle mutations in these genes or their control elements will be involved in some malignancies.

Since CSF action may often be highly localized and the expression of CSFs and their receptors is very difficult to measure in vivo, it is hoped that further studies on the controlling elements of their genes will yield clues as to how these molecules are regulated physiologically.

# 7

# Biological actions of the colony-stimulating factors in vitro

Each of the colony-stimulating factors can stimulate the proliferation of granulocyte-macrophage progenitor cells and their progeny. This is most readily demonstrated as the formation by these progenitor cells of granulocytic and/or macrophage colonies in semisolid agar cultures. This was the original biological action noted for the CSFs and was used as the bioassay to monitor their purification. However, it is now recognized that each CSF can exert other actions on granulocyte-macrophage populations (Metcalf, 1991a). These include (a) differentiation commitment, (b) maturation induction, (c) maintenance of membrane transport and cell viability, and (d) stimulation of mature cell functional activity.

Each of these major functions will be discussed separately. Because no functional differences have been noted in vitro between native or recombinant CSFs, either glycosylated or nonglycosylated, the type of molecule used in particular studies will not necessarily be identified.

## Proliferative stimulation

When single CSFs are used as the stimulus for granulocyte-macrophage colony formation, cell separation studies have shown that the cells generating the colonies are committed granulocyte-macrophage progenitor cells (Nicola et al., 1980; Metcalf, 1984). Analysis using the glucose-6-phosphate dehydrogenase marker (Singer et al., 1979) and the use of single cell cultures have shown that colonies are the clonal progeny of individual progenitor cells. If care is taken to avoid significant colony overcrowding in agar cultures (fewer than 50 colonies per 1 ml culture), then the cells within any one colony can be safely accepted as being the clonal progeny of that progenitor cell. This generalization is subject to certain qualifications: (a) Methylcellulose cultures allow significant cell and clonal movement and are less reliable than the more solid agar cultures in ensuring that clones remain distinct. (b) In most hemopoietic cultures, nonclonogenic cells die in the culture and do not present a problem for interpreting populations found in colonies. Significant exceptions are found in cultures of peripheral blood or peritoneal cells, where numerous monocyte-macrophages may persist and become incorporated in developing colonies. (c) Each CSF also stimulates the formation of clones of subcolony size. These are formed by the initial progeny of progenitor cells. They are not usually recorded but do constitute an additional source of cells potentially contaminating developing colonies.

The formation of granulocyte-macrophage colonies in semisolid cultures of marrow cells is absolutely dependent on the addition of CSF unless the cultures prepared contain an excessive number of cells, in which case apparently spontaneous colony formation can occur. Spontaneous colony formation is due to the local production of CSF by adherent monocyte-macrophages and occasional endothelial or fibroblast cells in the cultures, and is highly dependent on the number of cells cultured (Moore and Williams, 1972). Thus, in cultures of 25,000 mouse or human bone marrow cells, usually no colony formation occurs in unstimulated cultures, and at most a few clusters of granulocytes or macrophages may develop. "Spontaneous" colony formation in crowded cultures is reduced in cultures of marrow cells from mice with inactivation of either the GM-CSF or the G-CSF gene, so endogenous production of both these CSFs in crowded cultures is partly responsible for the phenomenon of spontaneous colony formation.

The inclusion of CSF in increasing concentrations in cultures of bone marrow cells stimulates colony formation with a sigmoid dose–response curve (Figure 7.1). The ascending linear portion of the dose–response curve reflects the activation of progressively less responsive progenitor cells to commence cell division. Colony numbers reach a plateau when all available progenitor cells are actively proliferating.

It will be noted that in cultures of mouse bone marrow cells, GM-CSF, M-CSF, and Multi-CSF stimulate the formation of an approximately equal maximal number of colonies as scored after 7 days of incubation, although the actual cellular composition of these colonies differs markedly with the three CSFs. In sharp contrast, G-CSF stimulates the formation of a much lower total number of colonies, and these are of much smaller size.

The same phenomenon is observed in cultures of human marrow cells, where the number of colonies stimulated by GM-CSF is approximately

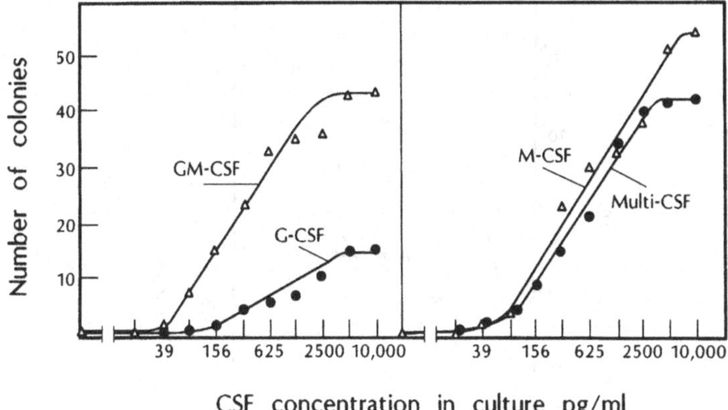


Figure 7.1. Colony formation in cultures of 25,000 mouse bone marrow cells stimulated by purified recombinant GM-CSF, G-CSF, M-CSF, or Multi-CSF. Colony formation was scored after 7 days of incubation.

equal to the number stimulated by Multi-CSF after 7 or 14 days of incubation. In contrast, the maximal number of colonies stimulated by G-CSF tends to be lower, and characteristically many of these colonies disappear during the second week of incubation due to dispersion and/or death of mature granulocytic cells in the colonies. M-CSF has essentially no colony-stimulating activity for human cells in conventional agar cultures but is active in cultures prepared using agarose and incubated in low oxygen concentrations (Broxmeyer et al., 1990).

The CSF concentration range required to stimulate colony formation is shown for murine CSFs in Figure 7.1, and the range is essentially similar for human CSFs acting on human marrow cells. Using the conventional unit system that assigns 50 U/ml to the concentration stimulating a half-maximal number of colonies to develop, this gives an estimate of biological activity for each purified murine CSF of approximately $10^8$ U/mg protein, with 400–800 U/ml (4–8 ng/ml) stimulating a maximal number of colonies to develop.

It should be recognized that this method of monitoring induced cell proliferation is a little misleading, since colony size continues to increase progressively with increasing CSF concentrations. As a consequence, total cell production actually rises progressively throughout such a dose curve, as shown in Figure 7.2.

A similar type of dose–response curve can be obtained using colony formation by appropriate CSF-responsive cell lines, as shown in Figure 7.2. Suspension cultures of marrow cells, purified progenitor cells, or CSF-

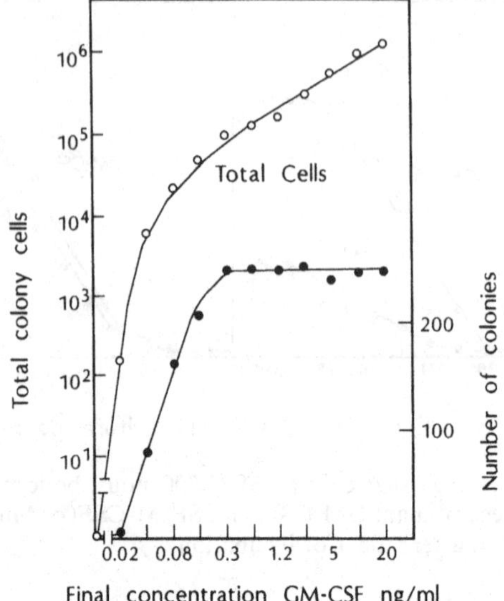


Figure 7.2. Assays of the proliferative action of CSFs by enumerating colonies obscure the fact that colony size increases progressively with increasing CSF concentrations. If the average number of cells per colony is considered, total cell production rises progressively as CSF concentrations are increased. The cultures were initiated using 300 GM-CSF-dependent FDC-P1 cells per culture, and the colonies were analyzed after 7 days of incubation.

responsive cell lines can be used to obtain similar dose–response curves based on either tritiated thymidine uptake or the visual counting of cells in microwell cultures.

It is important to emphasize that when CSF concentrations are increased even a thousandfold beyond those stimulating the formation of a maximal number of colonies, no inhibition of cell proliferation is observed. Thus, the CSFs are not regulators of the type exhibiting a biphasic concentration effect, and regardless of the concentration involved, CSFs are never inhibitory for cell division.

Artificial CSF-responsive cell lines can be generated by insertion of cDNAs encoding the appropriate receptor chains. Cloned cell lines can then be selected that express a large number of receptors, which can demonstrate exceptionally high responsiveness to stimulation by CSF, as shown in Figure 7.3. Use of such lines can provide a bioassay that is at least as sensitive as the best immunoassay and has the additional advantages that the CSF being detected is certified as being functionally active by its capacity to stimulate cell proliferation and that the responses are specific because of the insertion of a single type of receptor.

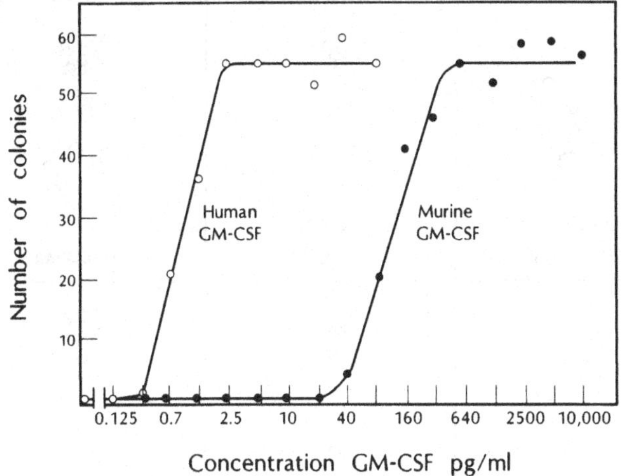


Figure 7.3. Hyperresponsive cell lines can be created by insertion of appropriate receptors. This figure illustrates the responsiveness of a murine FDC-P1 cell line after insertion and expression of the $\alpha$- and $\beta$-chains for the human GM-CSF receptor. The resulting cell line exhibits a detectable proliferative response to less than 1 pg/ml human GM-CSF, greater responsiveness than exhibited to murine GM-CSF, a normal regulator of this cell line. Each culture was initiated using 100 cells.

A variety of evidence indicates that even in cultures of marrow cells that contain many other cell types, the CSFs act directly on the responding progenitor cells and their clonal progeny: (a) The progenitor cells express receptors for CSF, as do their maturing progeny (Nicola and Metcalf, 1985b, 1986). (b) Colony formation is linear with respect to cultured cell numbers, with the linear relationship passing through zero. (c) Clones initiated by CSF continue to proliferate when transferred to CSF-containing cultures lacking other cultured cells (Metcalf and Burgess, 1982; Metcalf and Nicola, 1983). (d) FACS-purified progenitor cells respond to CSF stimulation (Nicola et al., 1980). (e) Single cells, whether progenitor cells or their early progeny, can be stimulated to proliferate by CSF in conventional or serum-free cultures (Metcalf and Burgess, 1982; Peleraux and Eliason, 1989).

### *Heterogeneity of proliferative responses*

In cultures of bone marrow cells being stimulated by a CSF, there is remarkable heterogeneity in the appearance of the developing clones and colonies. There are a number of reasons underlying this complex heterogeneity.

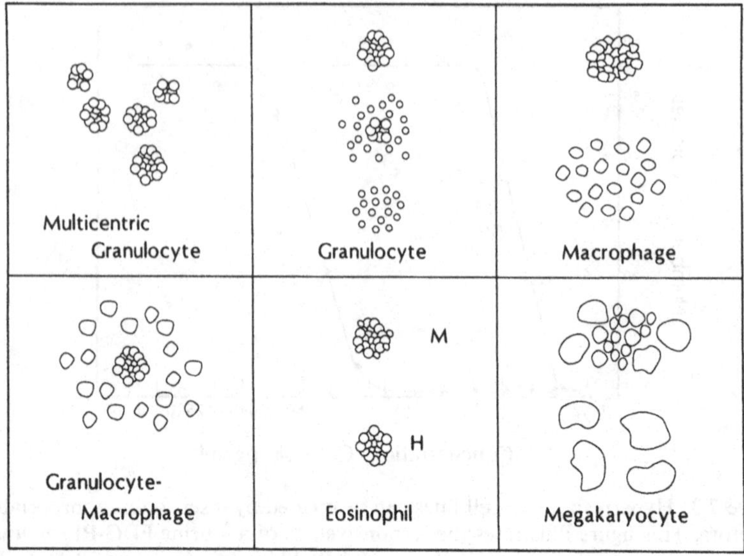


Figure 7.4. Schematic representation of the variety of colonies of different shapes and sizes that can develop side by side in a culture of bone marrow cells. Human eosinophil colonies (H) are characteristically compact, but colonies of other types can vary widely in size and shape.

First, each CSF can stimulate the proliferation of cells in more than one lineage, and colonies composed of cells in these various lineages can exhibit characteristic differences in shape and size (Figure 7.4). Colonies wholly composed of immature granulocytes are compact. When maturation commences in these colonies, the mature granulocytes are smaller than the immature cells and more motile in the agar medium, so a corona of mature cells tends to form around a central core of immature cells (Figure 1.1). Colonies wholly composed of mature granulocytes can consist of widely dispersed cells with no remaining central region. Macrophage colonies can either be compact aggregates of cells (if stimulated by M-CSF) or be loosely dispersed in structure (if stimulated by GM-CSF; Metcalf and Nicola, 1992). Granulocyte-macrophage colonies often have a central region of granulocytes surrounded by a corona of dispersed macrophages. Murine eosinophil colonies have a general resemblance to granulocytic colonies but are usually slightly more compact. Human eosinophil colonies in 14-day cultures are characteristically small and very compact. The cells in megakaryocytic colonies are very large and tend to be widely dispersed if the colonies are formed by mature precursors. With colonies formed by less mature precursors, there can be a compact central region, and the colonies will contain cells of widely varying size and may contain cells of other lineages. The precise identification of these various colony types requires an analysis of appropriately stained cultures.

Second, cultured bone marrow populations contain progenitor cells that vary in their differentiation stage within any one lineage. The least-mature progenitors have the greatest proliferative potential and will form larger colonies than their slightly more mature progeny. At the other extreme, the progeny of the most mature progenitor cells have the potential to form only clones (clusters) of subcolony size, and such clones inevitably outnumber colonies developing in the culture.

Third, there is a characteristic asynchrony in the onset of proliferation by progenitor cells in a semisolid culture. Because of this, the number of developing clones increases linearly in such cultures over a period of 4–5 days (Metcalf, 1970) (Figure 7.5). The reasons for this asynchrony have not been defined, but it is not based on the cell cycle status of the cells at the time of commencing the culture (Metcalf, 1972). To some degree, the duration of the asynchronous onset of proliferation can be reduced by increasing the CSF concentration, but some asynchrony persists, regardless of the CSF concentration used. It is obvious that late-initiating clones

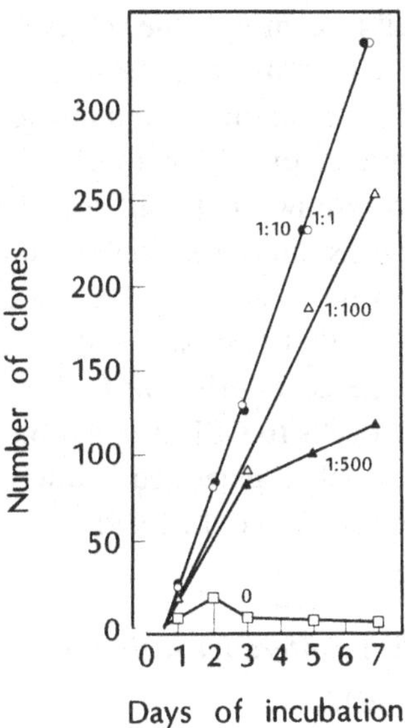


Figure 7.5. In cultures of marrow cells being stimulated by a CSF, there is a characteristic asynchrony in the initiation of clones (defined as three or more cells) during the incubation period. To some degree this asynchrony can be reduced by increasing the concentration of CSF. (Reproduced with permission from Metcalf, 1970.)

only achieve a smaller size than early-initiating clones, even after a total incubation time of 7–14 days.

Fourth, there are marked quantitative differences in responsiveness to CSF stimulation exhibited by different progenitor cells, differences that are inherited to some degree by the progeny of such cells. This can contribute to the size heterogeneity of colonies at any one CSF concentration and is independent of the maturation stage of the progentor cells or any other cells in the colony.

Fifth, in cultures of normal marrow cells, the maturation of some colony cells occurs while cell division is continuing. At any one time in a culture, some colonies can be composed wholly of immature cells, some wholly of mature cells, and others of a mixture of both types. There is no synchrony of maturation within a culture, so widely differing colonies of these types can be located side by side in the same culture. This strongly suggests that maturing cells in one colony cannot influence the maturation of cells in adjacent colonies. This heterogeneity based on maturation asynchrony is not significantly influenced by the CSF concentration present in the cultures.

Transfer of dividing cells from a CSF-stimulated culture to a culture lacking CSF leads to cessation of cell division. How quickly this occurs depends on the cells under study. With suitable CSF-dependent cell lines, the majority of cells fail to complete the cell cycle in progress and never generate two daughter cells (Metcalf, 1985). At the other extreme, approximately one-third of immature granulocytic cells from developing mouse colonies can produce one further cell division and, less often, a second following CSF withdrawal (Metcalf and Merchav, 1982). In serum-free cultures of murine cells, up to four cell divisions were sometimes observed following CSF withdrawal (Peleraux and Eliason, 1989).

There is some evidence that CSF stimulation may not be mandatory throughout the cell cycle, except during the $G_1$ phase (Pluznik et al., 1984). Intermittent exposure of cells to CSF stimulation does result in cell proliferation, but the cell number generated is lower than that achieved by continuous stimulation (Begley et al., 1988).

### *The proliferative action of CSFs*

During early work on the biology of CSF action, the view was repeatedly expressed that hemopoietic cells did not require active proliferative stimulation because they possess an intrinsic, unaided capacity for cell division. The suggestion made by these critics was that the CSFs are merely factors allowing the cells to remain in good health in vitro; such cells can then exhibit their intrinsic capacity for division. The subsequent demonstration (see later) that CSFs are indeed necessary for cell survival in vitro gave substance to this otherwise improbable proposal. That the CSFs stimulate cell division has required proof.

There are several lines of evidence indicating that the CSFs play an active role in stimulating cell division. First, the CSFs force cells to enter the S phase of the cell cycle. With M-CSF-dependent cell lines from which M-CSF had been withdrawn, the readdition of M-CSF rapidly initiated DNA synthesis (Tushinski et al., 1982). Similarly, if normal progenitor cells are noncycling ($G_0$), as is the case with progenitor cells in the liver during midtrimester fetal development in larger animals, stimulation by CSF forces entry of a significant proportion of such cells into the S phase of the cell cycle within 3 hours (Moore and Williams, 1973).

Second, the molecular basis of this action has been defined by studies on M-CSF-responsive cell lines, where, after initial M-CSF withdrawal, stimulation by M-CSF results in a rapid rise in cyclin D1 early in the $G_1$ period, followed later by a rise in cyclin D2 (Roussel and Sherr 1993). The passage of cells through the cell cycle is now recognized to be mediated by members of the cyclin family, and the prominent action of M-CSF in elevating cyclin D1 agrees with the requirement for CSF stimulation during $G_1$ and indicates the need for the CSF to achieve a specific activation of the intracellular regulatory machinery controlling cell division.

Third, when murine peritoneal exudate cells are cultured in agar medium, delays of up to 14 days occur before cell division commences (Lin and Stewart, 1974). The survival of cells during this lag period is not CSF-dependent, but the subsequent cell division is wholly CSF-dependent, providing an example in which the proliferative effects of the CSF are not ascribable simply to an action supporting cell survival in vitro.

Fourth, the viability of some CSF-dependent cell lines can similarly be sustained after withdrawal of CSF by maintaining high ATP levels. This maneuver permits cell survival but does not result in any cell division (Whetton and Dexter, 1983). Cell lines engineered to overexpress *bcl*-2 can also exhibit extended cell survival in the absence of CSF, but again such cells do not undergo division (Vaux et al., 1988, Nunez et al., 1990).

Fifth, a quantitative relationship can be demonstrated between CSF concentration and the *rate* of cell division as determined by the length of the cell cycle. Although an obvious relationship is evident between CSF concentration and the average number of cells in developing colonies, this by itself does not prove a relationship between CSF concentration and cell cycle times, for two general reasons: (a) Continuous maturation to nondividing end cells occurs in normal hemopoietic colonies, and a significant number of cells maturing in the presence of low CSF concentrations would have a major effect in restricting the capacity of colony cell numbers to increase, giving an end result that would resemble slowing of cell cycle times. (b) A major heterogeneity exists in the quantitative responsiveness of cells to stimulation by CSF, and higher concentrations of CSF might be activating cells that, upon activation, had more rapid cell cycle times than those of other clonogenic cells. These problems were resolved by studies comparing the cell cycle times of separated daughter or granddaughter cells of individual precursor cells when these were subsequently cultured with differing concentrations of CSF. Such studies were performed with both normal progenitor cells (Metcalf, 1980) and clonogenic cell lines (Metcalf, 1985), the latter eliminating the problem of possible maturation-induced truncation of further cell proliferation. Both studies showed that cell cycle times were directly influenced by CSF concentration and thus that CSF was playing a role in determining cell cycle times.

Sixth, a specific region of the intracytoplasmic domain of hemopoietin receptors has been identified as being necessary to enable the receptor to stimulate cell division as distinct from other functions (Nakamura et al., 1992; Sakamaki et al., 1992). Extension of this molecular dissection of the receptor structure should eventually allow a complete refutation of the suggestion that CSFs act merely to permit cell survival.

When a CSF binds to high-affinity receptors on a responding cell, the CSF–receptor complex is rapidly internalized (Tushinski et al., 1982; Nicola et al., 1988). This leads to degradation of the internalized CSF with a net loss of CSF. Where the number of CSF receptors is large on a responding cell population and the amounts of CSF available are relatively limited, CSF consumption by responding cells can result in the loss of a high proportion of the CSF (Tushinski et al., 1982) (Figure 7.6). Under these conditions, the total number of available CSF molecules, rather than CSF concentration, can become important (Nicola and Metcalf, 1988), and CSF depletion can lead to the cessation of proliferative stimulation.

The prominent heterogeneity in responsiveness of normal progenitor cells (Metcalf and MacDonald, 1975) or cell lines (Metcalf, 1992) to proliferative stimulation by the CSFs is not unique to the CSFs and is seen with other growth factors. Its cellular basis remains largely unresolved. Precursor cells vary in the number of receptors they express at any one time for the various CSFs, and one possibility is that the number of receptors

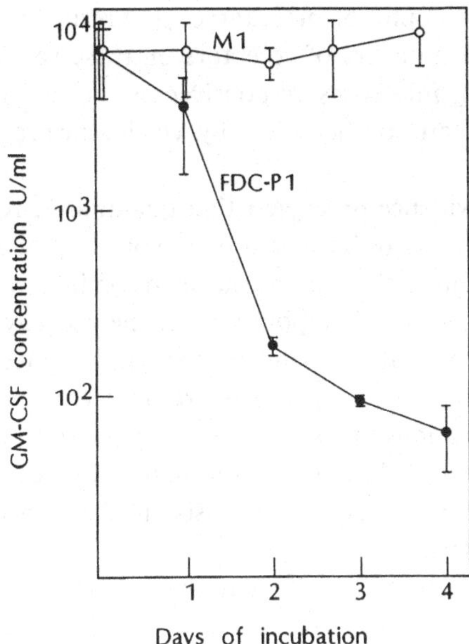


Figure 7.6. Incubation of receptor-bearing cells can deplete the medium of a growth factor. FDC-P1 cells, exhibiting receptors for GM-CSF, are responsive to stimulation by GM-CSF and deplete the medium of GM-CSF during this response. Culture of similar numbers ($0.5 \times 10^6$ cells/ml) of M1 cells, lacking receptors for GM-CSF, does not deplete GM-CSF.

may determine quantitative responsiveness. Such a relationship has been documented between IL-2 receptor expression on T-lymphocytes and their responsiveness to proliferative stimulation by IL-2 (Cantrell and Smith, 1984). However, data from studies with GM-CSF have not supported such a simple relationship. It has proved possible to induce responsiveness of the murine cell line FDC-P1 to proliferative stimulation by the non-cross-reactive human GM-CSF by insertion of human GM-CSF receptor $\alpha$-subunit cDNA, with or without human GM-CSF receptor $\beta$-subunit cDNA, into these cells. Major variations in quantitative responsiveness of such cloned cell lines to stimulation by human GM-CSF have been observed, but they did not correlate well with corresponding differences in the number of expressed high- or low-affinity GM-CSF receptors (Metcalf et al., 1990; Lock et al., 1994).

A correlation has also been observed between CSF responsiveness and the lineage of cells responding. This phenomenon is most evident for murine GM-CSF (Metcalf et al., 1986c), where macrophage precursors are more responsive than granulocyte precursors, and both are much more responsive than eosinophil or megakaryocyte precursors (see Tables 7.5 and 7.6). Since the numbers of receptors on these various cells do not show corresponding differences, responsiveness may in part be dictated by the differentiation status of the cells or by which gene programs are active at a particular time.

There is some evidence to suggest that quantitative responsiveness is a heritable trait tending to be shared by the progeny of a particular cell (Metcalf, 1992). Thus, although progeny clonogenic cells within a colony also exhibit hereogeneity of responsiveness, the progeny of a highly responsive cell tend to exhibit a higher average quantitative responsiveness to stimulation than do progeny of a less responsive clonogenic cell (Figure 7.7). Such a relationship can also be inferred from the capacity of a colony to develop with a low concentration of CSF, because the progeny within such a clone must also be responsive to that concentration or the colony could not develop.

The design of the granulocyte-macrophage progenitor cell population is such that individual cells co-express receptors for more than one CSF and possibly for certain other growth factors. This has raised the general question of how many distinct mitotic signaling pathways a cell might possess. It seems reasonable to assume that only a single control mechanism exists for directing the passage of cells through a cell cycle, even though this may be a complex process requiring the activation of a number of genes. If, as has already been discussed, there are major differences between the cytoplasmic signaling domains of different receptors, differences probably exist in the initial events elicited after binding of these regulators to their unique receptors. Does this indicate the existence of multiple possible mitotic signaling pathways from membrane receptors to the appropriate nuclear genes, or do initially distinct pathways activate a *common* final signaling pathway impinging on the nucleus?

One biological approach to this question is to insert various receptors into appropriate cell lines to determine whether all can function as initiators of mitotic signaling. We used the FDC-P1 murine cell line for such a purpose. This cell line depends for cell division on stimulation either by GM-CSF or Multi-CSF but can also respond transiently to stimulation by IL-4 and interferon $\gamma$. The insertion of cDNAs with expression of the receptors for M-CSF, Epo, SCF, human GM-CSF, and $\beta$-fibroblast growth factor permits these cells to respond by proliferation after stimulation by the appropriate regulator. This mitotic responsiveness to nine different activated receptors makes it improbable that nine completely independent signaling systems would exist in the single cell type – least of all for a foreign inserted receptor such as the human GM-CSF receptor.

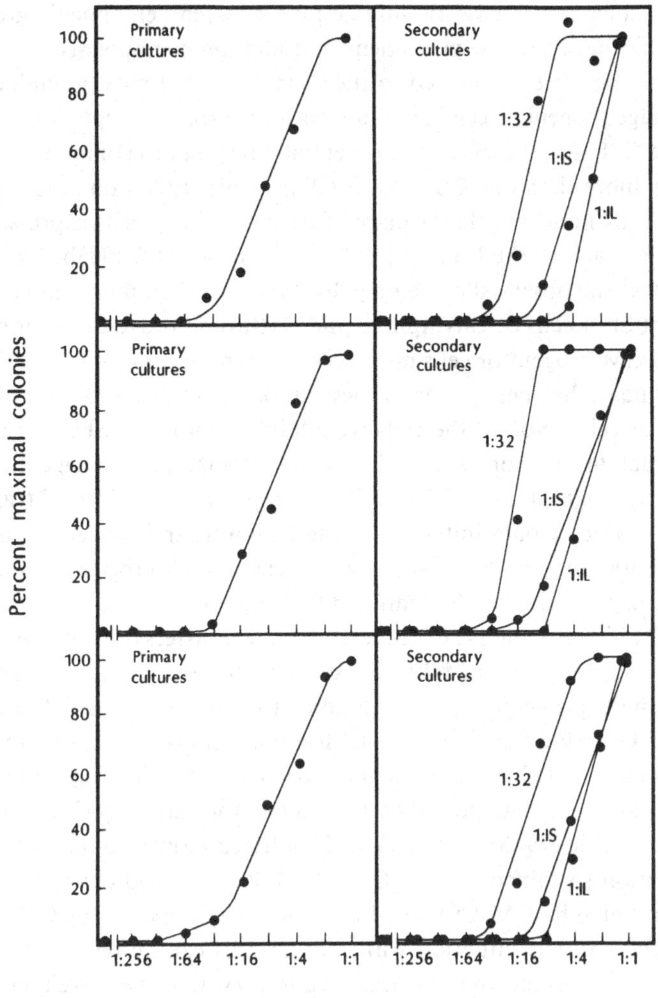


Figure 7.7. Heterogeneous responsiveness of 32D cells forming colonies after stimulation by spleen-conditioned medium (SCM) containing Multi-CSF. If colonies developing in cultures stimulated by low concentrations of Multi-CSF (1:32) are recloned, the overall responsiveness of the cells in the secondary cultures is again heterogeneous, but the cells are more responsive than those from either large (1:1L) or small (1:1S) colonies that required high concentrations of Multi-CSF (1:1) to develop. (Reproduced with permission from Metcalf, 1992.)

The responsiveness of these murine cells not only indicates the permissiveness or promiscuity of available signaling pathways, but strongly favors the conclusion that initially disparate signaling pathways ultimately funnel into a single final mitotic signaling pathway. This conclusion, if valid, is of relevance for synergistic interactions between hemopoietic growth factors that have become prominent in studies on hemopoiesis.

Several lines of evidence led to the conclusion that most granulocyte-macrophage progenitor cells simultaneously co-express receptors for more than one CSF and therefore can potentially respond to combined stimulation by more than one CSF. Autoradiographic studies on mouse bone marrow cells indicated that a major fraction of blast cells expresses receptors for each of the four CSFs (Nicola and Metcalf, 1985b, 1986). In no case was the observed percentage 100%, but such populations contain irrelevant blast cells of B-lymphoid and erythroid lineages, so that many if not all GM progenitor cells must co-express receptors for each CSF. A similar finding has been made in these laboratories using FACS-purified progenitor cells. Not all the cells were labeled with all CSFs, but again not all such progenitor cells are in the granulocyte-macrophage lineage. The autoradiographic studies have been supported by reciprocal transfer studies in which clones initiated by one CSF were transferred to culture dishes containing another CSF, in which case a high proportion showed continuing proliferation (Metcalf and Burgess, 1982; Metcalf and Nicola, 1983). The high percentage of successful cross-transfers of clones initiated by GM-CSF, M-CSF, or Multi-CSF strongly suggests that there is a broad overlap in the progenitor cells responding to these three CSFs. The situation with G-CSF differs in that G-CSF could stimulate an approximately similar number of clones to commence proliferation, but only a minority of these clones were supported to final colony formation by G-CSF (Metcalf and Nicola, 1983). Many G-CSF-initiated clones could have their proliferation sustained by GM-CSF or Multi-CSF, and conversely, few clones initiated by GM-CSF or Multi-CSF were supported by G-CSF.

The approximate situation with murine cells can be represented diagrammatically, as shown in Figures 7.8 and 7.9 with respect to either granulocyte or macrophage colony-forming cells. At least with murine cells, the number of clonogenic cells responding to M-CSF can vary widely according to the serum used in the cultures. With supplemented newborn calf serum, the number of clones can be about twice as large as those stimulated by other CSFs. The most likely explanation of this phenomenon is that such sera allow expression of the usually latent proliferative potential of relatively mature macrophages.

Confirmation of the conclusion that most progenitor cells co-express receptors for more than one CSF and therefore can be stimulated by more than one CSF has come from culture experiments in which combinations of CSFs are used to stimulate colony formation. In one experiment (Figure 7.10), mouse bone marrow cells were stimulated to proliferate by GM-CSF,

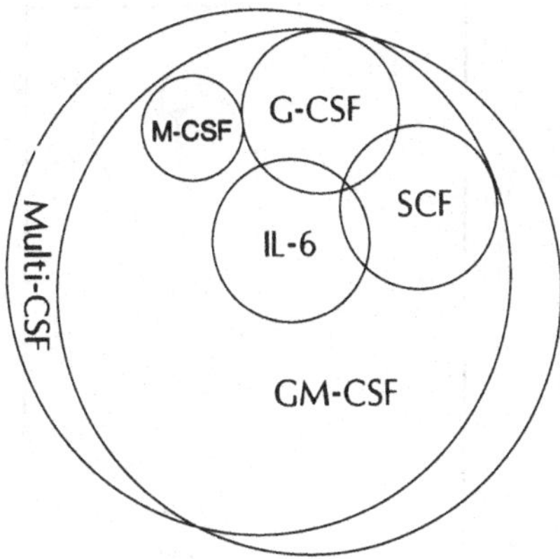


Figure 7.8. Schematic diagram representing murine granulocyte progenitor cell populations and the relative number of such cells that exhibit sustained proliferation when stimulated by various growth factors.

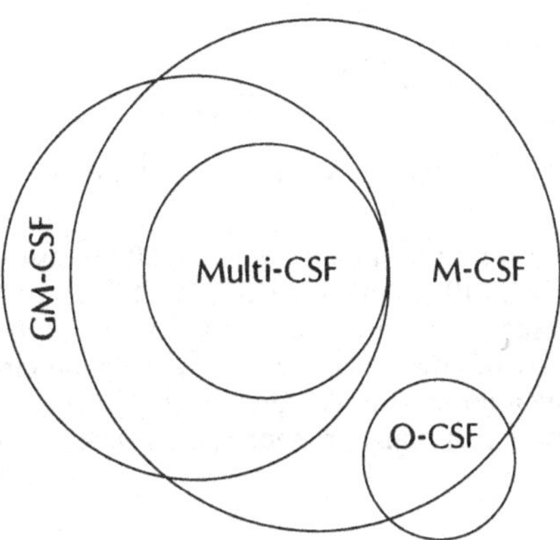


Figure 7.9. Schematic diagram representing murine macrophage progenitor cell populations and the relative number of such cells that exhibit sustained proliferation when stimulated by various growth factors. The size of the population responding to osteoclast CSF (O-CSF) is not yet known and its representation is arbitrary.

M-CSF, or G-CSF acting alone or in combination. If each CSF stimulated a distinct subset of progenitor cells, the figure shows that, in combination, a high number of colonies should result. What is observed, however, is that the combination stimulates the formation of a considerably smaller number of colonies than expected by the simple sum of colonies stimulated by each CSF acting alone. The conclusion is that many of the colony-forming cells would have responded to stimulation by any one of the three CSFs.

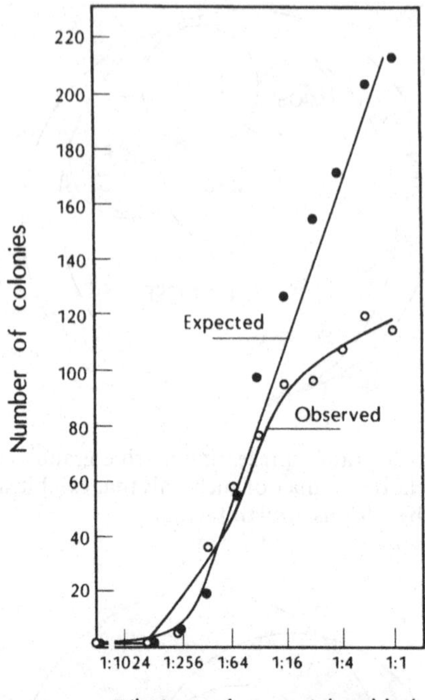


Figure 7.10. Colony formation in cultures of 50,000 mouse bone marrow cells stimulated by a mixture of 10 ng/ml GM-CSF, G-CSF, and M-CSF. If each CSF stimulated distinct subsets of progenitor cells, the mixture of the three CSFs should stimulate the formation of colonies indicated by the solid circles. However, the actual observed colony number stimulated by the CSF combination (open circles) is much lower, indicating that many progenitor cells were responsive to more than one CSF.

### *Synergistic proliferative responses*

Co-expression of CSF receptors on individual progenitor cells and their progeny makes possible the interactions noted earlier between CSF receptors following ligand binding (Chapter 5) and leads to the expectation that altered proliferative responses might occur with the use of combinations of CSFs to stimulate cell populations.

In cultures of mouse or human bone marrow cells prepared using combinations of two or more CSFs, enhanced proliferation occurs (McNiece et al., 1988; Bot et al., 1990b; Metcalf and Nicola, 1992). For CSF pairs at equivalent concentrations, a greater number of progeny cells is generated than following the use of twice the concentration of either CSF alone

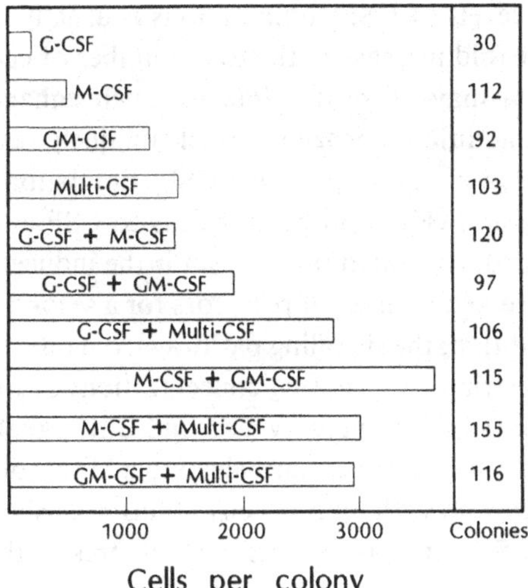


Figure 7.11. Cultures of mouse bone marrow cells stimulated by 10 ng/ml of murine CSFs alone or in combination. The combination of CSFs does not result in additive responses in terms of the number of colonies but does result in an increased average cell number per colony.

(Metcalf and Nicola, 1992). While there is some increase in the number of colonies, the enhanced response does not involve the formation of an additive number of colonies (Figure 7.11), since, as just discussed, for the most part the progenitor cells responding to each CSF are the same population. The increased cell production is therefore achieved mainly by an increase in the number of progeny cells produced by individual progenitor cells. As best exemplified by the combination of GM-CSF plus M-CSF, this increase does not occur uniformly, and indeed the size of most colonies remains unaltered in cultures containing the combined stimuli. Rather, there are certain progenitors whose proliferation is very strongly enhanced to form macroscopically visible colonies, and these are responsible for much of the observed overall increased cell production (Metcalf and Nicola, 1992). The data strongly suggest that there are some granulocyte-macrophage progenitors whose proliferation, or optimal proliferation, requires co-stimulation by two or more CSFs, a behavior resembling that of stem cells and providing further evidence of the heterogeneity of granulocyte-macrophage progenitor cells.

These synergistic responses to CSF combinations vary in magnitude with the concentrations of CSFs used and are more evident when lower concentrations are used. As shown in Figure 7.11, enhanced cell production by relatively high levels of CSF combinations is usually only moderate, with a two- to fourfold increase in the total number of cells formed.

Two phenomena may be responsible for such enhanced responses: (a) recruitment of additional progenitor cells uniquely responsive to one CSF or another or else requiring double CSF stimulation and (b) synergistic responses by individual progenitor cells to CSF combinations. In the latter case, one documented mechanism is the induced expression by one CSF of an increased number of receptors for a second CSF (Jacobsen et al., 1992). In addition, the signaling pathway from one type of occupied receptor may be restricted by limiting concentrations of a signaling intermediate that can be supplemented by a second CSF signaling pathway.

Not all CSF combinations necessarily lead to additive or enhanced proliferative responses, and with murine cells, it has been shown that a combination of GM-CSF with M-CSF actually suppresses the proliferation of a subset of macrophage progenitor cells, even though a rise occurs in total cell production as a result of the combination (Metcalf and Nicola, 1992). This unusual response can be duplicated using FDC-P1 cells that normally express GM-CSF or Multi-CSF receptors and in which a retrovirus has been used to insert the cDNA for the M-CSF receptor with subsequent expression on the membrane of M-CSF receptors (Metcalf et al., 1992b). With such cells, the combination of either GM-CSF or Multi-CSF with M-CSF severely reduced the number of clonogenic cells and restricted their capacity for cell production (Figure 7.12). The phenomenon was not due simply to activation of a tyrosine kinase signaling pathway together with a non–tyrosine kinase pathway, since control cells with an inserted tyrosine kinase receptor for fibroblast growth factor (FGF) did not show inhibition when FGF was combined with either GM-CSF or Multi-CSF. Studies have shown that the phenomenon may be based in part on the capacity of both GM-CSF and Multi-CSF to cause degradation of the mRNA for the M-CSF receptor (Gliniak and Rohrschneider, 1990), although this would not explain why a response at least equal in magnitude to what could be induced by GM-CSF (or Multi-CSF) alone failed to occur.

### *Stimulation of stem cell proliferation*

When purified stem cells became available from FACS sorting for analysis in vitro, such cells failed to proliferate in semisolid cultures when stimulated by individual CSFs (Li and Johnson, 1992). This observation could

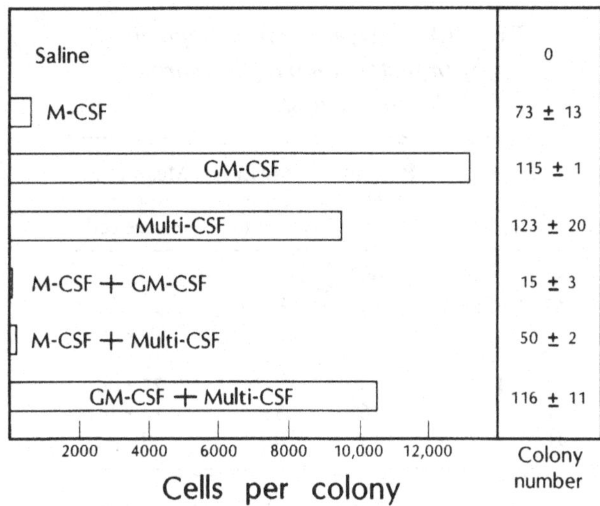


Figure 7.12. Colony formation by FDC-P1 cells expressing inserted M-CSF receptors. When acting alone, M-CSF, GM-CSF, and Multi-CSF all stimulate colony formation. However, the combination of GM-CSF or Multi-CSF with M-CSF results in a marked suppression of colony formation. (Reproduced with permission from Metcalf et al., 1992b.)

have indicated either that the cells could not survive in agar cultures of this type or that CSFs had no proliferative action on stem cells.

Subsequent observations with SCF (Zsebo et al., 1990; Williams et al., 1990a) and then with IL-11 (Musashi et al., 1991) and IL-12 (Jacobsen et al., 1993) have required a revision of both of these conclusions. Purified stem cells can proliferate with high cloning efficiency (up to 100%) in agar cultures, but adequate cell proliferation in either agar or liquid cultures is wholly dependent on the use of combinations of growth factors (Migliaccio et al., 1991; Li and Johnson, 1992; Meunch et al., 1992; Miura et al., 1993). In combinations including SCF, the SCF seems to ensure cell survival, but *proliferation* depends on the combination of SCF with other factors that include IL-1, IL-6, IL-11, IL-12, and the four CSFs. None of these combinations can stimulate self-generation by the stem cells, but the amplified proliferation resulting from the use of combinations of growth factors can be documented either in suspension culture by monitoring the total number of cells or total number of progeny progenitor cells, or in clonal cultures by measuring any increased size of the resulting blast colonies.

Table 7.1. *Receptors for hemopoietic growth factors on purified murine hemopoietic stem cells*

| Factor | Percent labeled cells | Mean grain count | Mean grain count reference cells |
|---|---|---|---|
| SCF | 100 | — | 130 |
| Multi-CSF | 56 | 8±6 | 26±20 |
| G-CSF | 60 | 26±21 | 120±30 |
| GM-CSF | 0 | — | 36±9 |
| M-CSF | 0 | — | 27±20 |
| IL-1 | 56 | 5±2 | 14±10 |
| IL-6 | 13 | 10±2 | 59±32 |

*Note:* Analysis performed on FACS-fractionated stem cells using $^{125}$I-labeled growth factors and autoradiography. Grain counts reflect the number of receptors on individual cells but must be multiplied by 10–15 to give actual receptor numbers. Reference cells analyzed in parallel were murine bone marrow granulocytes and/or monocytes.
*Source:* W. J. McKinstry, G. R. Johnson, C. L. Li, and D. Metcalf (unpublished data).

Purified stem cells that can repopulate irradiated recipients express the c-*kit* product, which is the receptor for SCF (*kit*-ligand, Steel factor). This membrane marker is used in the final purification of murine stem cells, and receptors for SCF are therefore present on all stem cells. Analysis of the expression on murine stem cells of receptors for other hemopoietic regulators indicates that a proportion of stem cells express receptors for IL-6, IL-1, and G-CSF, although the number of receptors is relatively small (Table 7.1). These cells do not express receptors for GM-CSF or M-CSF, and the capacity of these factors to co-stimulate stem cell proliferation requires these cells to commence expression of these receptors at some stage in the culture.

Indeed, the initiation of stem cell proliferation occurs after a distinct delay, which, in part, may be based on the initial low-level expression of receptors for many growth factors on these cells. The delay in onset of proliferation may represent the time required for an agent like SCF to increase the level of expression of receptors for these other growth factors, which are necessary to stimulate cell division.

Essentially similar results have been obtained with cultures of enriched populations of human $CD34^+$ cells, which contain cells equivalent to murine stem cells. Proliferation depends on co-stimulation by a combination of factors, and the more factors included, the greater the cell proliferation (McNiece et al., 1991; Smith et al., 1993). Extremely high levels of proliferation are probably achieved at the expense of the population of stem cells, since these become progressively expended in forming maturing progeny.

In combination with SCF or IL-12, Multi-CSF appears to have stronger actions in stimulating cell production by stem cells than the other CSFs, but all four CSFs clearly enhance cell production. Unlike the stimulating action of CSF combinations on progenitor cells, the enhancing actions of growth factor combinations on stem cells greatly increase cell production (Metcalf and Nicola, 1991).

In early experiments, a striking enhancement of colony formation, resulting in the formation of macroscopic colonies, was noted when IL-1 and M-CSF were used to co-stimulate immature marrow precursors surviving 5-fluorouracil pretreatment (Bradley et al., 1980; Jubinsky and Stanley, 1985). Although, when fully developed, such colonies were composed exclusively of macrophages, the formation of comparable giant colonies can also be achieved with combinations including GM-CSF or Multi-CSF, in which case the developing colonies also contain cells of other lineages (Stanley et al., 1986; Lorimore et al., 1990). HPPC forming giant colonies in vitro are likely to be stem cells; hence, combinations of factors are required for proliferative stimulation.

While SCF in combination with other factors has a major effect in enhancing progenitor cell formation by stem cells with a resulting major increase in mature cell production, it was not initially regarded as having the capacity to stimulate colony formation when acting alone. However, analysis has shown that at relatively high concentrations (25–200 ng/ml), SCF can stimulate by direct action the formation by murine cells of mainly two types of small colonies – composed entirely of either blast cells or typical granulocytic cells (Metcalf and Nicola, 1991) (Table 7.2). The cells generating the blast colonies are probably a mixture of stem cells and the least-mature progenitor cells, and from 50 to 100% of the cells in such colonies are committed progenitor cells. When G-CSF, GM-CSF, or Multi-CSF (but not M-CSF) is combined with SCF in cultures of mouse bone marrow cells, the size of these blast colonies can be amplified 10- to 30-fold (Table 7.3). In contrast, there is relatively little size amplification of the granulocytic colonies formed in the same cultures by committed

Table 7.2. *Stimulation by purified recombinant SCF of colony formation by mouse bone marrow cells*

| Concentration in culture (ng/ml) | Number of colonies | | | |
|---|---|---|---|---|
| | G | GM | M | Blast |
| 100 | 61 | 13 | 7 | 22 |
| 50 | 38 | 3 | 8 | 16 |
| 25 | 33 | 10 | 4 | 14 |
| 12 | 25 | 4 | 4 | 4 |
| 6 | 10 | 7 | 6 | 2 |
| 3 | 1 | 1 | 0 | 0 |

*Note:* Cultures contained 50,000 (C57BL × SJL)$F_1$ bone marrow cells and were scored after 7 days of incubation using cultures stained with acetylcholinesterase, Luxol Fast Blue–hematoxylin.
*Source:* D. Metcalf (unpublished data).

Table 7.3. *Mean cell content of colonies and blast colonies in cultures of mouse bone marrow cells stimulated by SCF with or without added CSF*

| Stimulus | Mean cell count | |
|---|---|---|
| | Blast colonies | All colonies |
| SCF | 250 | 190 |
| SCF + G-CSF | 3,130 | 1,720 |
| SCF + GM-CSF | 5,650 | 3,430 |
| SCF + Multi-CSF | 6,500 | 5,060 |

*Note:* Cultures were prepared containing 75,000 C57BL bone marrow cells and stimulated by 100 ng/ml SCF with or without 10 ng/ml CSF. Colonies were analyzed after 7 days of incubation.

progenitor cells. The conclusion is that SCF–CSF interactions have their major effect by amplifying the formation of progenitor cells by stem cells but have a relatively minor effect on the subsequent proliferation of these progenitor cells.

The notable synergistic effect of combining SCF with GM-CSF, G-CSF, or Multi-CSF whereby the number of maturing progeny is greatly increased cannot be viewed simply as a maneuver resulting in an increase in the CSF concentration. The special effect on blast cell colonies has just been noted. However, an equally revealing observation comes from an analysis of colonies stimulated by SCF plus GM-CSF. If the consequence of the synergy was merely to increase the effective concentration of GM-CSF, a major increase in the number of megakaryocytic colonies should have occurred (see the section on GM-CSF). However, no such increase is observed, which implies that the effects of such combinations depend on certain cells, such as stem cells, requiring two simultaneous but qualitatively different signals.

This conclusion could be at odds with the data discussed earlier from an analysis of FDC-P1 cells; those data suggested the existence of a single, final, common mitotic signaling pathway. It may therefore be that for certain cells like stem cells and some progenitor cells, the situation is more complex and that at least two sets of signals are required.

A notable feature of the generation of blast cell colonies by the combined action of SCF with the CSFs and other regulators has been the demonstration that many of the progenitor cells formed cannot be further stimulated to proliferate by the growth factor combination used to generate them (Metcalf, 1993a). For example, as shown in Table 7.4, the combination of SCF plus G-CSF generated an expanded number of progenitor cells, more than half of which could not be further stimulated to proliferate by this combination. The same feature was noted with SCF plus IL-6. This abortive formation of progenitor cells was less evident with the broader-acting GM-CSF and Multi-CSF, where most of the progenitor cells generated responded to stimulation by the factor combination initiating their formation.

These data indicate that with combinations such as SCF plus G-CSF, it becomes necessary to include other regulators if all the progenitor cells formed are then to be stimulated to produce maturing progeny.

These findings suggest that the phenomenon of synergistic interactions between CSFs and other growth factors is not merely a curious laboratory phenomenon; it actually documents a basic aspect of the design of the regulatory control system used in the body, a design in which combinations of growth factors not only enhance but are mandatory for the most effective generation of mature cells. This conclusion is supported by in vivo data in animals and humans, to be discussed later.

Table 7.4. *Inability of the factor combination used to generate blast cell colonies to stimulate the continued proliferation of progenitor cells present in such colonies*

| Stimulus used to generate blast colonies | Number of colonies analyzed | Progenitor cells per colony stimulated using | |
|---|---|---|---|
| | | SCM | Original factor combination |
| SCF + G-CSF | 43 | 522 ± 374 | 91 ± 140 |
| SCF + IL-6 | 46 | 483 ± 414 | 51 ± 87 |
| SCF + Multi-CSF | 41 | 518 ± 450 | 210 ± 240 |
| SCF + GM-CSF | 32 | 337 ± 236 | 393 ± 246 |

*Note:* Primary cultures were initiated using 75,000 C57BL marrow cells and 100 ng SCF plus 10 ng G-CSF, 500 ng IL-6, 10 ng Multi-SCF, or 10 ng GM-CSF. After 7 days of incubation, individual blast colonies were resuspended and recultured in secondary cultures using either 0.1 ml of SCM or 100 ng SCF plus the second stimulus used in the initiation of the primary colonies. Figures represent the calculated mean colony content of progenitor cells ± SD.
*Source:* Metcalf (1993a, Table 4).

## Proliferative actions of specific CSFs

### *GM-CSF*

Although characterized initially as a strong proliferative stimulus for granulocytic and macrophage cells in cultures of mouse bone marrow cells, GM-CSF in fact acts on a broader range of responding cells (Metcalf et al., 1986c) (Table 7.5). At concentrations below 1 ng/ml, the actions of GM-CSF are restricted to macrophage and granulocytic populations, with macrophage progenitors being more responsive than granulocytic progenitors. The macrophage colonies stimulated are characteristically dispersed in morphology, which is due to the direct action of GM-CSF, presumably affecting cell motility in agar (Metcalf and Nicola, 1992). Above 2 ng/ml, GM-CSF becomes an effective proliferative stimulus for eosinophil progenitors and, above 16 ng/ml, for megakaryocytic precursors. At these high concentrations, GM-CSF can also stimulate some colony formation by less mature erythroid and multipotential precursors (Metcalf et al., 1986c) (Table 7.6). When combined with erythropoietin, this action on erythroid precursors becomes more prominent and is confined to the

Table 7.5. *Colony formation by mouse bone marrow cells stimulated by purified native GM-CSF*

| GM-CSF concentration (ng/ml) | Mean number of colonies per culture | Percentage of colonies | | | |
|---|---|---|---|---|---|
| | | G | GM | M | Eo |
| 32 | 136 | 32 | 33 | 30 | 5 |
| 16 | 140 | 32 | 37 | 29 | 2 |
| 8 | 138 | 32 | 24 | 36 | 8 |
| 4 | 124 | 40 | 23 | 34 | 3 |
| 2 | 115 | 14 | 27 | 58 | 1 |
| 1 | 91 | 19 | 14 | 67 | 0 |
| 0.5 | 77 | 21 | 21 | 58 | 0 |
| 0.25 | 54 | 12 | 21 | 67 | 0 |
| 0.125 | 48 | 13 | 13 | 74 | 0 |
| 0.06 | 20 | 12 | 7 | 81 | 0 |

*Note:* Replicate cultures contained 75,000 C57BL marrow cells and 0.1 ml of serial twofold dilutions of purified native GM-CSF. Colonies scored on day 7. Cultures were fixed and then stained with Luxol Fast Blue-hematoxylin and differential colony counts performed. Colony counts are means of duplicate cultures. G denotes granulocyte; GM, granulocyte-macrophage; M, macrophage; Eo, eosinophil.
*Source:* Metcalf et al. (1986c, Table 1).

immature BFU-E precursors (Metcalf and Johnson, 1979; Metcalf et al., 1980).

Similar findings have been made with human GM-CSF acting on human marrow cells. GM-CSF stimulates the development of a maximal number of granulocytic and macrophage colonies at a concentration of 1–4 ng/ml, is an effective proliferative stimulus for eosinophil precursors (Metcalf et al., 1986b), and can have at least some proliferative effects on megakaryocytic precursors (Mazur et al., 1987) as well as multipotential and erythroid precursors (Bot et al., 1989). For a satisfactory stimulation of the growth of BFU-E, GM-CSF must be combined with erythropoietin (Migliaccio et al., 1987). It is characteristic in human cultures stimulated by GM-CSF that eosinophil colonies are slower to develop than are granulocytic or macrophage colonies and become obvious only in the second week of incubation. The actions of human GM-CSF on these populations have been documented to be direct effects on the responding cells (Metcalf et al., 1986b).

GM-CSF can also strongly stimulate progenitor cell formation by murine stem cells when acting in association with SCF and biases the formation

Table 7.6. *Stimulation of megakaryocytic and mixed erythroid colony formation in mouse bone marrow cultures by high concentrations of recombinant GM-CSF*

| GM-CSF concentration in culture (ng/ml) | Mean number of colonies | | |
|---|---|---|---|
| | Megakaryocyte | Pure erythroid | Mixed erythroid |
| 4,096 | 14 | 0 | 3 ± 1 |
| 2,048 | 15 | 1 ± 1 | 4 ± 3 |
| 1,024 | 10 | 0 | 1 ± 1 |
| 512 | 8 | 1 ± 1 | 4 ± 3 |
| 256 | 8 | 0 | 3 ± 1 |
| 128 | 6 | 1 ± 1 | 3 ± 3 |
| 64 | 5 | 0 | 3 ± 2 |
| 32 | 4 | 0 | 2 ± 1 |
| 16 | 2 | 0 | 0 |
| 8 | 1 | 0 | 0 |
| 4 | 1 | 0 | 0 |
| 2 | 0 | 0 | 0 |
| 1 | 0 | 0 | 0 |

*Note:* Cultures contained 75,000 C57BL bone marrow cells in agar for megakaryocytic colony formation and methylcellulose for erythroid colony formation. CSF concentrations shown are the final concentrations in the culture dish and were calculated in units on the basis of prior assays on granulocyte-macrophage colony formation by bone marrow cells. Mean colony counts from duplicate cultures for megakaryocytic colonies and mean colony counts ± SD of four replicate cultures for erythroid colonies.
*Source:* Metcalf (1986c, Table 2).

of progenitor cells slightly in the direction of granulocytic progenitor cell formation (Metcalf, 1991b).

GM-CSF has strong but anomalous interactions with M-CSF. With murine cells, this combination strongly potentiates the proliferation of some granulocytic and macrophage progenitor cells but at the same time inhibits the proliferation of some macrophage progenitor cells (Metcalf and Nicola, 1992). With human cells, very low concentrations of GM-CSF exert a powerful synergistic action on M-CSF, allowing it to become an effective colony-forming stimulus (Caracciolo et al., 1987).

GM-CSF has been reported to be an exclusive proliferative stimulus for dendritic cell formation from marrow precursors (Inaba et al., 1992b).

Such dendritic cells appear as a subset of cells within developing macrophage and granulocyte-macrophage colonies, which were, presumably, merely characterized as macrophage or granulocyte-macrophage in composition previously. GM-CSF is reported to be the only one of the four CSFs with this action, but whether it also has actions on the formation of dendritic cells in other locations is not yet known.

There have been reports that GM-CSF has the capacity to stimulate the proliferation of some nonhemopoietic cells. GM-CSF has been reported to increase placental size and reduce the frequency of spontaneous abortions in certain mice (Clark et al., 1994), as well as to stimulate the proliferation of placenta-derived cells (Athanassakis et al., 1987). High-affinity receptors for GM-CSF have been described on rat oligodendrocytes, and GM-CSF was observed to stimulate the proliferation of these cells (Baldwin et al., 1993). This is part of an expanding body of evidence suggesting functional cross-reactions between the regulators controlling hemopoiesis and those controlling cells of neural crest origin (Giulian and Ingeman, 1988; Balkwill and Burke, 1989; Suzumura et al., 1990). GM-CSF has also been reported to stimulate endothelial cell proliferation (Bussolino et al., 1989) and, at high concentrations, the proliferation of some nonhemopoietic tumors, particularly those of neural crest origin, such as small-cell lung cancers and melanomas that express receptors for GM-CSF (Dedhar et al., 1988; Baldwin et al., 1989; Berdel et al., 1990). At more physiological concentrations, no actions of GM-CSF have been noted on such tumor cells in cloning or metabolic assays (Salmon and Lui, 1989; Foulke et al., 1990; Twentyman and Wright, 1991).

## *G-CSF*

In cultures of mouse bone marrow, G-CSF predominantly stimulates the formation of a relatively small number of small, well-differentiated granulocytic colonies (Metcalf and Nicola, 1983) (Table 7.7). This pattern of colony formation is characteristically different from that stimulated by the other CSFs. The nature of such colonies might suggest that G-CSF is a highly selective stimulus for neutrophilic-granulocytic cells. Furthermore, because the number of G-CSF-stimulated colonies is smaller than those stimulated by GM-CSF or Multi-CSF, as well as the fact that such colonies are typically smaller and more mature than the latter colonies, this might suggest that G-CSF is a proliferative stimulus for only a subset of granulocytic progenitor cells at a relatively late stage in differentiation. The restriction of G-CSF receptors to cells of the granulocytic lineage is

Table 7.7. *Colony formation by mouse bone marrow cells after stimulation by purified recombinant G-CSF*

| Concentration in culture (ng/ml) | Total colonies | Colonies G | GM | M | Eo |
|---|---|---|---|---|---|
| 10 | 21 | 18 | 1 | 2 | 0 |
| 5 | 22 | 18 | 2 | 2 | 0 |
| 2.5 | 19 | 17 | 0 | 2 | 0 |
| 1.25 | 16 | 15 | 1 | 0 | 0 |
| 0.6 | 11 | 11 | 0 | 0 | 0 |
| 0.3 | 10 | 9 | 1 | 0 | 0 |
| 0.125 | 6 | 6 | 0 | 0 | 0 |
| 0.08 | 4 | 4 | 0 | 0 | 0 |
| 0.04 | 2 | 2 | 0 | 0 | 0 |
| 0.02 | 1 | 1 | 0 | 0 | 0 |

*Note:* Cultures of 25,000 mouse bone marrow cells were incubated for 7 days before analysis. G-CSF used was purified nonglycosylated recombinant human G-CSF. G denotes granulocyte; GM, granulocyte-macrophage; M, macrophage; Eo, eosinophil.
*Source:* D. Metcalf (unpublished data).

in accord with this interpretation, with the puzzling exception that receptors are also present on some murine monocytes (Nicola and Metcalf, 1985b).

These general conclusions are supported by the behavior of G-CSF in cultures of human marrow cells. Again, the dominant form of colony stimulated is composed of granulocytes (Nicola et al., 1979b; Strife et al., 1987; Kannourakis and Johnson, 1990). Cell separation studies have suggested that the human progenitor cells responding to G-CSF may be more mature than those responding to other CSFs. This conclusion is supported by the observations that the colonies are relatively small and their number becomes maximal after 7 days of incubation, after which they tend to disappear by cell dispersion and death more rapidly than do colonies stimulated by other types of CSF (Begley et al., 1985).

However, the actions of G-CSF are broader than apparent from scoring semisolid cultures of marrow cells after a conventional 7-day period of incubation. Although the dominant colony type in cultures of both species is granulocytic, a smaller number of granulocyte-macrophage and macrophage colonies are also stimulated to develop by G-CSF. The significance of such colonies is uncertain because, in serum-free cultures of mouse cells, G-CSF has been reported to stimulate granulocytic colony formation almost exclusively (Eliason, 1986).

More convincing evidence of the broader action of G-CSF has come from an analysis of early events in clonal cultures. In cultures of mouse marrow or fetal liver, G-CSF can *initiate* the proliferation of a relatively large number of progenitor cells in both the granulocytic and macrophage lineages but cannot sustain the proliferation of most of these clones (Metcalf and Nicola, 1983). When G-CSF is used to stimulate crowded cultures enriched for stem cells, but possibly also containing cells capable of the endogenous production of other factors, blast colonies form that contain progenitor cells that can then respond to G-CSF alone (Suda et al., 1987). The combination of G-CSF with SCF in cultures of murine marrow cells can clearly enhance the generation of cells by stem cells, causing a major 7- to 10-fold increase in the number of cells in blast colonies formed by such cells (Metcalf and Nicola, 1991). In line with the observations on early clone formation stimulated by G-CSF alone, a large proportion of these blast colony cells were committed macrophage progenitors (Metcalf, 1991b), which, however, could not be stimulated by SCF plus G-CSF to proliferate further, as was the case with many of the committed granulocytic progenitors (Metcalf, 1993a). With human cells enriched for $CD34^+$ cells, co-stimulation by SCF and G-CSF also strongly enhanced progenitor cell formation (Migliaccio et al., 1992b).

Thus, particularly when acting on stem cells in concert with other regulators, G-CSF has a broader range of actions in generating progenitor cells of various types than implied by its fairly selective ultimate actions on mature granulocyte-committed progenitor cells.

There is little evidence of proliferative actions of G-CSF on nonhemopoietic cells, but one group has claimed a proliferative action of G-CSF on endothelial cells or cell lines (Bussolino et al., 1989; Bocchietto et al., 1993).

## *M-CSF*

In agar cultures of mouse marrow or fetal liver cells, or in agarose cultures of human marrow cells, M-CSF stimulates the predominant formation of macrophage colonies. The cells in such colonies are often tightly clumped, a direct action of M-CSF on the behavior of macrophages in such colonies (Metcalf and Nicola, 1992). Curiously, human M-CSF is almost inactive as a CSF in agar cultures of human marrow cells, although

Table 7.8. *Colony formation by mouse bone marrow cells after stimulation by purified recombinant M-CSF*

| Concentration in culture (ng/ml) | Total colonies | Colonies G | GM | M | Eo |
|---|---|---|---|---|---|
| 10 | 63 | 4 | 7 | 52 | 0 |
| 5 | 59 | 3 | 7 | 49 | 0 |
| 2.5 | 63 | 6 | 10 | 49 | 0 |
| 1.25 | 72 | 1 | 6 | 65 | 0 |
| 0.6 | 36 | 4 | 2 | 30 | 0 |
| 0.3 | 28 | 2 | 0 | 26 | 0 |
| 0.15 | 9 | 1 | 1 | 7 | 0 |
| 0.08 | 4 | 0 | 0 | 4 | 0 |

*Note:* Cultures of 25,000 mouse bone marrow cells were incubated for 7 days before analysis. M-CSF used was purified recombinant murine M-CSF produced in a yeast expression system. G denotes granulocyte; GM, granulocyte-macrophage; M, macrophage; Eo, eosinophil.
*Source:* D. Metcalf (unpublished data).

it does demonstrate activity in agarose cultures (Broxmeyer et al., 1990). The basis for this phenomenon is not understood, but the addition of low concentrations of GM-CSF to agar cultures allows the M-CSF to function effectively as a stimulus for human cells (Caracciolo et al., 1987).

M-CSF-stimulated colony formation is not exclusively of a macrophage type, and in cultures of both species, a smaller number of granulocyte-macrophage and granulocytic colonies also develops (Table 7.8). In view of the cross-lineage actions of other CSFs, it is unclear why there has been resistance to the conclusion that M-CSF also has a limited capacity to stimulate granulocytic colony formation. One possibility raised was that M-CSF might induce the formation of G-CSF or GM-CSF in the culture dish. However, M-CSF also stimulates some granulocytic colony formation in marrow cultures from mice with homozygous inactivation of either the G-CSF or GM-CSF gene, so this explanation seems improbable. It has also been suggested that the apparent action of M-CSF in stimulating granulocytic colony formation may be due to the presence of G-CSF or IL-6 in the serum used in the cultures, the more so since the combination of even a low concentration of M-CSF with G-CSF strongly enhances granulocytic colony formation. However, M-CSF can stimulate equivalent granulocytic colony formation in serum-free marrow cultures (Eliason, 1986). Furthermore, there are receptors for M-CSF on murine granulocytic cells, so a direct proliferative action is possible. In addition, at least some progenitor cells precommitted by GM-CSF to the granulocytic lineage can continue to proliferate and generate large granulocytic colonies when clones initiated by GM-CSF are transferred to cultures containing M-CSF (Metcalf and Burgess, 1982).

Although one study failed to demonstrate enhancement by M-CSF of SCF-stimulated blast colony formation (Metcalf and Nicola, 1991), other experiments indicate that M-CSF can co-stimulate the proliferation of early precursor cells when acting with SCF, IL-1, and other factors. This is the likely basis for the original description of at least some of the high-proliferative-potential colony formation stimulated by IL-1 plus M-CSF (Bradley et al., 1980).

From in vivo studies on osteopetrotic mice, lacking a capacity to produce M-CSF, it is evident that M-CSF is necessary for the formation of osteoclasts by a subset of macrophage precursors (Wiktor-Jedrzejczak et al., 1991). In in vitro studies, M-CSF was shown to be necessary for both the proliferation of osteoclast precursors and their subsequent maturation (Tanaka et al., 1993). M-CSF may not be an exclusive stimulus for osteoclast formation, since a different osteoclast CSF has been reported (Lee et al., 1991). It is not yet clear whether both agents act on the same population of precursors or whether distinct subsets of such precursor cells exist.

It has become evident that M-CSF most likely plays an important role in the biology of placental tissue. Trophoblast cells are stimulated to proliferate by M-CSF (Athanassakis et al., 1987). M-CSF receptor levels are high on trophoblast cells, and large amounts of M-CSF mRNA are produced in adjacent uterine cells (Arceci et al., 1989). This rise in the uterine production of CSF is hormonally controlled (Pollard et al., 1987), and unlike the stiuation with the other CSFs, plasma M-CSF levels are elevated in mice during pregnancy (Bartocci et al., 1986). The proliferative actions of M-CSF on trophoblast cells are therefore not likely to be an incidental action of this regulator but to represent a major nonhemopoietic aspect of the biology of M-CSF.

M-CSF receptors have been described on a variety of nonhemopoietic tumor cells, with some evidence that M-CSF might enhance the invasiveness of such cells (Filderman et al., 1992), but it is unclear whether M-CSF has any proliferative action on such cells, although this remains a possibility (Malik and Balkwill, 1991). When M-CSF receptors are inserted into fibroblasts, M-CSF can then stimulate the proliferation of such cells (Roussel and Sherr, 1989), but data of this type merely indicate the permissiveness of cellular signaling pathways rather than document a physiological action of M-CSF on fibroblasts.

## *Multi-CSF (IL-3)*

Multi-CSF stimulates the proliferation of an extremely broad range of hemopoietic cells. In agar cultures of adult mouse marrow cells, Multi-CSF stimulates the formation of macrophage, granulocytic, eosinophil, megakaryocytic, multipotential, and blast colonies (Table 7.9), and in cultures of mouse fetal liver cells, it is a strong stimulus for BFU-E-derived erythroid colony formation (Metcalf et al., 1987a). In cultures of human cells, Multi-CSF stimulates the formation of granulocytic, macrophage, and eosinophil colonies and, when combined with erythropoietin, is a powerful stimulus for erythroid colony formation by the early erythroid BFU-E precursors (Kannourakis and Johnson, 1990). Multi-CSF has little or no proliferative action on mature erythroid precursors (CFU-E) (Sawada et al., 1991). With megakaryocytic precursors, Multi-CSF can stimulate the proliferation of all types, from the least-mature cells forming mixed megakaryocytic colonies containing cells of other lineages to the mature precursors forming only a small number of mature megakaryocytes. When combined with IL-6, SCF, IL-11, or LIF, Multi-CSF can stimulate the formation of an increased number of megakaryocytic colonies of all sizes (D. Metcalf, unpublished data). This suggests that some megakaryocytic precursors may require co-stimulation by two or more factors. In suspension cultures of marrow cells or cultures of mast cell lines, Multi-CSF also has a strong capacity to stimulate mast cell proliferation (Clark-Lewis and Schrader, 1988; Moore, 1988).

The cells most highly responsive to Multi-CSF are mast cells and a type of progenitor cell in mouse marrow that forms characteristic, uniformly dispersed colonies possibly composed of natural cytotoxic cells (Claesson et al., 1982; Metcalf et al., 1987a). The responsiveness of other types of progenitor cells in general follows the pattern of responsiveness to GM-CSF higher concentrations being required to stimulate erythroid and megakaryocytic colony formation (Metcalf et al., 1987a).

A variety of evidence, based either on the frequency of responding clonogenic cells or on the size of the colonies generated, indicates that Multi-CSF has the strongest actions of the four CSFs in stimulating early hemopoietic precursor cells. When acting alone, it stimulates the formation of the largest number of blast colonies, multipotential colonies, and

Table 7.9. *Colony-stimulating activity of purified native Multi-CSF in agar cultures of C57BL mouse bone marrow cells*

| Concentration in culture (ng/ml) | Total colonies | Absolute number of colonies | | | | | | | |
|---|---|---|---|---|---|---|---|---|---|
| | | G | GM | M | Eo | Meg | Mix | Blast | Disp |
| 256 | 180 | 45 | 54 | 24 | 4 | 26 | 24 | 2 | 1 |
| 128 | 185 | 40 | 52 | 31 | 15 | 23 | 15 | 4 | 5 |
| 64 | 178 | 35 | 61 | 34 | 12 | 22 | 10 | 2 | 2 |
| 32 | 171 | 23 | 71 | 32 | 6 | 24 | 12 | 0 | 3 |
| 16 | 143 | 27 | 48 | 42 | 4 | 11 | 6 | 3 | 2 |
| 8 | 180 | 26 | 64 | 54 | 8 | 18 | 6 | 0 | 4 |
| 4 | 138 | 28 | 46 | 36 | 5 | 14 | 5 | 0 | 4 |
| 2 | 146 | 23 | 43 | 43 | 17 | 14 | 2 | 0 | 4 |
| 1 | 99 | 17 | 33 | 35 | 1 | 10 | 0 | 0 | 3 |
| 0.5 | 76 | 12 | 24 | 27 | 1 | 4 | 1 | 0 | 7 |
| 0.25 | 51 | 8 | 19 | 15 | 0 | 4 | 1 | 0 | 4 |
| 0.125 | 17 | 3 | 6 | 2 | 0 | 3 | 0 | 0 | 3 |
| 0.06 | 4 | 0 | 1 | 0 | 0 | 0 | 0 | 0 | 3 |
| 0.03 | 3 | 0 | 0 | 0 | 0 | 0 | 0 | 0 | 3 |

*Note:* A total of 75,000 C57BL bone marrow cells were cultured in agar medium for 7 days. Mean colony counts are from duplicate cultures. Colonies were typed from cultures stained with acetylcholinesterase/Luxol Fast Blue–hematoxylin. G denotes granulocyte; GM, granulocyte-macrophage; M, macrophage; Eo, eosinophil; Meg, megakaryocyte; Mix, mixed lineage with or without erythroid cells; Blast, blast cell; Disp, dispersed cell colonies.
*Source:* Metcalf et al. (1987a, Table 2).

immature megakaryocytic colonies and, in combination with erythropoietin, the largest number of burst erythroid colonies. Similarly, its presence in regulator combinations is essential for obtaining good proliferative responses by stem cells.

This feature of the proliferative action of Multi-CSF has led some researchers to conclude that it is an early-acting regulator that must be combined with late-acting CSFs to produce fully mature progeny. This view is mistaken, since Multi-CSF, acting alone, is quite capable of stimulating the formation of fully mature granulocytic, macrophage, or megakaryocytic colonies. The data do indicate, however, that Multi-CSF has an exceptional skewing of its proliferative actions, being clearly superior to the other CSFs in its actions on early cells in these lineages.

When acting on stem cells in association with SCF, IL-11 or IL-12, Multi-CSF strongly enhances blast cell proliferation with the formation of progenitor cells (de Vries et al., 1991; Metcalf, 1991b; Musashi et al., 1991; Ploemacher et al., 1993). Analysis of murine blast cell colonies has shown that Multi-CSF in combination with SCF increases the relative frequency of granulocytic progenitors formed and has the largest capacity of all four CSFs to induce the formation of eosinophil progenitors (Metcalf and Nicola, 1992; Metcalf, 1993a).

A curious feature of the action of Multi-CSF on murine bone marrow cells is a very marked difference in responsiveness exhibited by cells from mice of different strains. Thus, cells from NZB, NZC, Rf, and A/J strain mice respond very poorly to proliferative stimulation by Multi-CSF (Kincade et al., 1979; Moore, 1988; Hapel et al., 1992) while responding normally to other CSFs. The molecular basis for this anomalous behavior has not been established, but comparable genetic-based refractoriness has not been noted with the other CSFs.

Multi-CSF has been reported to stimulate the formation of at least some types of B-lymphocytes (Palacios et al., 1984; Kinashi et al., 1988; Clayberger et al., 1992) and of pre-T-cells, particularly when in combination with SCF (Chervanak et al., 1992). Proliferative actions on nonhemopoietic cells have not been noted.

## *Discussion*

The patterns of colony formation stimulated by the four CSFs in cultures of murine marrow cells can readily be distinguished from one another by simple inspection of the cultures (Figure 7.13). GM-CSF and Multi-CSF stimulate cultures containing a dominant population of approximately equal numbers of granulocytic, granulocyte-macrophage, and macrophage colonies, but Multi-CSF also stimulates the formation of characteristically loosely dispersed colonies possibly composed of natural cytotoxic cells. M-CSF stimulates the formation of a dominant population of macrophage colonies and G-CSF the formation of a notably smaller number of colonies of small size and almost exclusive granulocytic composition. All colony formation is stimulated over an apparently similar concentration range.

This familiar pattern of colony formation underestimates the true range of activities of each CSF, which also includes strong actions on stem cell proliferation with the formation of new progenitor cells. In no case is the action of the CSFs on progenitor cells exclusive to one lineage, and thus the CSFs form an overlapping series of regulators, each with dominant actions on granulocyte-macrophage populations (Figure 7.13). GM-CSF and Multi-CSF also have strong actions on eosinophil, megakaryocytic, and erythroid populations, while Multi-CSF is the only CSF with actions on mast cells and B-lymphocytes.

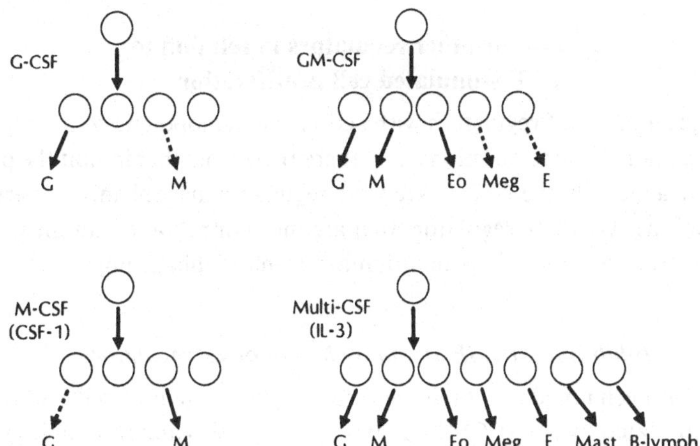


Figure 7.13. Diagram summarizing the actions of the four CSFs on murine progenitor cells and their formation by stem cells. Solid arrows indicate strong actions, and dashed arrows indicate either weak actions or those requiring high CSF concentrations. G denotes granulocytes; M, macrophages; Eo, eosinophils; Meg, megakaryocytes; E, erythroid cells; B-lymph, B-lymphocytes.

Based on the number and cellular content of colonies developing in clonal mouse marrow cultures, GM-CSF and Multi-CSF appear to be by far the strongest stimuli for granulocytic cell formation. For example, GM-CSF- or Multi-CSF-stimulated granulocytic colonies contain up to 5,000 cells, whereas G-CSF-stimulated colonies typically contain only 200–400 cells at most. On this basis, G-CSF would be predicted to be a relatively weak stimulus for granulocytic formation in vivo. Similarly, M-CSF would be assessed to be a stronger stimulus for macrophage formation than either GM-CSF or Multi-CSF.

From this discussion of the proliferative actions of the CSFs in vitro, two general points should be reiterated: (a) Progenitor cells are a transit population, and the proliferative actions of any one CSF would deplete this pool unless new progenitor cells were generated from stem cells. This new cell formation is in fact accomplished by CSF stimulation but requires the collaboration of other factors. (b) Synergistic interactions are readily demonstrable in vitro between the CSFs, on the one hand, and between the CSFs and other regulators, on the other. As a consequence of both phenomena, when a single CSF is injected in vivo and elicits a proliferative response, that response will almost certainly involve significant interactions with other growth factors in the body.

## Actions of other regulators in relation to CSF-stimulated cell proliferation

The large number of regulators with actions on hemopoietic cells requires consideration of three questions: Are there regulators that inhibit the proliferative actions of the CSFs? Are there regulators that enhance or permit CSF action? Are there regulators that are more important than the CSFs in their proliferative actions on granulocyte-macrophage populations?

### *Inhibition of CSF action by hemopoietic regulators*

TGF$\beta$ has been noted to inhibit megakaryocytic progenitor cell proliferation stimulated by Multi-CSF (Ishibashi et al., 1987) and to inhibit granulocyte-macrophage colony formation stimulated by GM-CSF, M-CSF, or Multi-CSF (Ohta et al., 1987). However, under different culture conditions, TGF$\beta$ can enhance GM-CSF action (Keller et al., 1991). In a study of TGF$\beta$ action on FDC-P1 cells expressing receptors for M-CSF, the action of M-CSF was strongly inhibited, but not that of GM-CSF. Although TGF$\beta$ increased transcription of mRNA for the M-CSF receptor, it blocked the induction by M-CSF of c-*myc* but had no action on the induction of c-*myc* by GM-CSF (Chen and Rohrschneider, 1993). The inhibitory actions of TGF$\beta$ on GM-CSF-stimulated colony formation were significantly blocked by basic fibroblast growth factor (Gabrilove et al., 1993).

IL-4 also has a curious effect of enhancing granulocytic or macrophage colony formation stimulated, respectively, by G-CSF or M-CSF but of inhibiting granulocyte-macrophage colony formation stimulated by Multi-CSF (Rennick et al., 1987b). Similarly, IL-4 inhibited the generation of progenitor cells by IL-3 but enhanced IL-3-stimulated mast cell formation.

The CSFs themselves have been observed to have some inhibitory actions. As noted already, the combination of GM-CSF and M-CSF can suppress some types of macrophage colony formation. Similarly, G-CSF has a weak but reproducible capacity to suppress megakaryocytic colony formation stimulated by IL-6 (D. Metcalf, unpublished data).

### *Enhancement of CSF actions*

There are numerous regulators that enhance CSF action. The most extensively described is SCF, which, as already noted, strongly enhances the actions of CSFs on stem and early progenitor cells. In the same general category are IL-11 and IL-12, which strongly enhances the actions of certain

CSFs (Musashi et al., 1991; Jacobsen et al., 1993). IL-4 enhances the actions of G-CSF and M-CSF and some of the actions of Multi-CSF. Similarly, IL-6 enhances megakaryocytic colony formation stimulated by Multi-CSF, as do IL-11 and LIF.

Although the mechanisms responsible are still uncharacterized, it should be pointed out that colony crowding can strongly enhance CSF-stimulated colony formation. This phenomenon was observed in early studies on the CSFs (Metcalf, 1968) and is a consistent, though rarely commented upon, phenomenon in cultures stimulated by purified CSFs. Cells of multiple differentiation lineages are involved in the crowding enhancement phenomenon, which suggests that the mechanisms involved may be nonspecific or trivial, even though the magnitude of the enhancement is far from trivial. Possibilities range from CSF-induced colony cell production of important co-factors or regulators to the production by such cells of useful metabolites for cell growth or even to alterations in pH or the removal of potentially inhibitory products from the medium. The phenomenon warrants further investigation, even though it may potentially be no more than an in vitro artifact.

Curiously, certain regulator combinations might be expected to be mutually enhancing but little evidence of enhancement has been observed in studies in this laboratory. Thus, IL-6 can stimulate granulocytic colony formation by mouse bone marrow cells which superficially resembles that stimulated by G-CSF. However, combination of IL-6 with G-CSF produces no enhancement of colony size and only a minor increase in colony number. A similar lack of enhancement has been noted with eosinophil colony formation when IL-5 is combined with GM-CSF.

Megakaryocytic colony formation by murine cells is stimulated rather weakly by either SCF or IL-6 alone. The combination of both factors does not strongly enhance megakaryocytic colony formation, and the presence of Multi-CSF appears to be mandatory for major enhancement to be observed with either SCF or IL-6. The failure of the combination of SCF and IL-6 to enhance megakaryocytic colony formation strongly is in sharp contrast to the major enhancement of blast colony size occurring in the same cultures and emphasizes the fact that the outcome of combining regulators is determined mainly by the nature of the responding cell.

### *The existence and relative importance of other factors active in stimulating granulocyte formation*

Apart from documenting a major difference between the growth factor requirements of stem cells versus typical single-lineage progenitor cells, the recent work on stem cell populations has drawn attention to three regulators not initially considered to play much of a role in the regulation of granulocyte-macrophage formation – SCF, IL-6, and IL-11.

The direct colony-stimulating effects of SCF were noted in an earlier section (Table 7.2), and in cultures of murine cells, SCF induces the formation mainly of small blast colonies or colonies of granulocytes.

In the purification studies of Sachs and his colleagues on embryo-conditioned medium, and later on other types of media, active factors were noted that were termed macrophage-granulocyte inducers (MGI), and in retrospect, those grouped as MGI-1 seem likely to have included M-CSF (MGI-1M), G-CSF (MGI-1G), and GM-CSF (MGI-1GM) (see the review by Sachs, 1990). MGI-2 was active in inducing differentiation in the M1 leukemic cell line, but its actions on normal marrow cells were described as mainly differentiation-inducing. Sequencing of MGI-2A revealed it to be IL-6 (Shabo et al., 1988), a factor originally characterized as having actions on B-lymphocytes (Hirano et al., 1986).

It was subsequently shown that IL-6 could stimulate the formation of mature megakaryocytic colonies (Ishibashi et al., 1989b) and, in combination with IL-3, could enhance the proliferation of multipotential precursors (Ikebuchi et al., 1987). Reexamination of the actions of IL-6 in clonal cultures of mouse marrow cells showed that, at high concentrations (20–200 ng/ml), it also stimulated, at least in part by direct action, the formation mainly of small granulocytic colonies resembling those stimulated by G-CSF (Metcalf, 1989) (Figure 7.14, Table 7.10). As noted earlier, IL-6 is also active in combination with other factors in stimulating progenitor cell formation by stem cells. The apparently direct actions of IL-6 in stimulating some granulocytic colony formation remain puzzling since no high-affinity IL-6 receptors have so far been demonstrated by autoradiography on immature or mature granulocytes, and IL-6 might have some capacity to stimulate such cells by forming an IL-6-soluble receptor complex that may then activate the gp 130 chain of the receptor (Taga et al., 1989).

Preliminary studies in this laboratory indicate that, at relatively high concentrations, IL-11 and the flk-2 ligand (Lyman et al., 1993) also have some capacity to stimulate granulocytic colony formation in cultures of mouse bone marrow cells.

Are CSFs the major regulators of granulocyte and macrophage production? This question can be discussed using both in vitro and in vivo data, but here only the in vitro data will be considered.

In clonal cultures of mouse bone marrow cells, only GM-CSF, M-CSF, and Multi-CSF have a well-documented capacity to stimulate macrophage

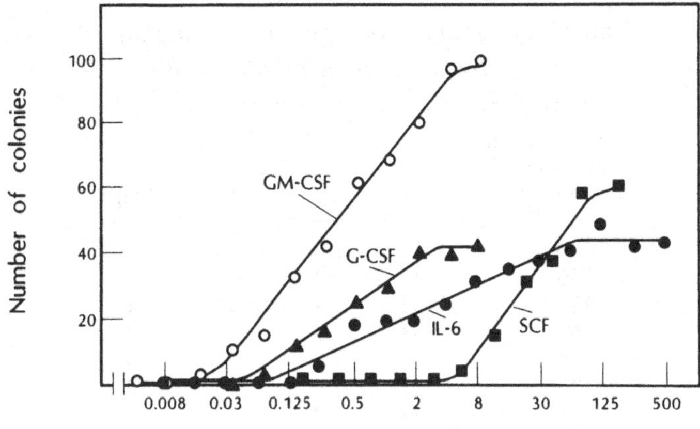


Figure 7.14. Colony formation in 7-day cultures of 50,000 mouse bone marrow cells stimulated by purified recombinant GM-CSF, G-CSF, IL-6, or SCF. Note that stimulation of colony formation by either IL-6 or SCF requires the use of higher concentrations than those for the CSFs.

colony formation. The properties of osteoclast colony–stimulating factor (O-CSF; Lee et al., 1993) are not yet well documented, and from the data available the CSFs would appear to be the major regulators of macrophage formation.

The situation is different for granulocytic colony formation because, with murine cells, at least four other agents, IL-6 (Metcalf, 1989), SCF (Metcalf and Nicola, 1991), IL-11, and the ligand for the flk-2 receptor (D. Metcalf, unpublished data), have some capacity to stimulate granulocytic colony formation by direct action on granulocyte precursors. In principle, therefore, these four agents could play at least some role in controlling granulocyte formation in vivo. However, three features of stimulation by these latter regulators tend to downgrade their possible importance: (a) The number of colonies stimulated by each is relatively low (Figure 7.14); (b) the colonies formed are quite small, unlike the very large colonies that are stimulated by GM-CSF or Multi-CSF; and (c) the concentrations of IL-6, SCF, and IL-11 required to stimulate colony formation are higher than those required for the CSFs, although in the case of SCF it could be argued that soluble SCF is probably less efficient than membrane-displayed SCF.

The in vitro data therefore suggest that, when acting in isolation, IL-6, SCF, and IL-11 are likely to be less effective stimuli of granulocyte

Table 7.10. *Stimulation of colony formation by IL-6 by mouse bone marrow cells*

| Concentration in culture (ng/ml) | Total colonies | | | |
|---|---|---|---|---|
| | G | GM | M | Meg |
| 500 | 34 | 4 | 14 | 3 |
| 250 | 30 | 4 | 9 | 4 |
| 125 | 32 | 8 | 13 | 4 |
| 64 | 33 | 5 | 13 | 0 |
| 32 | 29 | 8 | 7 | 0 |
| 16 | 22 | 9 | 6 | 2 |
| 8 | 18 | 7 | 12 | 0 |
| 4 | — | — | — | — |
| 2 | 5 | 6 | 9 | 0 |
| 1 | 5 | 1 | 5 | 0 |
| 0.5 | 6 | 1 | 10 | 0 |
| 0.25 | 3 | 4 | 3 | 0 |

*Note:* Cultures contained 50,000 (C57BL × SJL)$F_1$ marrow cells and were stimulated by purified recombinant human IL-6. Cultures were scored after 7 days of incubation.
*Source:* D. Metcalf (unpublished data).

proliferation than are the CSFs and are likely to contribute in only a relatively minor way to the stimulation of granulocyte formation in vivo.

However, as has already been discussed, regulators do not exist in vivo in isolation from one another, and interactions of major dimensions might occur. It bears repeating that the combination of SCF with IL-6 is a very strong proliferative stimulus for blast cell and granulocytic colony formation, not greatly different from that of SCF with G-CSF. The final assessment of the relative importance of SCF, IL-6, IL-11, and the flk-2 ligand therefore depends on a reassessment of the situation from in vivo studies.

For cells in other lineages, a final assessment also requires in vivo studies, but the in vitro data do provide some initial information. GM-CSF, Multi-CSF, and IL-5 appear equally efficient in vitro in stimulating eosinophil colony formation, a not particularly unexpected conclusion since each agent acts through receptors containing a common $\beta$-chain from which most mitotic signaling probably originates. Assessment of the relative importance of the known megakaryocyte-stimulating factors is more difficult. As a single agent, Multi-CSF is by far the most active agent in terms of concentration required, the number of colonies developing, and colony size compared with SCF or IL-6. However, combinations of Multi-CSF with SCF, IL-6, or IL-11 stimulate a larger number of colonies than does Multi-CSF alone. The relative importance of these factors and the possible consequences of their interactions again require in vivo assessment, using parameters such as the number of megakaryocytes or platelets. Multi-CSF is the only one of the CSFs with mast cell–stimulating activity, but other mast cell–stimulating regulators are known, such as SCF and IL-9, so similar problems of assessment exist.

A crucial consideration in assessing the likely importance of each of these regulators in vivo is the concentration of each in appropriate locations. Thus, the apparent inefficiency of SCF or IL-6 when assessed in vitro will require reassessment if concentrations of these agents are far higher in vivo than are those of the CSFs. Furthermore, if, as seems likely, Multi-CSF is rarely present in vivo, its importance as a possible regulator in vivo again requires careful assessment.

## Differentiation commitment

Differentiation commitment is defined as the irreversible step occurring in a cell that leads either to restriction of certain existing potentialities or to the acquisition of new capabilities.

In hemopoietic populations there are several situations in which differentiation commitment occurs: (a) in multipotential stem cells, where differentiation commitment reduces or abolishes a preexisting capacity for self-generation and leads to the formation of committed progenitor cell progeny restricted to the formation of a limited number of cell lineages or, more often, a single lineage; (b) in bipotential granulocyte-macrophage progenitor cells, where commitment can determine the future capacity of the cells to form only granulocytic or macrophage progeny; and (c) in immortalized or leukemic cell lines, where differentiation commitment again restricts the capacity for self-renewal divisions and leads the cells to undergo a variety of other fates - death, maturation, or limited proliferative capacity, with or without obvious maturation.

These various examples have several common features. Differentiation commitment appears to be an irreversible process, restricted in occurrence to cells in cell cycle, and, where analyzed, probably occurring mainly at the end of $G_1$ or at the $G_1$–S interface (Metcalf, 1982a; Metcalf and Burgess, 1982; Boyd and Metcalf, 1984; von Melchner and Hoffken, 1985). The process is commonly asymmetrical with one daughter cell exhibiting commitment and the other either no commitment or an alternative type of commitment. In general, commitment results in a reduction in proliferative potential of the cells concerned, either through the loss of self-renewal capacity or because the altered genetic program in the affected cell permits only a reduced capacity for further cell division.

Commitment differs from the subsequent process of maturation induction in its irreversibility and because there is usually no obvious immediate change in the morphology of the affected cell. Despite the usual absence of obvious morphological changes, it is likely that major changes have occurred during commitment that suppress certain transcriptional events and activate others. This can sometimes be detected by changes in the membrane expression of certain proteins and by the expression of receptors for various regulators.

The question of what happens to the expression of membrane receptors for regulators during commitment has long been a subject of controversy. Multipotential cells have been postulated as perhaps expressing receptors for all regulatory factors and commitment as an event associated with restriction of receptor expression to those regulators then relevant to a single hemopoietic lineage. The contrary view is that stem cells express no receptors for lineage-active regulators and that the commitment event itself results in the first expression of receptors for the required regulator. Current data on receptor expression on stem and committed progenitor cells fit neither model, because an intermediate situation has been observed. Thus, stem cells clearly have receptors for some regulators like SCF, G-CSF, and IL-6, but not for others such as erythropoietin, GM-CSF, and M-CSF (Table 7.1). Committed progenitor cells lack certain, now-irrelevant receptors; for example, granulocyte-macrophage progenitors do not have erythropoietin receptors. Thus, there are some examples of receptor loss with differentiation commitment and some examples of receptor gain. Whether a particular regulator can influence differentiation commitment in a cell will obviously be determined by whether or not the cell is currently expressing receptors for that regulator.

To analyze differentiation commitment in hemopoietic cells, it is mandatory to examine the progeny of the cell in question by clonal assays that make it possible to identify the cell populations generated by each of the progeny cells. The use of suspension cultures is usually not suitable for such a purpose, since the progeny of individual cells are mixed together, and there is no way to recognize death or failure to proliferate as the fate of certain committed cells.

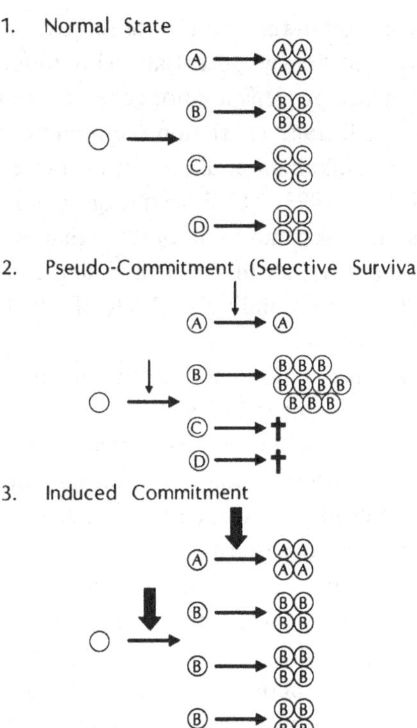


Figure 7.15. Schematic representation of differentiation commitment – for example, in the formation by stem cells of progenitor cells committed to different lineages. An agent may appear to induce selective commitment if particular subsets of progenitor cells die during the experiment. For true commitment to be documented, all the initial progeny must be accounted for.

As shown diagrammatically in Figure 7.15, it is necessary to account for all the progeny under analysis. If selective death of certain of the progeny occurs, it is easy to obtain evidence suggesting perturbed commitment that is in fact spurious, because it merely documents selective survival and proliferation. This basic problem is technically difficult to overcome, and the inability to account for the behavior of all progeny casts doubt on the validity of some information that superficially represents strong evidence for the capacity of CSFs to influence differentiation commitment.

Clonal analysis of the daughter and granddaughter cells of normal hemopoietic cells has documented two types of situation: (a) With stem cells or multipotential cells, most data indicate that the progeny can be quite variable in their lineage commitment and proliferative capacity, with virtually any combination of lineage potentials being observable. The data indicate that single-lineage progeny are not generated in a fixed sequence and that the process of lineage restriction (commitment) appears to be stochastic, or random (Nakahata et al., 1982; Ogawa et al., 1983; Suda et al., 1984; Mayani et al., 1993). (b) With lineage-committed progenitor cells, on the other hand, it is common to observe that both daughter cells generate colonies that are similar in size, shape, and composition if both are cultured under the same conditions (Metcalf, 1980; Mayani et al., 1993).

The question at issue for hemopoietic regulators, and the CSFs in particular, is whether they can reproducibly alter these parameters in normal cells or cultured cell lines. For normal hemopoietic cells, it is obvious that multipotential or stem cells offer a potentially ideal model for analysis because progeny in multiple lineages can be generated. The specific question at issue is whether the usual pattern of stochastic commitment can be reproducibly biased or skewed by the action of a particular CSF. Unfortunately, stem cells and early multipotential cells require co-stimulation by factor combinations to obtain cell proliferation, which makes it very difficult to detect the possible action of a single factor under examination. Possibly for this reason, one study using stimulation by complex combinations of factors failed to reveal evidence of induced lineage commitment (Mayani et al., 1993).

One of the striking features of normal granulocyte-macrophage colonies is the absence of colony-forming (progenitor) cells with a capacity to generate secondary colonies resembling the original colony. Such colonies may contain cells with some clonogenic proliferative capacity, but the clones generated are always much smaller than the original colony. Thus, CSFs cannot stimulate self-generation by granulocyte-macrophage progenitor cells, regardless of the concentration used. This may imply that CSFs have a powerful action in inducing differentiation commitment in all responding granulocyte-macrophage progenitor cells, as defined by an immediate loss of genuine self-renewal potential. However, a more likely explanation is that these progenitor cells have already lost their self-renewal potential during their formation by stem cells, in which case the phenomenon does not necessarily indicate any particular action of the CSFs on differentiation commitment.

However, there do appear to be four examples of differentiation commitment where the CSF involved appears to have been responsible for the observed commitment.

First, when stem cells generate progenitor cell progeny under the action of SCF, co-stimulation by CSFs enhances progenitor cell formation with no evidence of cell death occurring in such expanding blast colonies. Analysis of the relative frequency of progenitor cells committed to various lineages indicated that both GM-CSF and Multi-CSF differed from G-CSF in leading to the development of a significantly higher percentage of committed granulocytic progenitors (Metcalf, 1991b). Multi-CSF was exceptional in stimulating the formation of a higher proportion of committed eosinophil progenitor cells (Metcalf, 1993a).

Second, somewhat similar observations on a nonclonal level have been made on the actions of the CSFs on CSF-dependent, multipotential cell lines that exhibit no differentiation commitment under basal culture conditions. Here, progenitor cell commitment could be inferred from the development of maturing progeny in a particular lineage. The addition of GM-CSF or G-CSF led to granulocyte formation and the addition of M-CSF to macrophage formation, the implication being that these regulators had achieved differing patterns of progenitor cell commitment (Valtieri et al., 1987; Heyworth et al., 1990). In this experimental model, selective survival of appropriate progenitors cannot be excluded.

Third, with bipotential granulocyte-macrophage progenitors, initial stimulation by GM-CSF or M-CSF appeared to lead to selective production of daughter or granddaughter cells committed, respectively, either to granulocyte or macrophage formation, and their subsequent cell production was then uninfluenced by the type of CSF used to stimulate further cell divisions (Metcalf and Burgess, 1982).

Fourth, what, in principle, is a similar commitment event is observed in the action of G-CSF on the WEHI-3BD$^+$ myelomonocytic leukemic cell line. The cells in this line normally exhibit no differentiation and a large (greater than 90%) capacity for self-generation of clonogenic cells. CSF induces irreversible differentiation commitment in a proportion of WEHI-3B cells, as established by clonal analysis of the behavior of daughter and granddaughter cells exposed to G-CSF (Metcalf, 1982a). When subsequently cultured in the absence of G-CSF, the affected cells had either lost their clonogenicity, remained clonogenic but formed differentiating colonies, or remained unaffected. In this analysis, differential survival could be ruled out as the basis of the phenomenon, and it exhibited the irreversible characteristic of differentiation commitment.

While the examples are not extensive, the implication is that CSFs can, to a degree, influence differentiation commitment in multipotential or bipotential precursors and thus bias the subsequent formation of maturing

Table 7.11. *Competitive commitment and the formation of colonies containing both granulocytic and macrophage cells stimulated by G-CSF with M-CSF*

| Stimulus | Number of colonies | Number of cells per colony | Absolute number of colonies | | |
|---|---|---|---|---|---|
| | | | G | GM | M |
| G-CSF | 11 ± 2 | 120 ± 100 | 7 | 2 | 2 |
| M-CSF | 45 ± 5 | 160 ± 90 | 0 | 1 | 44 |
| G-CSF + M-CSF | 68 ± 11 | 370 ± 220 | 7 | 18 | 43 |

*Note:* Cultures contained C57BL mouse bone marrow cells and were stimulated by 1 ng/ml G-CSF and/or 2 ng/ml M-CSF. Colonies were analyzed after 7 days of incubation. Mean values from quadruplicate cultures ± SD.
*Source:* Metcalf (1984, Table 16).

progeny. In this context, the actions of different CSFs can be potentially competitive and competitive commitment might be expected – for example, with a combination of GM-CSF and M-CSF acting on bipotential progenitor cells. This might well result in the formation of an unusual proportion of granulocyte-macrophage colonies containing subclones committed to the exclusive formation of either granulocytic or macrophage progeny. Such an outcome has been observed in cultures containing a mixture of a G-committing CSF and M-CSF, as shown in the example in Table 7.11 (Metcalf, 1984).

## Maturation induction

Maturation refers to the dramatic morphological and functional changes exhibited by hemopoietic cells as they progressively change from, for example, myeloblasts to promyelocytes, myelocytes, metamyelocytes, and then polymorphs. These changes clearly require many distinct transcriptional activations to generate proteins responsible for achieving changes in cell size and shape, granule formation, and special cell functions. Maturation is notable for its fidelity within any one lineage, so that neutrophil granules do not appear in erythroid cells or eosinophil granules in neutrophils. This remarkable fidelity almost certainly requires that the multiplicity of inductive events be tightly linked, probably in an autocatalytic cascade.

When CSFs stimulate single undifferentiated progenitor cells to form colonies of mature progeny, maturation is nearly complete, and the implication is compelling that the CSF concerned must have been involved in the maturation events. However, it is improbable that one set of CSF-initiated signals could achieve, by continuing direct action, the complex events required for maturation. CSF activation of maturation would be feasible, however, if maturation is an autoregulating series of events requiring only that a CSF have the capacity to *initiate* the activation of such a self-sustaining autocatalytic cascade. It could be argued, however, that, after differentiation commitment, maturation might be an automatic event based solely on transit of the cells through a necessary number of cell divisions, the whole process requiring no special maturation-initiating signals.

The evidence on this question is somewhat contradictory. Granulocyte maturation has been reported to be induced by G-CSF in two continuous cell lines normally proliferating as undifferentiated cells (Valtieri et al., 1987; Heyworth et al., 1990). This seems to be unequivocal evidence that CSF action can at least initiate maturation. However, a multipotential cell line normally requiring stimulation by Multi-CSF for continuous growth has been observed to undergo apparently spontaneous maturation following removal of the CSF, if extended cell survival in the absence of CSF is ensured by insertion and expression of the cDNA for *bcl*-2 (Fairbairn et al., 1993). In this system, maturation from undifferentiated cells to identifiable erythroid, granulocytic, or macrophage cells occurred without cell division, suggesting not only that cell division was not necessary to trigger maturation, but that the process could be CSF-independent. The problem with this system is that only a minority of the cells underwent maturation, and there remains the possibility that prior exposure of the cells to CSF had generated the signal required to subsequently initiate maturation, even if this did not occur while the cells were being stimulated to divide actively by continuing CSF stimulation – a default system where cessation of cell division achieved activation of a previously latent signal.

To complicate this question, it is clear that, with increasing CSF concentrations, colony size increases. Since maturation is occurring in such colonies, this will lead to passage of the cells to a postmitotic state that truncates the possibility of further population expansion. The implication is that high CSF concentrations might postpone or suppress maturation induction, permitting the cells to remain immature and capable of further cell division.

The typical highly mature nature of G-CSF-stimulated colonies and the obvious ability of G-CSF to initiate maturation in some cell lines has raised the possibility that the CSFs exhibit a certain hierarchy in their capacity to induce differentiation, with G-CSF and M-CSF exhibiting this capacity more strongly than Multi-CSF or GM-CSF (Nicola and Metcalf, 1985a). It has even been suggested that certain hemopoietic factors are only differentiative ("maturation-inducing"), while others are proliferative in their actions (Sachs, 1990). When applied to the CSFs, this categorization goes beyond established facts, since the CSFs unequivocably possess both actions.

The most compelling evidence indicating that CSFs can initiate maturation as an active process comes from the recent recognition that the G-CSF receptor contains a region near the C-terminus that is required for maturation to occur in responding cells (Fukunaga et al., 1993). In the absence of this receptor region, G-CSF can stimulate cell division, but not maturation, thus eliminating the possibility that maturation is passively linked to the occurrence of a certain number of cell divisions. The validity of this conclusion has been supported by analysis of G-CSF receptors in at least one patient with congenital neutropenia, a disease state in which there is a failure to produce a normal number of mature neutrophils associated with accumulation of cells in the marrow that are arrested at the promyelocytic stage of maturation (Dong et al., 1994). Analysis showed the cells to be heterozygous with respect to their G-CSF receptors - one allele of the G-CSFR gene encoding for a truncated version of the receptor that lacked the differentiation-inducing domain. This disease is corrected by relatively high doses of G-CSF, an outcome that could be based on the fact that the functioning G-CSFR is a homodimer and that, by random chance in such cells, a normal homodimer would form in one of four instances.

A proposal that may accommodate these conflicting observations is that CSFs might actively initiate maturation or make this process occur more effectively or more rapidly than otherwise. However, maturation induction may then be delayed in many cells if they are being subjected to high levels of CSF signaling, in which case proliferative responses dominate. Even if this proposal is valid, it is clear that the exact responses exhibited by the cell will be dictated by the active gene programs operating at the time in that cell. This is evident when cells reach a postmitotic state in differentiation where they can remain fully responsive to CSF signaling, but not in a proliferative manner. The converse of this situation may apply in less mature cells, where proliferative responses might suppress responsiveness to signals that would otherwise initiate maturation.

There is little current evidence that a regulator can interfere with the details of an integrated intracellular program of maturation. For example, GM-CSF can stimulate the formation of both neutrophilic granulocytes and eosinophils, but these cells execute their individual maturation programs with fidelity, and regardless of the GM-CSF concentration used, the neutrophils do not contain eosinophil granules or eosinophils contain neutrophilic granules. Similarly, when cDNA for the M-CSF receptor is inserted in erythroid precursors, M-CSF can then stimulate the formation of what appear to be normal erythroid colonies (McArthur et al., 1994). Conversely, insertion of cDNA for the erythropoietin receptor into macrophage precursors allows erythropoietin to stimulate macrophage colony formation.

On the other hand, the injection of G-CSF can result in the appearance of neutrophils that are larger than normal or can have "toxic" granules and abnormal lobulation (Kerrigan et al., 1989). It is unclear whether such changes represent the perturbation of a maturation program or are merely due to an acceleration of that program. This question has not so far been studied in much detail, and it seems to warrant further investigation using a variety of cell markers or functional tests to establish whether subtle changes can be induced in mature cells being formed in response to stimulation by individual regulators.

## Membrane transport and viability

It was recognized early that granulocyte-macrophage progenitor cells, when cultured in the absence of a CSF, rapidly lose their proliferative capacity and die. This process occurs with a half-life of 21 hours for adult murine cells, 9 hours for fetal murine cells, and 48 hours for human progenitor cells (Metcalf, 1984).

This phenomenon is more dramatic with continuous, CSF-dependent cell lines, where culture in the absence of CSF leads to arrest of cell cycles in progress and loss of clonogenic cells from the culture with a half-life of 8 hours (Metcalf, 1985). With such cells in suspension culture, there are typically no surviving cells present within 1–3 days after the initiation of culture – the basis of the zero background in microwell assays for CSFs.

The early progeny of normal granulocyte-macrophage progenitor cells exhibit a similar dependency on CSF for viability, and clones transferred to CSF-free cultures usually die within the next few days (Metcalf and Foster, 1967; Paran and Sachs, 1968). Somewhat surprisingly, mature granulocytes and eosinophils also exhibited a dependency on CSF for extended survival in vitro, and the addition of even very low concentrations of CSF to cultures of such cells increased their survival in vitro (Begley et al., 1986; Lopez et al., 1986).

The molecular basis for this action of the CSFs on cell survival in vitro has been established in general terms as being due to their capacity to maintain the transport integrity of cell membranes. Withdrawal of CSF from responsive cells leads to abnormalities in glucose transport, the $Na^+/K^+$ antiporter, and calcium transport, with falling intracellular ATP levels (Whetton and Dexter, 1983; Hamilton et al., 1988; Vairo and Hamilton, 1988). To a degree, this action of the CSFs can be substituted for by maintaining high extracellular ATP levels (Whetton and Dexter, 1983). The end consequence of the withdrawal of CSF from responding hemopoietic populations is the onset of death by apoptosis (Williams et al., 1990b), and on this basis, these CSF actions are now commonly referred to as preventing or delaying apoptotic death.

This in vitro action of the CSFs has made many studies on CSF function difficult to undertake. In essence, CSF-deprived cells cannot successfully be used as controls for CSF-stimulated cells because deprived cells are in fact dying, rather than unstimulated, cells. It has yet to be documented whether the CSFs exert a comparable survival function in vivo, but their in vitro action forms an essential background to all CSF actions such as proliferative stimulation and functional activation, because unless membrane transport remains intact, no effective responses are possible by such cells.

## Functional activation

Early documentation that mature granulocytes or macrophages continue to express membrane receptors for the CSFs raised the possibility that the CSFs might have functional effects on mature cells. There is now a very large literature documenting that the CSFs can indeed stimulate a wide variety of functional activities of mature granulocytes, monocytes, and eosinophils. This information for GM-CSF and G-CSF has been summarized in a number of reviews (Demetri and Griffin, 1991; Gasson, 1991; Hollingshead and Goa, 1991; Grant and Heel, 1992), and the salient points for all four CSFs are summarized in Tables 7.12, 7.13, 7.14, and 7.15.

Table 7.12. *Effector functions stimulated by GM-CSF*

| |
|---|
| *Neutrophils* |
| Increased or decreased chemotaxis |
| Increased cell adherence |
| Enhanced oxidative metabolism and expression of FMLP receptors |
| Increased phagocytosis and antibody-dependent cell-mediated cytotoxicity |
| Increased production of IL-1, G-CSF, M-CSF, CR1, CR3 |
| Increased production of cationic antimicrobial proteins |
| Priming of cells for PAF and $LTB_4$ production |
| *Eosinophils* |
| Chemotaxis |
| Enhanced responses to chemotactic agents |
| Enhanced cell adhesion |
| Enhanced phagocytosis |
| Enhanced cytotoxicity and antibody-dependent cytotoxicity |
| Priming for production or secretion of $LTC_4$, ECP, EDN |
| *Monocytes* |
| Chemoattractant effect |
| Enhanced adhesive and phagocytic activity |
| Decreased expression of M-CSF receptor |
| Increased production of G-CSF, M-CSF, TNF, IL-1, IL-6, PGE, plasminogen activator |
| Increased expression of macrophage surface antigens |
| Priming for increased oxidative metabolism |
| Increased tumoricidal action and antibody-dependent cell killing |
| Inhibition of growth of intracellular organisms - e.g., *Mycobacterium*, *Leishmania*, *Candida albicans* |
| Inhibition or enhancement of HIV replication |
| Suppression of complement factor synthesis |
| Induction of $\alpha_v\beta_3$ integrin expression |
| *Basophils* |
| Release of histamine from granules |

*Note:* PAF denotes platelet activating factor; $LTB_4$, leukotriene $B_4$; $LTC_4$, leukotriene $C_4$; ECP, eosinophil cationic protein; EDN, eosinophil-derived neurotoxin; PGE, prostaglandin E. For detailed referencing of these observations, see the reviews by Gasson (1991) and Grant and Heel (1992).

The comprehensiveness of CSF studies has not been uniform, and the information in the tables probably reflects this to some degree. Where comparative studies have been undertaken, one action, that of GM-CSF on neutrophils, appears to be stronger than those of G-CSF or Multi-CSF (Sullivan et al., 1993).

In stimulating cell functions, the lineage specificity of cellular responsiveness is maintained. For example, GM-CSF, but not G-CSF or M-CSF,

Table 7.13. *Neutrophil effector functions stimulated by G-CSF*

| |
|---|
| Enhanced survival in vitro |
| Priming for superoxide production elicited by FMLP |
| Induction of respiratory burst in adherent cells |
| Increased surface expression of CD11b (C3bi receptor) |
| Increased adherence |
| Increased affinity of homing receptor LAM-1 |
| Stimulation of antibody-dependent cytotoxicity |
| Induction of interferon $\alpha$ production |
| Increased chemotaxis |
| Enhanced release of arachidonic acid |

*Note:* LAM-1 denotes lymphocyte adhesion molecule 1. For detailed referencing of these observations, see the reviews by Demetri and Griffin (1991) and Hollingshead and Goa (1991).

Table 7.14. *Macrophage effector functions stimulated by M-CSF*

| |
|---|
| Enhanced survival in vitro |
| Stimulation of production of G-CSF, interferon, plasminogen activator inhibitors 1 and 2, plasminogen activator, thromboplastin, $\gamma$-glutamyl transpeptidase, thromboxane, superoxide |
| Enhanced killing of *Candida albicans* |
| Enhanced cytotoxicity for tumor cells with or without antibody |
| Stimulation of glucose uptake, $Na^+/K^+$-ATPase activity |
| Increased mRNA for *fos*, *myc* |
| Stimulation of tyrosine phosphorylation, kinase activation |
| Enhanced respiratory burst |
| Increased adhesion to endothelium |
| Induction of cholesterol esterases |
| Production of $\alpha_v\beta_5$ integrin |
| Induction of osteoclast differentiation, migration, and chemotaxis |
| Increased phagocytosis |
| Enhanced secretion of lipoprotein lipase |
| Enhanced replication of HIV |

*Note:* For references, see Nemunaitis (1993) and Van de Pol and Garnick (1991).

can stimulate eosinophil function, while M-CSF selectively stimulates macrophage function and G-CSF granulocytic function.

The concentrations of CSF required to stimulate functional activity are comparable to, or slightly lower than, those stimulating cell proliferation in corresponding immature cells. Although it has not been extensively

Table 7.15. *Effector functions stimulated by Multi-CSF*

| |
|---|
| *Mast cells* |
| Enhanced release of histamine and PAF induced by IL-8 or cross-linkers of IgE receptor |
| Enhanced granule formation |
| Enhanced chemotaxis |
| *Eosinophils* |
| Prolonged survival in vitro |
| Priming for chemotactic responses |
| Increased expression of ICAM-1 |
| Enhanced phagocytosis of *Candida albicans* |
| Enhanced formation of $LTC_4$ |
| Increased synthesis of eosinophil proteoglycan |
| Enhanced antibody-dependent cytotoxicity for *Schistosomula* |
| Enhanced antibody-dependent cytotoxicity for tumor cells |
| Increased superoxide production |
| *Macrophages* |
| Increased expression of class II histocompatibility antigens |
| Stimulated phagocytosis |
| Increased production of PGE |
| Increased production of G-CSF |
| Increased production of IL-1, IL-6, TNF |
| Increased killing of *Listeria monocytogenes* and *Candida albicans* |
| Inhibition of interferon $\gamma$ activation |
| *Neutrophils* (murine only) |
| Increased antibody-dependent cytotoxicity |
| Increased MHC class II expression |

*Note:* PAF denotes platelet activating factor; MHC class II, major histocompatibility complex class II; $LTC_4$, leukotriene $C_4$; PGE, prostaglandin E; ICAM-1, intercellular adhesion molecule 1. For references, see Frendl (1992) and Ziegler et al. (1993).

analyzed, it is likely that continuous stimulation is required to maintain heightened functional activity, and withdrawal of CSF leads to a rapid decline in such responses.

The types of response elicited are appropriate for each cell type and clearly depend on the gene program operating in the cell, but multiple effects seem to occur simultaneously. For example, when GM-CSF acts on macrophages, the cells simultaneously become more adherent and exhibit heightened phagocytic activity, as well as the production of superoxide and increased production of various cell products such as IL-1, interferon $\gamma$, TNF, and other regulators. Not all functions of mature cells are necessarily stimulated by CSF action, and some selectivity of responses has been noted – for example, in the action of GM-CSF on macrophages, where superoxide production is enhanced but cell-mediated killing is not (Elliott et al., 1991).

These CSF-induced responses seem best viewed as an *enhancement* of the various responses. In most cases other agents induce similar responses, which can be of greater magnitude. Some CSF-induced responses such as those on mature neutrophils clearly depend on subsequent stimulation by other agents such as the bacterial chemotactic peptide FMLP.

The various CSF actions on mature cells that have been documented from in vitro studies lead to certain expectations of the consequences of CSF action in vivo, particularly in situations where local infection or inflammation results in high local concentrations of CSF in a tissue. The overall effects of these CSF actions would most likely lead to increased margination of cells in local capillaries, enhanced exit of the cells into the affected region, accumulation and immobilization of cells in such sites, functional activation as evidenced by increased phagocytic and cytotoxic actions, increased tissue survival of the cells, and release either locally or systemically of a variety of proinflammatory agents.

The CSFs at present appear to be part of a regulatory network that interacts to control mature cell function rather than to exclusively stimulate such functions. Future studies may, however, identify situations and cell types in which the CSFs play a unique or dominant role for particular cells. For example, GM-CSF seems to have a special role in modulating the function of certain dendritic cells for which other regulators will not substitute.

Few studies have yet been reported on the interactions between CSFs in stimulating the functional activation of mature cells. This is an important question. Based on the information available for proliferative stimulation, it can be anticipated that combinations of CSFs might elicit additive or synergistic responses. However, there may also be some situations in which the responses are antagonistic. One example of such an antagonistic action is the inhibition by GM-CSF of G-CSF-initiated increases in neutrophil alkaline phosphatase (Teshima et al., 1990).

## General discussion

The in vitro studies on the biological actions of CSFs have revealed two interesting general aspects: (a) their pleiotropic actions on responding cells and (b) the overlapping actions of the four CSFs, leading some researchers to conclude that there is redundancy between the CSFs and, to a lesser degree, between CSFs and other hemopoietic regulators.

The pleiotropic actions of the CSFs became obvious during the late 1970s, and at that time, it was a novel concept that growth factors might also exhibit other, quite different actions on responding cells. Subsequent studies have made it evident that the CSFs are not peculiar in this regard, since most growth factors have at least some of the range of actions exhibited by the CSFs.

Some of the responses elicited by the CSFs require signals to enter the nucleus - for example, to control cell cycling, differentiation commitment, or maturation induction - but these signals must differ and have different target genes. Conversely, actions of the CSFs on membrane integrity or phagocytosis may merely require local actions adjacent to the activated receptors, while CSF-induced transcription and protein synthesis may involve actions in multiple locations within the cell.

Because only a single receptor type exists for each CSF, activation of the receptor by CSF binding could achieve the required multiple signaling events if (a) an early divergence of signaling occurred from the activated receptor, or (b) more readily, if different regions of the receptor interacted with and activated differing signaling intermediates. As discussed earlier, the analysis of mutated receptors is showing that the second alternative is the more likely, since, with the Epo, G-CSF, and GM-CSF receptors, data already indicate the occurrence of selective interactions of differing signaling intermediates with differing regions of the intracytoplasmic domain of the receptor. The fact that, in their high-affinity form, all the CSF receptors are dimers supports the additional possibility that differing signals may emanate from the two chains.

While the CSFs are capable of eliciting diverse cellular responses, it is likely that, to a large degree, any response they can elicit by individual cells is strictly dictated by the current gene program of the responding cell. The CSFs cannot force a postmitotic polymorph to become less mature and resume mitotic activity. Postmitotic cells certainly respond to CSF stimulation, but the responses are restricted to those more appropriate for a cell at that maturation stage.

The overlapping actions of CSFs on granulocytes and macrophages and to a lesser degree on eosinophils, megakaryocytes, and erythroid cells do raise the question of the significance of this apparent redundancy. While this question is better addressed after consideration of the in vivo actions of the CSFs, certain comments can be made on the basis of the cell biology observable in vitro.

Several molecular aspects of the CSF-receptor system suggest a common evolutionary origin of these CSFs and, therefore, the possibility of an incomplete and possibly fruitless divergence of functions from a common ancestral regulator. There is a close physical linkage of the GM-CSF and Multi-CSF genes, a general similarity in the structure and regulatory elements of the genes, a physical linkage at least in humans between the genes encoding the receptor $\alpha$-chains, and a sharing of $\beta$-chains by the two CSF receptors. A common origin of the receptors for GM-CSF, G-CSF, and Multi-CSF is also likely because of the shared regions of homology in the extracellular domains of these receptors, even if the regulators themselves have diverged in amino acid sequence. If the four CSFs have arisen by evolutionary divergence, it seems illogical to regard the present molecules as exhibiting redundancy. It would be more reasonable to expect that this evolutionary divergence had achieved certain functional advantages by the resulting specialization, even if overlapping actions persist.

The most likely examples of the advantages achieved by this subtle specialization will probably emerge from a more careful examination of the diversity of functional responses exhibited by mature cells after CSF stimulation, but the information is insufficient at present for critical discussion. However, a consideration of the proliferation elicited by CSF combinations suggests that, for several reasons, it is advantageous for the body to employ two or more CSFs with partly overlapping actions. A greater proliferative response can be achieved by CSF combinations than can be achieved by single CSFs and with lower CSF concentrations. This probably achieves a significant economy in terms of demands on the CSF-producing cell system and reduces the risk of side effects or adverse responses to any one of the CSFs involved because CSF concentrations can be kept lower.

The peculiar biology of stem cells in requiring stimulation by multiple regulators before proliferation occurs cannot be overcome simply by increasing the concentrations of a single regulator. This curious behavior would represent a desirable fail-safe system if it were of importance to preserve as many stem cells as possible in a noncycling state. This is indeed a necessary requirement, since these stem cells are finite in number and must sustain hemopoiesis for the life of the animal. Some situations, such as during acute infections, might require massive increases in granulocyte production and function. If this can be achieved by a single CSF (e.g., by G-CSF), it is highly desirable that excess levels of that CSF not activate all stem cells into cycle. If this were to occur, short-term survival would be ensured at the cost of future marrow aplasia. A system requiring multiple regulators to activate stem cells may help to avoid this potentially lethal sequence.

Very little information exists either on the exact range of leukocytes that is required to mount optimal responses to infections or on the optimal sequence in which these cells should enter such responses. Most inflammatory states obviously involve cells of more than one lineage, and the required cellular responses could be highly complex. The existence of four CSFs with overlapping but distinctive cellular actions provides a regulatory system that should allow a subtle adjustment of the relative number of cells from different lineages that could not be achieved simply by adjusting the concentrations of a single regulator.

# 8
# The biology of colony-stimulating factor production, degradation, and clearance

Although there have been numerous publications on cells that produce colony-stimulating factors, there are a number of reasons why our understanding of the situation in vivo is seriously incomplete.

Like other hemopoietic regulators, and unlike classical hormones, the CSFs are not the exclusive products of one cell type residing in a single organ but can be produced by a wide variety of cells dispersed throughout the body. This has made it impossible so far to determine the precise contribution of particular cell types or organs to the total body production of CSF and might allow a situation in which local CSF production and concentrations are widely different in different parts of the body, with circulating CSF levels providing a very imperfect measure of the situation.

To compound this complexity, the high specific activity of the CSFs requires their production in only small amounts, and the concentrations of CSFs in the serum or of those extractable from tissues typically are relatively low. While specific immunoassays are now sufficiently sensitive to monitor such concentrations, some reservations can be raised about the validity of these assays. Unless the antibody is directed against the binding domain, one cannot assume that the molecules detected are necessarily biologically active, and one may merely be detecting intact antigenic epitopes on functionally inactive molecules. Conversely, bioassays are often impeded by the presence of toxic or inhibitory material in plasma or tissue extracts, requiring fractionation procedures of possibly varying efficiency before the low levels of CSF present can begin to be detected. There is a major problem in assessing levels of CSF production by monitoring mRNA levels: Transcriptional activity does not necessarily parallel the production or secretion of active protein, and Northern analyses are not sufficiently sensitive for the detection of the low levels of mRNA often involved. RNase protection assays are more sensitive and reasonably reliable as quantitative estimates, but the most sensitive method using the PCR has an inherent problem in providing reliable quantification. None of these procedures can provide evidence on which cell type in a tissue is producing the CSF detected. The only current method for approaching this question in intact tissues is in situ hybridization. This technique has worked well for regulatory factors such as M-CSF that are produced in relative abundance but has proved insensitive in detecting more than the most active subset of cells producing GM-CSF or G-CSF in normal tissues. The same problem of sensitivity applies to the use of specific CSF antibodies in a histochemical approach.

Probably the most serious problem is that estimates of CSF production performed on cultured cells or tissues inevitably overestimate the production; a major induction of transcription and CSF production occurs rapidly in such cultures, even using normal tissues in serum-free medium. This problem is certainly not unique to the CSFs, for, as shown in Figure 8.1, it can occur with other regulators, such as LIF, and involve a continuous

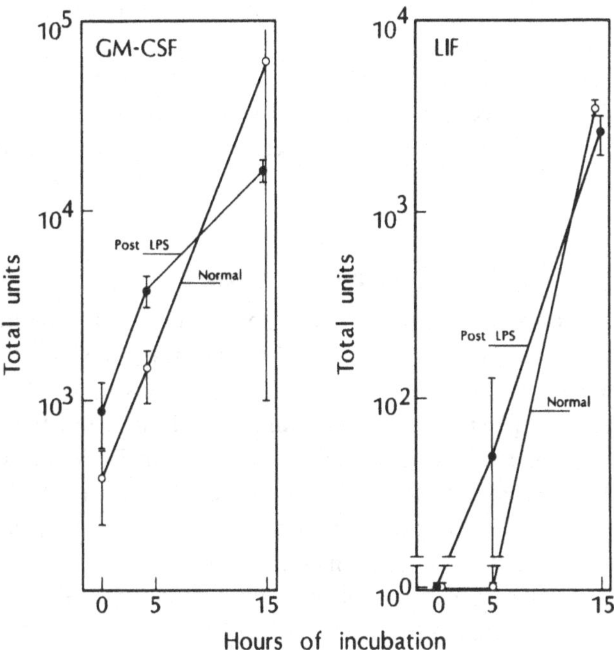


Figure 8.1. When lung tissue is incubated in vitro, levels of GM-CSF or LIF rise logarithmically during the incubation period, and the eventual levels can obscure differences existing in vivo (0 hour) between lung tissue from normal mice and mice preinjected with endotoxin (LPS).

logarithmic rise over an almost thousandfold range even within relatively short incubation periods. Figure 8.1 also indicates that this phenomenon of in vitro induction can obscure genuine differences between tissues. In the example shown, observations on extracted GM-CSF (0 hour) showed that the prior injection of endotoxin (LPS) had increased the lung content of GM-CSF. However, after 15 hours of incubation, levels of GM-CSF in and produced by the normal tissue had exceeded those from the tissue of endotoxin-injected mice, meaning that estimates based solely on incubated tissues would have given misleading data on the effects of endotoxin.

Most workers have learned not to trust established normal or neoplastic cell lines as necessarily giving valid information on the functional activity of the corresponding normal cells in vivo. To overcome this, a seemingly valid procedure, where technically possible, is to purify the normal cell type under study so that any information obtained can be related with confidence to that particular cell type. However, this well-intended approach has also run into problems because the use of even minor procedures such as density separation induces major increases in CSF transcription and thus can potentially result in quite misleading estimates of likely CSF production by such cells in vivo.

These cautionary remarks are not intended to discount published information on the subject, but merely to indicate that the information has profound limitations, even if the general picture emerging is probably broadly correct.

## Serum CSF levels

The introduction of more sensitive and specific immunoassays has begun to provide information on this issue, although still with some limitations due to the variable sensitivity of the available tests. CSF can be detected in the serum or plasma of normal humans and mice, but the situation differs according to the CSF involved. As shown in Table 8.1, M-CSF is detected in most normal adult human sera at the relatively high concentrations of 1,000–8,000 pg/ml (lower sensitivity of the assay, 660–5,000 pg/ml; Aihara et al., 1993; Cebon et al., 1994).

In contrast, GM-CSF was detected in only half of the samples analyzed, with levels ranging from 20 to 100 pg/ml (Cebon et al., 1994), using an assay with a lower sensitivity of 20 pg/ml. G-CSF was detected in normal serum at similarly low concentrations of $25 \pm 20$ pg/ml (Kawakimi et al., 1990). Multi-CSF has usually not been detected in normal serum, but in one report, levels of 25–40 pg were noted in 16% of samples (Verhoef et al., 1992).

Table 8.1. *CSF levels in normal human serum*

| Factor | Lowest sensitivity of assay (pg/ml) | CSF concentration in serum (pg/ml) | Reference |
|---|---|---|---|
| M-CSF | 660 | 2,400 ± 460 | Yong et al. (1992) |
| | NS[a] | 1,300 ± 300 (M)<br>1,500 ± 130 (F) | Aihara et al. (1993) |
| | 5,000 | 5,000–8,000 | Cebon et al. (1994) |
| GM-CSF | 20 | <20 (half); 20–100 (half) | Cebon et al. (1994) |
| | 5 | <5 (half); 5–25 (half) | Baiocchi et al. (1993) |
| G-CSF | NS[a] | 25 ± 20 | Kawakimi et al. (1990) |
| | 30 | <30 | Watari et al. (1989) |
| | 100 | <100 | Cebon et al. (1994) |
| Multi-CSF | 7 | <7 (21/25)<br>25–40 (4/25) | Verhoef et al. (1992) |

[a] Not stated.

The data from conventionally reared mice are somewhat comparable. M-CSF was detected in the serum by radioimmunoassay at levels of about 6 ng/ml (Bartocci et al., 1986), but by specific bioassay GM-CSF was not detected in most normal mice (lower sensitivity of detection, 100 pg/ml; Metcalf, 1988b). No Multi-CSF has been detected by specific bioassay in normal mouse sera (lower level of detection, 20 pg/ml; Metcalf, 1988b).

The potential significance of these levels can be assessed by comparing the levels with the in vitro dose–response curves for the CSFs (Figure 7.1). It is evident that M-CSF is present in serum in biologically relevant concentrations, while GM-CSF and G-CSF are present in concentrations that would be too low to exert significant proliferative effects unless acting in collaboration with other growth factors.

These observations suggest major differences in the biology of the CSFs. This has been reinforced by the observation that M-CSF levels rise two- to threefold in the serum of pregnant mice (Bartocci et al., 1986) and humans (Saito et al., 1992b; Yong et al., 1992) and are higher in cord blood and neonatal serum than in adult serum (Saito et al., 1992b). No pregnancy-related changes have been reported in GM-CSF or G-CSF levels.

The view has been expressed that while M-CSF is a circulating, hormone-like regulator, GM-CSF and, to a lesser degree, G-CSF are really paracrine factors not normally found in the circulation. While this probably oversimplifies the situation, there is a certain degree of truth in this view, at least under basal conditions.

In early biological studies using bone marrow colony-stimulating assays, CSF of uncharacterized type was detected in the serum of some normal animals, and levels of colony-stimulating activity were elevated in conventionally reared mice following whole-body irradiation (Hall, 1969) or the administration of cytotoxic drugs (Shadduck and Nanna, 1971). However, such responses were not detected in germ-free mice (Morley et al., 1972) or, in this laboratory, in specific pathogen-free mice following either irradiation or the administration of 5-fluorouracil. These observations imply that with the possible exception of M-CSF, the CSFs detected in earlier animal studies probably reflected exposure of these animals to microorganisms rather than responses simply to induced leukopenia.

Early studies on the effects of infections in humans and mice documented increases in CSF of an uncharacterized type in the sera of some patients with infections (Foster et al., 1968b; Metcalf and Wahren, 1968; Metcalf et al., 1971) and in animals with experiment-induced infections (Foster et al., 1968a; Trudgett et al., 1973). The injection of endotoxin represents a simpler model of some aspects of infections, and in mice a single intravenous injection of endotoxin elevates CSF levels 30,000-fold within 3 hours, with a return to preinjection levels usually occurring within 24–48 hours (Metcalf, 1971). A similar response to injected endotoxin has also been noted in humans (Golde and Cline, 1975). Subsequent analysis in this laboratory of the murine response showed that rises in GM-CSF levels represented only a minor component and that G-CSF is the major CSF involved in the rise. M-CSF levels were moderately elevated and remained elevated for longer than did those for G-CSF or GM-CSF. Multi-CSF was not detected in response to the injection of endotoxin.

A somewhat similar pattern was observed in mice in response to intravenous infection with *Listeria monocytogenes* (Cheers et al., 1988). At 24 hours after infection of susceptible mice, total CSF concentrations reached about 400 ng/ml, the approximate values for each CSF being as follows: GM-CSF, 500 pg/ml; M-CSF, >180 ng/ml; and G-CSF, 180 ng/ml, with again no Multi-CSF being detectable.

In two studies on patients with acute infections, G-CSF was elevated to 730 ± 895 pg/ml (Kawakami et al., 1990) and from 46 to more than 2,000 pg/ml (Watari et al., 1989). In an analysis of non-neutropenic patients with infections, G-CSF levels were elevated in half the serum samples analyzed, with levels of 100–10,000 pg/ml, but there were no significant rises in GM-CSF levels and a less marked but consistent rise in M-CSF levels to between 1,000 and 50,000 pg/ml. In this study, G-CSF levels fell promptly with resolution of the fever, but the rise in M-CSF levels was more sustained. Infections with gram-negative organisms were more effective in elevating CSF levels than were gram-positive infections (Cebon et al., 1994).

In patients with neutropenia but no detected infections, no elevations were noted in GM-CSF levels, but in some patients increased levels of G-CSF and M-CSF were observed (Cebon et al., 1994). Similarly in 82% of patients with aplastic anemia, G-CSF levels were elevated (mean value 260 pg/ml), and a similar situation was noted in Fanconi's anemia (Watari et al., 1989).

In one study of mice infected with *Mycobacterium lepraemurium,* elevated serum levels of Multi-CSF were reported 8–18 weeks after initial infection (Resnick et al., 1990).

Patients with leukemia or myelodysplasia present a further order of complexity in establishing the basis for abnormal CSF levels, but elevated levels of G-CSF have been observed in some patients with myeloid leukemia (Watari et al., 1989; Verhoef et al., 1992), while M-CSF levels were elevated in a large proportion of patients with lymphoid malignancies (Janowska-Wieczorek et al., 1991). A somewhat comparable situation has been observed in myelodysplastic patients (Watari et al., 1989; Janowska-Wieczorek et al., 1991; Verhoef et al., 1992).

The most complex clinical situation is found with patients following marrow transplantation, where leukopenia and possibly infections are present. In children who had received autologous peripheral blood transplants, elevated G-CSF levels (600–6,000 pg/ml) were observed 3–7 days post-transplantation in patients with lymphoid malignancies. A rise in GM-CSF levels was noted in some patients (150–500 pg/ml) without any change in M-CSF levels, and there was no detectable Multi-CSF (Kawano et al., 1993b). Similar changes in G-CSF and GM-CSF levels were observed in another study on adults following autologous peripheral blood transplants (Baiocchi et al., 1993) and in G-CSF levels following marrow transplantation (Cairo et al., 1992).

These studies in mice and humans have indicated that CSF levels can be rapidly and markedly elevated in response to endotoxin injection or infections and can be elevated in leukopenia in the absence of apparent infections and in regeneration following intensive cytotoxic drug therapy. Animal studies suggest that most of these responses are likely to have been triggered by the products of microorganisms, although changes in G-CSF levels may occur in response to leukopenia, and changes in M-CSF levels are evident during pregnancy. It is also possible that CSF levels are elevated in a variety of patients with myelodysplasia and leukemia in the apparent absence of infections.

The presence of high circulating CSF levels in some patients with leukemia or solid tumors requires a separate comment. In the case of myeloid leukemia, there are reasons to believe that autocrine CSF production by the leukemic cells may play a significant role in the pathogenesis and progression of these diseases, and such leukemic cells might well be one source of any additional CSF in the circulation. These considerations may not account for the high M-CSF levels noted in various lymphoid malignancies.

There are exceptional cancer patients with high white cell levels and high serum CSF levels, most frequently documented as G-CSF. Resection of tumors in such patients leads to restoration of normal CSF levels, and since the tumors can be shown to be actively producing CSF, the tumor tissue itself is likely to have contributed significantly to the elevated CSF levels (Asano et al., 1980; Nagata, 1990).

## Estimates of CSF concentrations available to act on hemopoietic cells

It would improve our understanding of the biology of the CSFs if estimates could be made of concentrations of the four CSFs actually present in the marrow or in local sites of inflammation. However, it is not technically possible to sample the resident fluid in such locations directly, and only the possible situation can be discussed.

It is logical to assume that the CSF concentrations in plasma are minimum estimates of what might be available to stimulate hemopoietic cells, provided only that circulating CSF can effectively penetrate tissue spaces in a tightly packed cell population like that in the marrow. From the changes induced by injected CSF, this ability can now be inferred. In one experiment, injected CSF did penetrate the marrow. In the mouse, a subset of lymphocyte-like cells in the bone marrow expresses an exceptionally large number of receptors for Multi-CSF. It was possible to show by autoradiography that intravenously injected radiolabeled Multi-CSF did bind to these cells in vivo (Metcalf and Nicola, 1988).

It can now be accepted, therefore, that plasma CSF can penetrate marrow populations and equilibrate with the fluid surrounding the cells. However, plasma CSF concentrations almost certainly underestimate those actually available to hemopoietic cells because of the capacity of marrow stromal and endothelial cells to locally produce at least G-CSF, GM-CSF, and M-CSF (Figure 8.2).

It is not yet clear whether all four CSFs can cross the placental barrier and enter the fetus and, if so, whether the CSF is produced locally in the

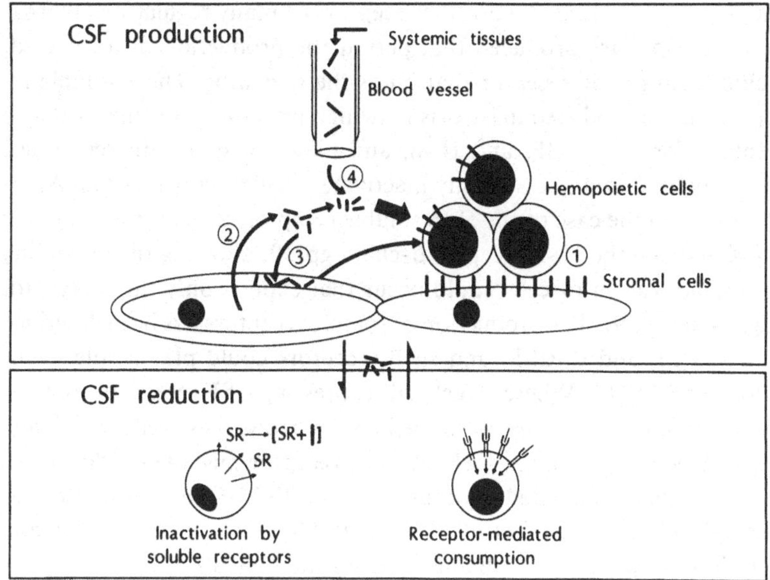


Figure 8.2. A dynamic equilibrium exists in the body between CSF production and consumption. CSFs can be produced in many locations and enter the marrow via the circulation (4). However, CSF can also be produced by local stromal cells and may be membrane-displayed (1) or secreted (2). Some CSF can be held in the glycocalyx of stromal cells (3). Consumption of CSF occurs mainly via receptor-mediated endocytosis by target hemopoietic cells, but complexing with secreted soluble receptors (SR) might be an alternative method of eliminating CSF.

placenta or reaches the placenta via the circulation. However, one study has documented that in rats injected subcutaneously with human G-CSF, at least some G-CSF did enter the fetal circulation and increase granulocyte levels (Medlock et al., 1993).

Four phenomena add complexity to attempts at assessing actual CSF concentrations impinging on hemopoietic cells (Figure 8.2). (a) Some regulators are produced by stromal cells in membrane-bound form that can activate cells making contact, without the need for secretion of the regulator in soluble form by the producing cells. This has been shown to be the case for M-CSF (Stein et al., 1990) and SCF (Toksoz et al., 1992). (b) The glycocalyx of stromal and possibly other cell types can loosely bind at least some CSFs in a location adjacent to responding cells (Gordon et al., 1987). The affinity of this binding is lower than that of CSF receptor binding, which suggests that such CSF can represent an unmeasurable reservoir of CSF, of whatever origin, that is available for use by local hemopoietic cells. (c) For the receptors of many regulators, alternative transcripts are produced that permit the production of a secreted, soluble form of the receptor that binds the regulator. These soluble receptors can be produced in surprisingly high amounts, as is the case with receptors for IL-2, LIF, and IL-6, and play two quite different roles. They may bind to and essentially inactivate circulating regulators. Alternatively, as in the case of the IL-6 soluble receptor, the complex can bind to and activate the IL-6 receptor $\beta$-chain gp130, allowing the possibility that the activation of cells could occur that express only the $\beta$-receptor (Taga et al., 1989). The production of soluble receptors has been described for GM-CSF and G-CSF, and such receptors could play a role in the biology of CSF. (d) Where target cells expressing CSF receptors are present in high concentrations, as in the bone marrow, these cells can significantly deplete extracellular CSF levels by receptor-mediated endocytosis. This has been documented to occur in vitro with M-CSF consumption by macrophages (Tushinski et al., 1982) and GM-CSF or Multi-CSF consumption by appropriate cell lines (Nicola and Metcalf, 1988). Consumption of G-CSF by neutrophils has been advanced as a possible basis for the inverse relationship noted between blood neutrophil levels and the serum levels of G-CSF achievable in humans by infusions of G-CSF (Layton et al., 1989) (Figure 8.3). The data in Figure 8.3 not only document the inability to maintain high G-CSF levels in the serum in the presence of a normal number of blood (and presumably marrow) granulocytes, but also demonstrate that the administration of CSF can achieve far higher serum concentrations of CSF than are encountered even in patients with active infections (10–50 vs. 0.5–10 ng/ml of G-CSF in infected patients). Data of this type should be kept in mind during the later discussion on the clinical uses of the CSFs. Although the body does respond to infections by elevating CSF levels, such levels are not as great as those achieved by injecting CSF, and therefore the resulting levels of granulocyte-macrophage formation achieved during a natural response to an infection can be increased by CSF administration.

Depending on the rate of CSF entry into, or local production of CSF in, hemopoietic regions, local consumption may outstrip the supply of new molecules, leading to decreased CSF concentrations. Indeed, studies with a model cell system indicated that, with cell crowding, CSF concentrations become of lesser importance in achieving cell stimulation than the actual supply (total number) of CSF molecules (Nicola and Metcalf, 1988).

The high circulating levels of CSF present in infections or states of spontaneous or induced aplasia suggest that, in these situations, CSF concentrations in the marrow would be well above those demonstrated to be

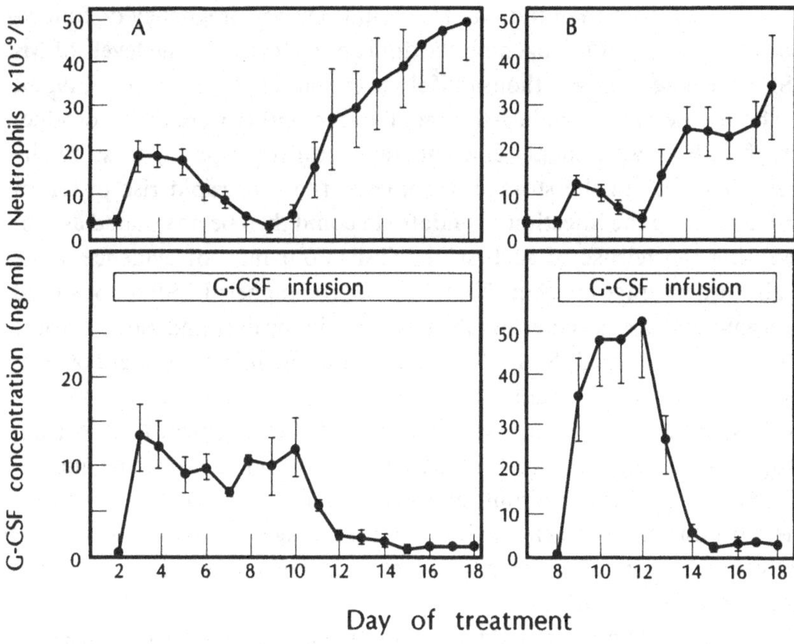


Figure 8.3. An inverse relationship is observable in humans between concentrations of serum G-CSF achieved by continuous infusion and levels of blood neutrophils, raising the possibility of significant consumption of G-CSF by neutrophils. (Reproduced with permission from Layton et al., 1989.)

necessary for biological activity in vitro. Similarly, in healthy adults, M-CSF is obviously present in the circulation in high enough concentrations and also presents no conceptual problems. In the case of G-CSF and GM-CSF, the actual concentrations available in the bone marrow remain a matter of speculation and in need of further investigation.

## Tissue and cellular sources of the CSFs

### *Tissue sources*

In early work, it was shown that CSF of uncharacterized type could be extracted from all tissues of the normal mouse in higher concentrations than those present in the serum (Sheridan and Stanley, 1971). In the mouse, certain organs, such as the salivary gland, lung, thymus, and kidney, have a two- to fourfold higher content of extractable CSFs than other organs, but the significance of this is unknown (Sheridan and Stanley, 1971). A subsequent study specifically measuring M-CSF indicated that M-CSF concentrations in the submaxillary gland, lung, spleen, kidney, and lymph nodes were higher than those in the serum. During pregnancy or following the injection of estrogen or chorionic gonadotropin, the levels of M-CSF were noted to rise a thousandfold in the uterus (Bartocci et al., 1986).

These observations indicated that all organs either were active producers of CSF or were highly efficient traps with the capacity to store circulating CSF. On the storage hypothesis, the very rapid rise in serum CSF following the injection of endotoxin could then be postulated as representing the release of such stored CSF. Four lines of evidence argue against this storage concept. First, injected radiolabeled CSF is not stored in organs and accumulates significantly only in the liver and kidney, where it is rapidly degraded. Second, in response to the injection of endotoxin, tissue CSF levels rise rather than fall, and these rises occur as rapidly as those in the serum (Sheridan and Metcalf, 1972). Third, mRNA transcripts have been observed for GM-CSF in lung and heart tissue and for G-CSF in heart tissue (Troutt and Lee, 1989). Fourth, and this is by far the most cogent argument against passive storage, is the fact that tissues actively generate CSF in vitro, a process that depends on active transcription and protein synthesis.

It is readily demonstrated that mouse tissues can actively produce CSF in vitro, most of which is then released to the medium. All tissues tested – including those from the salivary gland, thymus, heart, lung, muscle, spleen, liver, kidney, bladder, bone marrow, and bone shaft – produced CSF, the amounts produced being higher, at least initially, if the animal had been previously injected with endotoxin. Subsequent biochemical studies showed that both GM-CSF and G-CSF are present in such conditioned media (Nicola and Metcalf, 1981), as is M-CSF. Unfortunately, as noted earlier, these experiments overestimate the capacity of these tissues to produce CSF in normal health in vivo because a marked induction of GM-CSF and G-CSF transcription occurs in vitro, leading to enhanced CSF production in vitro. M-CSF transcription and production have not been noted to fluctuate in this manner during organ culture. In support of the general conclusion that organ production of CSFs in vivo normally occurs at a much lower level in normal health has been the difficulty in detecting mRNA for CSF in most organs.

In these experiments using whole tissues, the one CSF never encountered has been Multi-CSF. Even cultures of minced thymus and spleen tissue consistently fail to produce detectable Multi-CSF, which is in sharp contrast to the ready capacity of lymphoid cell suspensions to produce Multi-CSF in vitro following mitogenic stimulation.

Fewer studies have been reported using human tissues, but these have supported the more extensive information from the use of mouse tissues.

In particular, placental tissue has been found to be an exceptionally rich source of GM-CSF and G-CSF (Nicola et al., 1979b).

Less information is available about fetal and embryonic tissues, but both yolk sac and fetal liver in the mouse were found to produce significant amounts of CSF, with biochemical studies indicating that M-CSF was a major component of the observed CSF activity (Johnson and Burgess, 1978). High levels of M-CSF (17 ± 9 ng/ml) and G-CSF (1.9 ± 1.7 ng/ml) have been reported in human amniotic fluid, with immunohistochemical evidence suggesting production by epithelial cells of fetal membranes (Saito et al., 1992a).

These data on tissue content and production of CSFs probably indicate that no one organ is a dominant source of CSF. Even the amounts of CSF extracted from, or produced in vitro by, marrow or bone stroma are relatively low (Chan and Metcalf, 1972), suggesting that CSF production within the marrow might not be quantitatively outstanding. However, there are logical reasons for concluding that local CSF production within the marrow is an important biological process, which casts some doubt on the validity of evidence obtained by the present methods of estimating either CSF concentrations or the CSF production capacity of various tissues. Clearly, however, the evidence indicates that all organs can produce CSF and have the potential to increase such production rapidly when suitably induced, so the CSF-producing system should be visualized as being body-wide. Furthermore, in some situations CSF production may become dominated by a particular source. For example, during a lung infection, the lung might well become the major site of so much CSF production that the impact of this production also becomes significant elsewhere in the body (Nelson et al., 1994).

On this general question, one set of observations suggests that marrow-derived populations might be a major CSF source, whether the cells involved be hemopoietic or associated stromal cells. The injection of endotoxin into C3H/HeJ mice does not elevate serum or tissue CSF levels. However, if such mice are repopulated by responsive syngeneic C3H/GSF marrow cells, they subsequently exhibit nearly normal CSF responses following endotoxin challenge (Hultner et al., 1982). This suggests that marrow-derived cells may either be potent sources of CSF or be required in some circumstances to permit CSF responses by other cells.

### *Cellular sources*

The cell types shown to produce a particular CSF as identified by mRNA or specific bioassays are listed in Table 8.2. Fibroblast, macrophage, endo-

Table 8.2. *Cell types producing CSFs*

| Factor | Cell type | Reference |
|---|---|---|
| GM-CSF | T-Lymphocytes | Burgess et al. (1980); Chan et al. (1986); Kelso and Metcalf (1990) |
| | Macrophages | Rich (1986); Thorens et al. (1987) |
| | Endothelial cells | Quesenberry and Gimbrone (1980); Bagby et al. (1983); Broudy et al. (1986a, 1987); Seelentag et al. (1987); Sief et al. (1987) |
| | Fibroblasts | Munker et al. (1986); Zucali et al. (1986); Kaushansky et al. (1988) |
| | Stromal cells | Broudy et al. (1986b); Gualtieri et al. (1987); Rennick et al. (1987a) |
| | B-Lymphocytes | Pluznik et al. (1989) |
| | Mesothelial cells | Demetri et al. (1989) |
| | Osteoblasts | Horowitz et al. (1989) |
| | Mast cells | Plaut et al. (1989); Wodnar-Filipowicz et al. (1989) |
| | Eosinophils | Kita et al. (1991) |
| | Blast cells | Bot et al. (1990a) |
| G-CSF | Macrophages | Metcalf and Nicola (1985b); Lu et al. (1988); Vellenga et al. (1988) |
| | Fibroblasts | Koeffler et al. (1987); Kaushansky et al. (1988) |
| | Endothelial cells | Broudy et al. (1986a); Seelentag et al. (1987) |
| | Stromal cells | Rennick et al. (1987a); Fibbe et al. (1988); Migliaccio et al. (1992a) |
| M-CSF | Fibroblasts | Stanley and Heard (1977) |
| | Macrophages | Horiguchi et al. (1986); Rambaldi et al. (1987); Haskill et al. (1988) |
| | Endothelial cells | Seelentag et al. (1987); Seiff et al. (1987) |
| | Stromal cells | Lanotte et al. (1982) |
| | T-Lymphocytes (human) | Wong et al. (1987) |
| | Uterine decidual cells | Pollard et al. (1987) |
| Multi-CSF | T-Lymphocytes | Nabel et al. (1981); Kelso and Metcalf (1990) |
| | Mast cells | Wodnar-Filipowicz et al. (1989) |
| | Keratinocytes | Luger et al. (1985) |
| | Eosinophils | Kita et al. (1991) |
| | Stromal cells | Kittler et al. (1992) |

thelial, and stromal cells are prominent in having the capacity to produce GM-CSF, G-CSF, and M-CSF. The presence of such cells in most tissues may well account for much of the CSF extractable from all organs and the capacity of tissue from these organs to produce CSF in culture. The wide distribution of these cells and their likely accessibility to products of invading microorganisms also makes it evident that these cells are ideally located to initiate rapid changes in CSF production in response to infections.

This list of CSF-producing cell types also represents the only types readily obtainable in pure form for analysis in vitro. No studies have been reported on parenchymal cells such as hepatocytes or renal tubule cells, and it remains to be determined whether a much wider range of cell types has the capacity, when induced, to produce one or another CSF. It is still possible that the CSF-producing system may, on occasion, involve any tissue and any cell type.

The situation with Multi-CSF is quite different. Multi-CSF has never been detected in normal organ extracts or organ-conditioned media. Only T-lymphocytes and mast cells have been confirmed as producing Multi-CSF when suitably primed in vitro (Metcalf, 1984; Niemeyer et al., 1989), and only single reports have described Multi-CSF production by keratinocytes, eosinophils, and irradiated stromal cells (Luger et al., 1985; Kita et al., 1991; Kittler et al., 1992). The failure to detect Multi-CSF in vivo is puzzling in view of the presence of Multi-CSF receptors on hemopoietic cells and the strong proliferative effects of Multi-CSF in vitro on stem cells, megakaryocytes, and early erythroid cells.

The ability of a number of cell types to produce more than one CSF raises the possibility that individual cells may simultaneously exhibit these functions. This possibility has so far been confirmed only at the single-cell level for T-lymphocytes, where activated cells can clearly simultaneously produce not only GM-CSF and Multi-CSF, but also a number of other hemopoietic regulators (Kelso and Gough, 1988; Kelso and Metcalf, 1990).

The production of one type or another of CSF has been described for a number of tumor cell lines and primary tumors. Among nonhemopoietic tumors, these reports have involved cancers, sarcomas, and melanomas, but such activity appears to be exceptional for any one tumor type even though active tumors can produce high CSF concentrations. The exceptional nature of this CSF production and the fact that neoplastic, potentially derepressed cells are involved prevents such information from being used to draw any conclusions about the possible activity of corresponding normal cells.

So far no studies have attempted to compare quantitatively the relative amounts of various CSFs produced by individual cell types or the relative concentrations of different CSFs present in different tissues. However, the clear capacity of local cells within the marrow to produce GM-CSF and G-CSF must be taken into account when conclusions are drawn about the possible role of CSFs in the regulation of basal levels of hemopoiesis. The relatively low concentrations of these CSFs in the plasma do not argue against such a role if there is an adequate local source of these CSFs within the marrow itself.

## Inductive signaling of CSF production

The best-characterized natural inductions of CSF production have been the responses observed in acute infections, where elevated circulating levels strongly suggest that the responses were not confined to increased CSF production in the marrow. More direct evidence of the occurrence of body-wide increases in CSF production has come from the demonstration that following the intravenous injection of endotoxin, all organs developed a higher content of CSF and exhibited an increased capacity to produce CSF in vitro (Sheridan and Metcalf, 1972; D. Metcalf, unpublished data).

Several studies have documented that local tissue increases of CSF can occur in response to inflammation or infection. An analysis of sterile abscesses induced by carrageenan injection indicated increased CSF synthesis in the surrounding inflammatory tissue (Shikita et al., 1981). Similarly, in model renal infections induced by the introduction of *E. coli* into the bladder, heightened levels of GM-CSF and G-CSF mRNA were observed in the affected renal tissue (Rugo et al., 1992).

Macrophages recovered from the lungs of pneumonia patients were observed to produce G-CSF spontaneously and in higher concentrations than those produced by normal alveolar macrophages, the latter requiring priming by endotoxin before producing detectable G-CSF (Tazi et al., 1991). Similar observations were made in model pneumonia infections in rats. G-CSF was detected in the normal lung but not the serum. Following infection, lung G-CSF levels rose rapidly and preceded a rise in serum G-CSF levels (Nelson et al., 1994).

In an analysis of M-CSF concentrations in the cerebrospinal fluid, elevated levels were noted in patients with bacterial meningitis, without a corresponding elevation of M-CSF levels in the serum (Shimoda et al., 1993).

Increased levels of GM-CSF and Multi-CSF mRNA were observed in skin biopsies from allergic patients with late-phase cutaneous reactions (Kay et al., 1991), and in inflammatory and noninflammatory arthritis the affected joint fluid contained detectable CSF (Williamson et al., 1988). A higher than normal frequency of lymphocytes producing GM-CSF or Multi-CSF was observed in cells from the spleen and lymph nodes of mice undergoing graft-versus-host reactions (Troutt and Kelso, 1992).

Table 8.3. *Inductive signals for CSF production by various cells*

| Factor | Cell type | Inducer |
|---|---|---|
| GM-CSF | Fibroblasts | TNF, IL-1, TPA |
| | Endothelial cells | TNF, IL-1, TPA |
| | Macrophages | LPS, FCS, phagocytosis, adherence |
| | T-Lymphocytes | Antigens, lectins, CD28, IL-1, HTLV, IL-2 |
| | B-Lymphocytes | LPS, TPA |
| | Mesothelial cells | EGF + TNF |
| | Osteoblasts | PTH, LPS |
| | Mast cells | IgE, calcium ionophore |
| G-CSF | Macrophages | GM-CSF, Multi-CSF, interferon $\gamma$, LPS, IL-4 |
| | Endothelial cells | TNF, IL-1 |
| | Fibroblasts | TNF, IL-1 |
| | Stromal cells | IL-1 |
| M-CSF | Uterine cells | Pregnancy, chorionic gonadotropin, estrogen |
| Multi-CSF | T-Lymphocytes | Antigen, lectins, CD28, IL-1, IL-2 |

*Abbreviations:* FCS, fetal calf serum; HTLV, human T leukemia virus; EGF, epidermal growth factor; PTH, parathyroid hormone; TNF, tumor necrosis factor; TPA, phorbol ester.

In the case of cultured cells, effective inductive signals vary according to the cell type (Table 8.3). For endothelial cells, stromal cells, and fibroblasts, endotoxin, IL-1, and tumor necrosis factor $\alpha$ (TNF$\alpha$) are highly active inducing signals. Following an LPS challenge, IL-1 is elevated slightly earlier than the CSFs, which has led to the proposal that although LPS can appear to act directly on CSF-producing cells, a more effective system may be for LPS first to induce IL-1 production and release, with IL-1 then being the major inducing signal for CSF production (Neta et al., 1988) (Figure 8.4).

For T-lymphocytes, natural inductive signals may come from foreign antigens that are involved in mixed leukocyte cultures. However, the most potent initiating signals in vitro come from mitogens such as phytohemagglutinin or pokeweed mitogen or antisera directed against the T-lymphocyte receptors (Kelso and Metcalf, 1990). For B-lymphocytes, *Staphylococcus aureus* also provides an effective inducing signal.

The mechanisms responsible for the rise in mRNA vary according to the cell type involved and possibly with the inducing signal. As discussed earlier, in some situations increased transcription of mRNA is responsible for the increase while in other cases it is achieved by a transient increase in the stability of the mRNA.

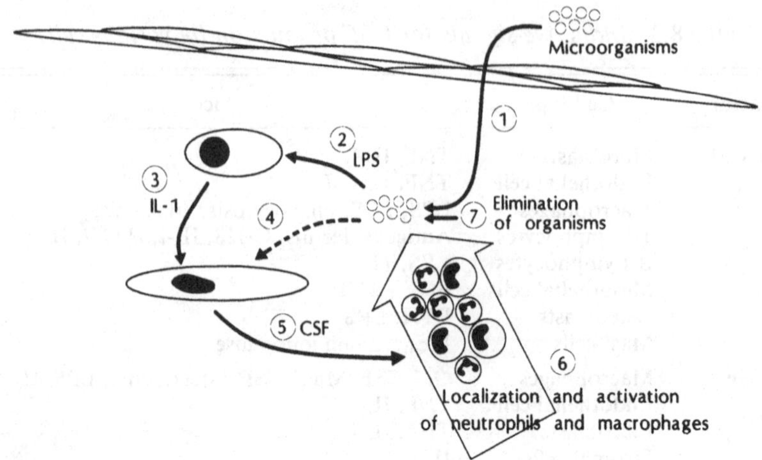


Figure 8.4. Schematic representation of possible events occurring in the rapid elimination of microorganisms entering the body (1). The microorganisms release endotoxin (LPS) that either directly activates CSF production (4) or first induces other cells (2) to produce IL-1 (3), which then initiates CSF production (5). The local CSF localizes and activates circulating neutrophils and macrophages (6) that eliminate the organisms.

The magnitude of the increases in mRNA and consequent CSF production also vary with the cell type involved. These range from two- to fourfold for endothelial cells to a thousandfold for T-lymphocytes. Increased CSF production usually begins to be detected within 3–6 hours, mRNA increases peaking usually within 15–24 hours, while CSF production can continue to rise logarithmically for at least 48 hours.

These data suggest two types of CSF response to infections. In response to a minor infection, LPS induces cells to produce IL-1, which then induces other local cells to produce CSF. This elevated CSF production is entirely local, and the low concentrations of CSFs are sufficient to control the required migration of existing cells to the local area and their subsequent activation, with elimination of the microorganisms. This whole process could be accomplished within minutes or hours with no or minimal evidence of a transient infection having occurred (Figure 8.4).

If the initial infection becomes established and results in a major local focus of infection and tissue damage, the CSF-based resistance system demonstrates its flexibility in coping with the problem. Following failure of the initial local response to suppress the infection, the local lesion provokes a massive local production of CSF that now enters the circulation. In addition, there is progressive entry of microbial products into the

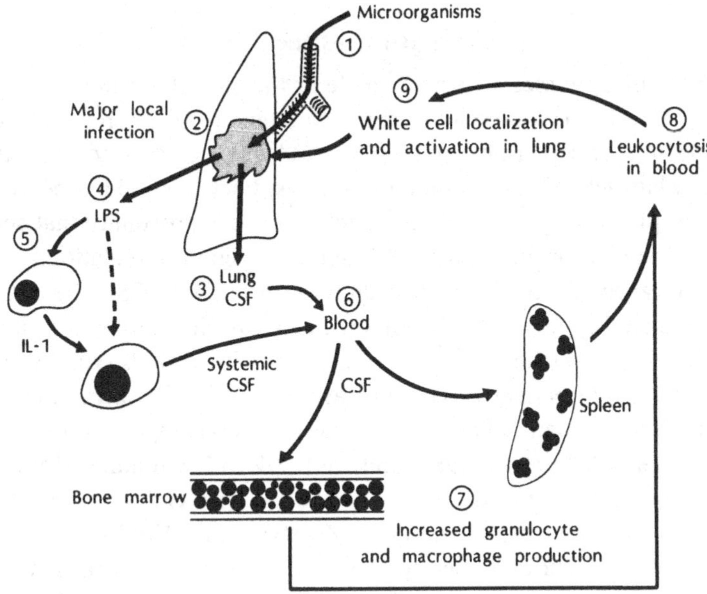


Figure 8.5. Schematic representation of possible events occurring during a major infection of lung tissue (2). Endotoxin (LPS) released by microorganisms (1) stimulates a major production of CSF in the lung (3) but LPS also enters the circulation (4) to stimulate directly, or via the induction of IL-1 (5), CSF production by many cell types. The elevated concentrations of CSF (6) stimulate the marrow and spleen to form an increased number of granulocytes and macrophages (7, 8) that are localized and activated by CSF action in the lung (9) to eliminate the infection.

circulation that would amplify the host response by stimulating the production of CSF in other tissues. This general rise in CSF levels would result in stimulation of the production of additional mature cells in the marrow and spleen. This results in a leukocytosis and the localization and activation of a massive number of neutrophils and macrophages in the local lesion to terminate the infection (Figure 8.5).

In principle, the same sequential amplification of responses might occur in immune or allergic responses or responses to tissue injury if these were of a type to initiate CSF production. The evidence from mice makes it rather unlikely that leukopenia, in the absence of infections, represents a significant inductive signal. However, if it does, the CSF responses again might either be localized in the marrow or be systemic from the outset, depending on the location of cells that monitor and respond to abnormally low white cell levels.

## Serum half-life of the CSFs

A number of estimates have been made of the half-life of intravenously injected CSF in the mouse and man. There tend to be discrepancies between estimates performed by bioassay and those performed using isotopically labeled CSF or radioimmunoassays. Each method has potential technical problems, but the discrepancies raise the possibility that some inactivation of macromolecular CSF may occur in the circulation.

In normal volunteers, after intravenous infusion of G-CSF, the G-CSF was eliminated by first-order kinetics with a mean elimination half-life of 163 minutes (Azuma et al., 1989). In patients with various types of neoplasm, some interpatient variability was noted following intravenous infusion, with elimination half-lifes in two reports ranging from 109 to 353 minutes (Gabrilove et al., 1988) and from 212 to 269 minutes (Morstyn et al., 1988). In patients injected intravenously with GM-CSF, the elimination half-life was 80–150 minutes (Morstyn et al., 1989b). The serum half-life of intravenously injected M-CSF in cancer patients ranged from 1.9 to 4.1 hours in one study (Sanda et al., 1992) and from 0.4 to 1.4 hours in another (Redman et al., 1992). In cancer patients, the elimination half-life of intravenously administered Multi-CSF was between 26 and 53 minutes (Biesma et al., 1993).

Similar results have been noted in mice injected with CSF. In mice injected with Multi-CSF, a serum half-life of 20 minutes was observed (Metcalf et al., 1986), and with GM-CSF a half-life of 35–95 minutes was observed (Metcalf et al., 1987a).

These data are in line with studies on comparable hormonal glycoproteins in indicating that the CSFs have relatively short half-lives in the circulation. Thus, there are two mechanisms allowing rapid restoration of normal hemopoiesis following removal of an inductive signal: (a) a rapid decline in mRNA levels and CSF production and (b) a relatively short serum half-life of the CSFs. Both mechanisms permit a rapid restoration of normal levels of hemopoiesis following resolution of an inducing situation.

## Clearance and degradation of the CSFs

Studies on the clearance and degradation of the CSFs have so far been performed only in mice and with suboptimal and potentially misleading $^{125}$I-labeled CSF.

A high proportion of intravenously injected radiolabeled GM-CSF, Multi-CSF, and M-CSF accumulates rapidly in the liver (Burgess and Metcalf, 1977; Bartocci et al., 1987; Metcalf and Nicola, 1988). However, the cells involved in this probable clearance and degradation may differ according to the type of CSF involved. With Multi-CSF, autoradiographic studies showed that the parenchymal cells were involved (Metcalf and Nicola, 1988), whereas with M-CSF most labeling was observed over Kupffer cells (Bartocci et al., 1987). After the intravenous injection of Multi-CSF, radiolabeled material also accumulated rapidly in the kidney with heavy labeling of Bowman's capsule cells of the glomerulus and certain renal tubule cells (Metcalf and Nicola, 1988), and these cells may play a significant role in the degradation and clearance of this factor.

As noted earlier, in vitro studies have indicated that significant consumption of M-CSF can occur by receptor-mediated internalization by macrophages, and it has been suggested that this process may be a major degradation pathway for M-CSF (Tushinski et al., 1982; Bartocci et al., 1987). Similarly, in humans the inverse relationship between the serum G-CSF levels and the number of neutrophils in the peripheral blood (Layton et al., 1989) has also suggested that receptor-mediated internalization and degradation of G-CSF by neutrophils may be significant in determining the serum half-life of G-CSF.

If most CSF production normally occurs locally and does not reach the circulation, it may be that target cell–mediated internalization is a significant component in the turnover of most CSF produced in the body (Nicola and Metcalf, 1988) (Figure 8.6). This would clearly be of major relevance in the bone marrow, where an exceptionally high number of receptor-expressing cells are located. Certainly, in cultures of bone marrow cells, added CSF is depleted relatively rapidly. If a comparable receptor-based consumption occurs in vivo, estimates of serum half-lives of CSF may have little relevance for the turnover times of CSF being produced, utilized, or degraded in local tissues such as the marrow.

On this basis, the consumption/degradation/clearance of CSF might be mainly mediated under basal conditions by receptor-mediated consumption by local target hemopoietic cells. Where significant levels of CSF circulate, as is the case for M-CSF under basal conditions, and for the other CSFs when levels are elevated in response to infections, degradation in the liver and kidney may then play a major role in eliminating CSF (Figure 8.6).

## Urine CSF levels

CSF is detected in low concentrations in the urine of normal humans. For reasons yet to be established but possibly related to the relatively high levels of plasma M-CSF, most of the CSF present in human urine appears

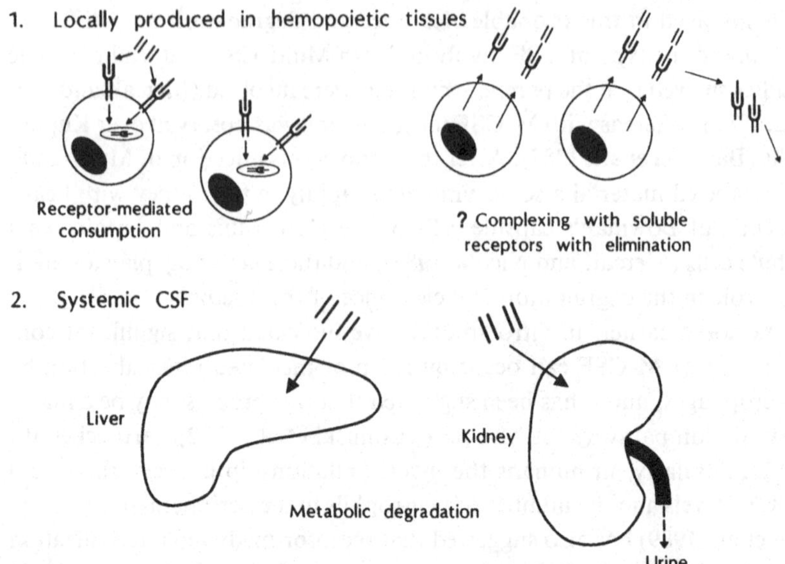


Figure 8.6. The degradation and consumption of CSF produced locally in hemopoietic tissues may occur mainly by receptor-mediated endocytosis or by complexing with secreted soluble receptors. In addition, CSF present in the circulation may also be degraded metabolically in the liver and kidney, with minor amounts being cleared to the urine.

to be M-CSF, although of lower molecular weight than the fully glycosylated form (Stanley et al., 1975). In leukemia, urinary CSF levels can be grossly elevated, but usually only in the presence of obvious systemic infections (Metcalf et al., 1971; Metcalf, 1984). In these situations, plasma and urine CSF concentrations tend to parallel each other, leading to the expectation that the kidney might clear CSF from the plasma to the urine. Bilateral nephrectomy or ureteral ligation did result in an elevation of serum CSF levels in either conventional or germ-free mice (Foster and Mirand, 1970; Sheridan and Metcalf, 1973b), but nephrectomy did not alter the basic pattern of a rise and then fall in serum CSF levels following the injection of endotoxin into mice, suggesting that renal clearance was not a major factor in determining the fall in serum CSF levels during this response (Sheridan and Metcalf, 1973b).

Urine CSF is elevated in humans in old age in the absence of an associated proteinuria (Stanley et al., 1972), but in renal disease urinary CSF levels are normal or subnormal despite elevated plasma CSF levels (Chan, 1972; Kawano et al., 1993a). Similarly, intravenously injected native GM-

CSF was detected in the urine of mice, but the amount cleared was only 0.5% of the amount injected, so clearance by the kidney appears to be only a minor pathway in determining the short half-life of plasma CSF (Metcalf, 1988b). Kidney and bladder tissue do have a capacity to produce CSF (Bradley and Metcalf, 1986; Nicola et al., 1979b; Metcalf, 1988b), so that CSF in the urine may, in part at least, be locally produced in the urinary tract.

The origin of the CSF appearing in the urine remains an unresolved problem in the basic biology of the CSFs.

## Comment

There is a general need for much more information on the physiology of hemopoietic growth factors such as the CSFs. In a situation where significant local production of CSFs occurs, information on serum CSF levels and the possible clearance of CSFs from the serum may have some value, but is likely to provide a very incomplete and often misleading picture of the concentrations of CSF available to target cells either in the marrow or in other local tissues.

It is unsatisfactory to administer CSFs clinically when information on existing tissue levels of the CSFs is so incomplete, both in normal health and in any disease state. It is beyond our present level of technology to obtain much of this information, and this aspect of the biology of hemopoietic regulators seems to have little appeal for most investigators. However, until precise information is available on these questions, we will not really understand how hemopoietic populations are actually regulated in vivo.

# 9
# Actions of the colony-stimulating factors in vivo

Two early studies were conducted on the effects of injecting into mice either embryo-conditioned medium containing CSF or semipurified human urinary M-CSF (Bradley et al., 1969; Metcalf and Stanley, 1971). The results suggested that granulocyte and macrophage formation might have been stimulated, but since the injected material was impure, the responses could not be ascribed unequivocally to the injected CSF.

Beginning in the late 1970s, extensive information was accumulated on the in vitro actions of pure CSFs before sufficient purified recombinant CSF was available for testing in vivo. These experiments produced clear expectations of the types of response that might be observed in vivo. The in vitro studies could not, of course, predict the possible occurrence of such responses as the release of cells from the marrow or population shifts between hemopoietic organs. From the in vitro data, GM-CSF and Multi-CSF were expected to be the strongest stimuli for granulocyte formation in vivo and M-CSF to be a strong stimulus for monocyte and macrophage formation.

In the long period before in vivo testing could be commenced, many critics predicted that injected CSFs would elicit no measurable responses for a variety of reasons. Some held that the CSFs were not likely to be genuine regulators, since CSF levels were very low in normal health and became elevated only during infections. Others doubted whether injected CSF could penetrate the tightly packed hemopoietic tissues of the marrow or whether the injection of a single CSF could hope to perturb significantly a homeostatic control system of obvious complexity involving many interacting regulators. It was also predicted that if CSF did elicit responses in vivo, such responses would terminate rapidly when available progenitor cells became depleted and, further, that by placing proliferative pressure on granulocyte and macrophage formation, available stem cells might become preoccupied with the formation of precursors for these cells, leading to the development of anemia or thrombocytopenia.

In retrospect, these criticisms may seem fanciful. However, when the first in vivo tests on CSFs were undertaken in the mid-1980s, there had been little experience with the consequences of injecting hemopoietic regulators in vivo, other than with erythropoietin, and there was a generally skeptical attitude, at least among those not likely to undertake the initial experiments.

## Routes of injection

Initially, the intravenous route was used in both mice and humans, in part to establish the half-life of the injected CSF and thereby establish a suitable dosage schedule. However, the intraperitoneal injection of mice is more easily accomplished when repeated injections are required, and these achieved somewhat more sustained elevations of circulating CSF (Metcalf et al., 1986a).

Ultimately, in both mice and humans, subcutaneous injections were superior in producing even more sustained elevations, based on the slower entry of the injected CSF into the circulation (Morstyn et al., 1989b; Cebon et al., 1990a). Although intraperitoneal injections are still sometimes used for convenience in mice, subcutaneous injections have become the most common method for administering CSF in larger animals and humans.

It was recognized that a single injection of CSF, even by the subcutaneous route, achieved high, circulating CSF levels for only 4–6 hours. In most studies with humans or animals, one or two injections per day have been practicable, if suboptimal, for delivering CSF. Some studies have been performed on animals with implanted osmotic pumps, although the continuing effectiveness of these after placement in vivo has been difficult to establish, and their large size has made them somewhat unpopular.

## Type of CSF for injection

The demonstration that both glycosylated and nonglycosylated recombinant CSFs had the same range of biological actions in vitro and, in general the same specific biological activity per milligram protein, as the native CSFs allowed in vivo studies using recombinant CSFs to be initiated. It was known by this point that nonglycosylated erythropoietin was ineffective in stimulating erythropoiesis in vivo because of accelerated clearance of the material, which raised the concern that recombinant CSF of bacterial origin might be inactive in vivo. In the event, all of the initial studies were performed with nonglycosylated recombinant CSF, and no differences have subsequently been noted between the in vivo actions of glycosylated and nonglycosylated forms. Even the half-lives of the two types of recombinant material have been surprisingly similar.

## In vivo effects of injected CSF

The first in vivo studies were performed in mice using murine Multi-CSF and GM-CSF and in humans using GM-CSF and G-CSF. These were followed by studies in both species using the other CSFs. It is more convenient to describe the in vivo effects by organ system rather than by the individual type of CSF.

### *Blood cell changes*

Injection of each CSF elevates the levels of mature cells in the peripheral blood. These elevations are dose-related in magnitude and can be sustained for as long as CSF injections are continued. Following cessation of injections, white cell levels usually fall to preinjection levels within 24–48 hours.

The types of blood cells elevated vary with the CSF used and qualitatively closely follow expectations from their actions in stimulating colony formation in vitro. However, contrary to expectations from its low in vitro colony-stimulating activity, G-CSF proved to be the most potent elevator of granulocyte levels in terms of both activity per dose injected and the absolute number achieved. Thus, in the dose range of 5–30 μg/kg per day in humans, it is possible for G-CSF injections to achieve neutrophil levels of 20,000–50,000 per microliter (Morstyn et al., 1988; Lindemann et al., 1989), whereas GM-CSF and Multi-CSF, when administered in comparable dose ranges, more typically elevate granulocytes to only lower levels (Lieschke et al., 1989; Ganser et al., 1990a,b) (Figure 9.1).

G-CSF has a weak capacity to elevate monocyte levels but has no effect on eosinophil, erythroid, or platelet levels. Both GM-CSF and Multi-CSF can elevate granulocyte, monocyte, and eosinophil levels.

Responses in mice to the injection of CSF follow a similar pattern to that seen in humans. Injection of G-CSF induces a clear dose-related neutrophil leukocytosis (Fujisawa et al., 1986; Tamura et al., 1987; Welte et al., 1987) (Figure 9.2), and the injection of similar doses of GM-CSF or Multi-CSF, while inducing quantitatively smaller neutrophil responses, in addition has some effect on the levels of eosinophils and monocytes (Metcalf et al., 1986a; Metcalf et al., 1987a,b). Daily injections in mice

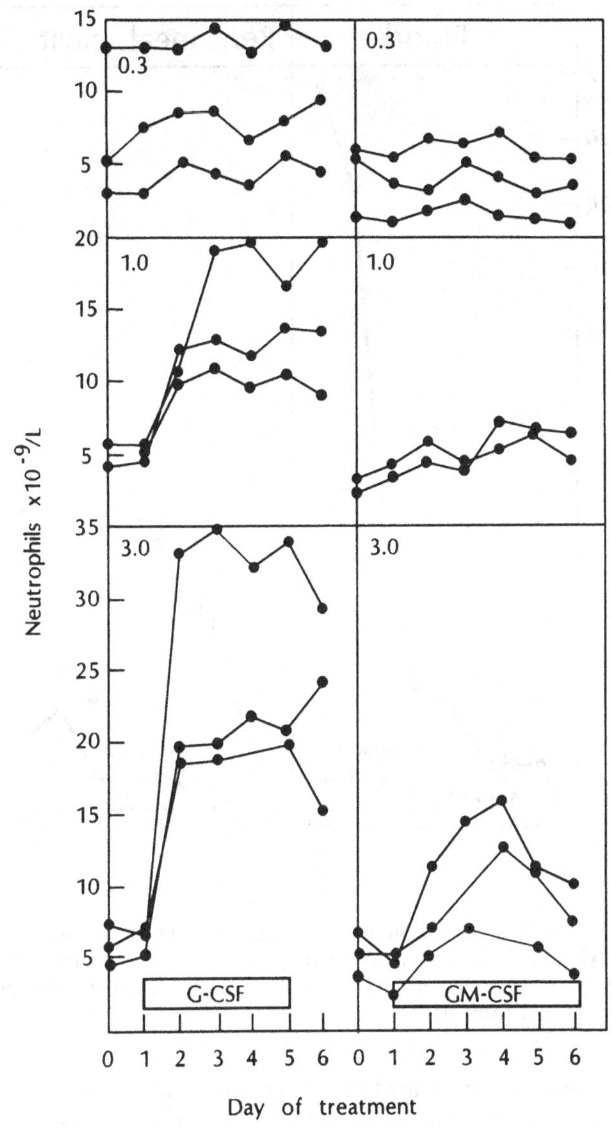


Figure 9.1. Changes in neutrophil levels in groups of three patients receiving 5 days of injections of 0.3, 1.0, or 3.0 $\mu$g/kg of G-CSF or GM-CSF. Note that G-CSF is more effective than GM-CSF in increasing neutrophil levels at comparable doses. (Reproduced with permission from Morstyn et al., 1989a.)

of up to 1 $\mu$g M-CSF did not alter the number of peripheral blood cells, but with doses above 10 $\mu$g daily a selective monocytosis was stimulated (Hume et al., 1988; Chikkappa et al., 1989). A similar selective monocytic response to M-CSF has been described in humans (Redman et al., 1992).

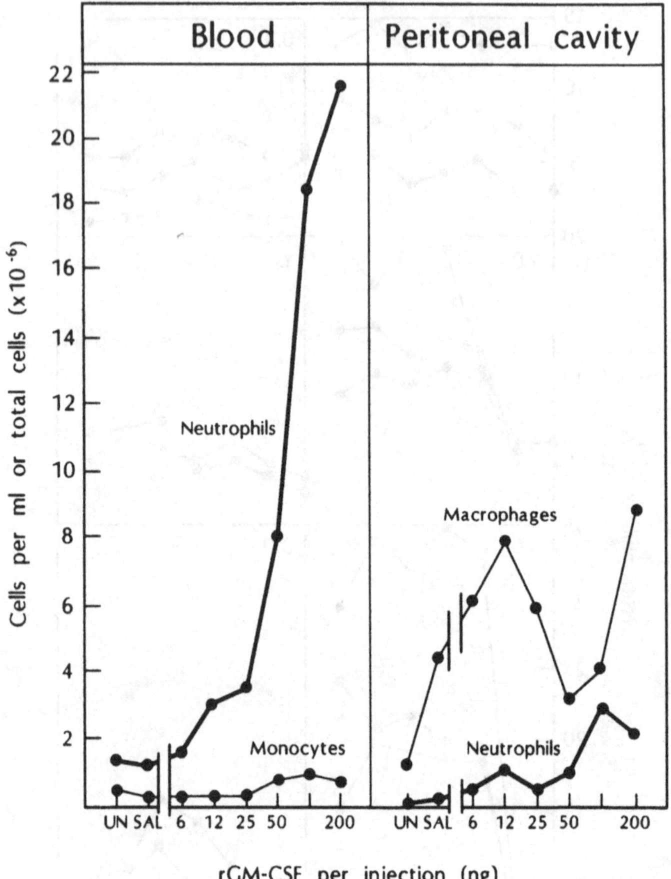


Figure 9.2. Dose-related elevation of neutrophils in mice receiving intraperitoneal injections of G-CSF for 6 days. Note the only minor increase of monocytes in the blood and at the site of injection in the peritoneal cavity. UN denotes uninjected; SAL, saline-injected controls.

The early sequence of events following the injection of CSF is best documented from studies in humans. Initially after the injection of G-CSF or GM-CSF, there is a transient fall in granulocyte levels (Morstyn et al., 1988; Lieschke et al., 1989), possibly based on an associated increased expression or affinity of various adhesion molecules such as CD11b or LAM-1 (Socinski et al., 1988b; Spertini et al., 1991). This fall would probably then be due to margination of circulating cells by adherence to the vascular endothelium, possibly with some enhanced exit of cells to the tissues.

This initial phase is superseded within 4–5 hours by a rise in granulocyte levels above preinjection values, based on CSF-accelerated release

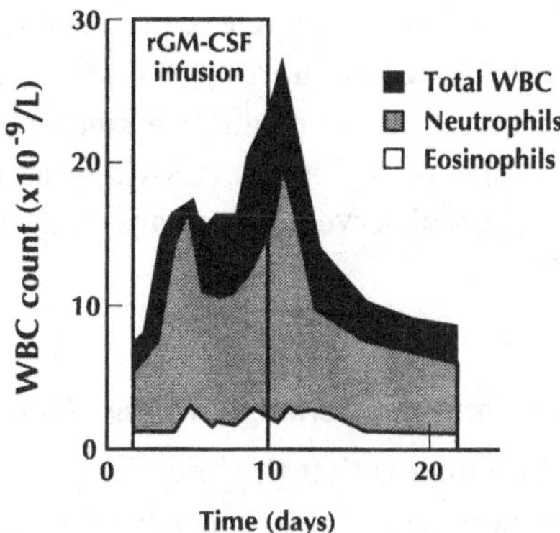


Figure 9.3. Sequential changes in blood cell levels induced in patients by the intravenous infusion of GM-CSF. Note the biphasic response of neutrophil levels as well as some rise in eosinophil levels. WBC denotes white blood cells. (Reproduced with permission from Steward et al., 1989.)

of mature cells from the marrow coupled with an acceleration of maturation (Lord et al., 1989). Thereafter, a definitive rise occurs based on a CSF-stimulated increase in the total number and cycling status of granulocyte-macrophage populations in the marrow and spleen with a consequent absolute increase in the production of mature cells. In some cases this sequence results in a double peak in the curve of increasing granulocyte levels in the peripheral blood (Steward et al., 1989) (Figure 9.3). No change has been observed in the half-life of mature neutrophils in the blood after the administration of G-CSF, and this seems not to be a mechanism contributing to the increase in peripheral blood neutrophils.

The rise in granulocyte and monocyte levels in humans usually reaches a plateau within 5–10 days, the absolute level of the plateau depending on the CSF dose used. With continuing CSF injections, levels of white cells are maintained for as long as injections are continued.

Responsiveness to G-CSF is similar in humans and in mice, but responses to GM-CSF and Multi-CSF at corresponding dose levels appear to be greater in primates and humans than in mice (Metcalf et al., 1986a,b).

It is more apparent with G-CSF than with the other three CSFs that CSFs do not simply elevate the number of fully mature cells in the peripheral blood. Some enlargement of the granulocytes appearing in the peripheral blood, with some abnormality in granules and nuclear lobulation, has been noted in responses to G-CSF (Kerrigan et al., 1989); immature band forms, metamyelocytes, and, less frequently, myelocytes can also appear in the blood during CSF-induced responses (Morstyn et al., 1988).

No significant changes occur in platelet or red cell levels following the injection of G-CSF or GM-CSF in short-term studies in mice and humans. The injection of Multi-CSF in mice causes a small elevation in platelet levels evident after 5 days of injections (Carrington et al., 1991), and a similar response has been observed in humans (Ganser et al., 1990a,b; D'Hondt et al., 1993).

### *Progenitor cell changes in the blood*

It was first observed in humans that the injection of G-CSF or GM-CSF causes a remarkable increase in the frequency of progenitor cells in the peripheral blood, in which normally few progenitors are present. In response to G-CSF, levels can rise more than a hundredfold, so that the frequency of granulocyte-macrophage progenitor cells can equal or exceed that in the bone marrow (Dührsen et al., 1988). Similar but smaller increases have been observed in response to the injection of GM-CSF or Multi-CSF (Socinski et al., 1988a; Ottmann et al., 1990; Villeval et al., 1990).

Peak levels of progenitor cells are achieved in response to G-CSF within 5–6 days with a possible decline occurring after this time (DeLuca et al., 1992) (Figure 9.4). The remarkable feature of this response is that it is not restricted to progenitor cells whose further proliferation is responsive to stimulation by G-CSF. Instead, comparable increases occur in committed

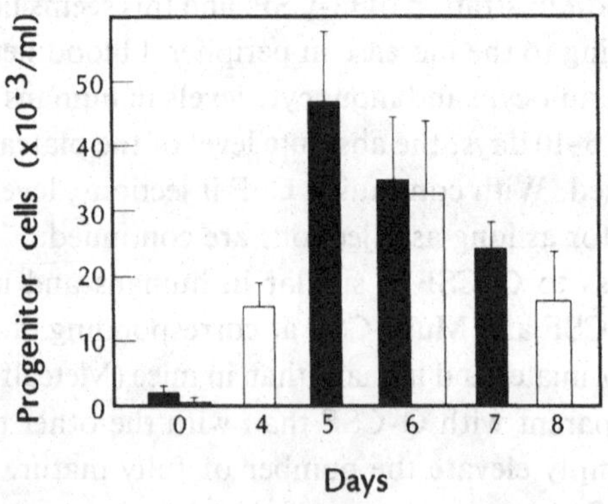


Figure 9.4. Increases in the progenitor cell content of the blood of patients injected with 12 $\mu$g/kg per day of G-CSF for 8 days. Solid columns represent data from sequential aphoreses performed on days 5, 6, and 7. Open columns are data from aphoreses performed on days 4, 6, and 8. (Reproduced with permission from DeLuca et al., 1992.)

macrophage, eosinophil, megakaryocytic, and erythroid progenitors, as well as in multipotential progenitors and blast colony-forming cells. Studies in mice injected with G-CSF have confirmed increases in the number of progenitor cells, as well as in CFU-S and the repopulating capacity in the blood (Bungart et al., 1990; Molineux et al., 1990a,b). However, studies in this laboratory have indicated that the various progenitor cells appearing in the blood are not a random sample of those in the marrow – megakaryocytic colony-forming cells being overrepresented and the relative frequency of other progenitors varying widely with time during the response (Roberts and Metcalf, in press). The exact mechanisms responsible for the increase in peripheral blood progenitor cells are unknown, but it is not likely to be due simply to an induced random egress of precursors from the bone marrow.

### *Bone marrow changes*

The changes induced by injected CSF have been documented in more detail in the mouse, where the absolute number of marrow cells can be determined. The injection of 200 ng daily for 6 days (a dose of ~8 μg/kg in humans) of GM-CSF or Multi-CSF slightly reduces the total number of bone marrow cells (Metcalf et al., 1986a, 1987b). This effect is more marked with the administration of G-CSF, where a 50% reduction in the total number of cells is observed after 5 days (Pojda et al., 1990). These decreases are to some extent compensated for by an increase in the relative frequency of granulocytes and monocytes, seen in most extreme form in mice injected with G-CSF, where the percentage of granulocytes increases from a norm of 20–50% to 80–90% (Pojda et al., 1990) (Figure 9.5). This rise in the relative frequency of granulocytes occurs at the expense of marrow lymphocytes and nucleated erythroid cells, which fall, particularly in G-CSF-injected mice, to very low levels. The injection of comparable doses of M-CSF induces relatively little change in marrow cellularity or composition.

Changes in the number of progenitor cells tend to parallel those in total cell number, remaining relatively constant in mice injected with Multi-CSF or GM-CSF but falling almost fivefold in mice injected with very high G-CSF doses. In mice injected with G-CSF, there is also a significant decrease in the marrow content of CFU-S (Pojda et al., 1990).

No data are available from normal humans on changes in absolute cell number in the marrow following the injection of CSF, and the increased cellularity observed in patients injected with G-CSF or GM-CSF

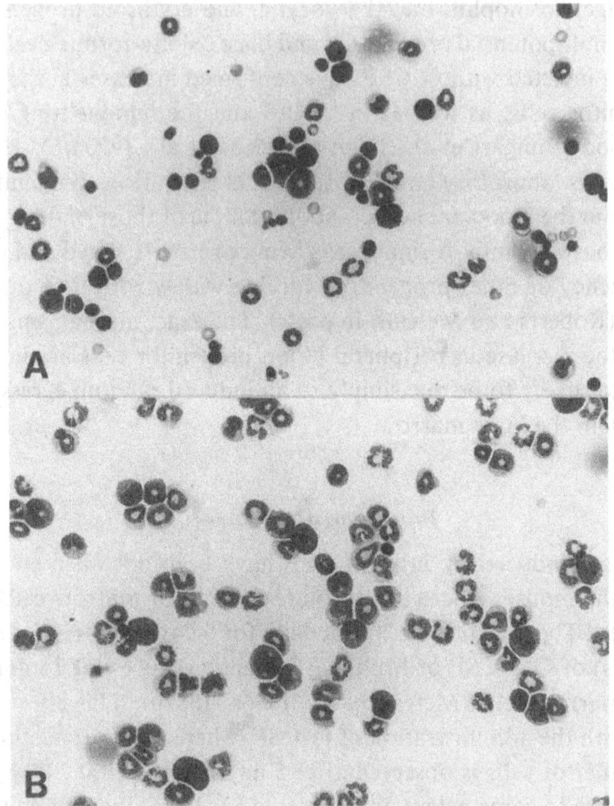


Figure 9.5. Morphology of bone marrow populations from (A) control mice and (B) mice injected daily for 5 days with 5 $\mu$g G-CSF. Note that G-CSF induces a marked increase in the frequency of immature and mature granulocytes and depletes the population of lymphocytes and nucleated erythroid cells. Cytocentrifuge preparations were stained with May Grunwald-Giemsa.

(see clinical section later) is a response observed in marrow-depleted patients where the CSF is accelerating regeneration. In patients injected with G-CSF, the frequency of committed progenitor cells in marrow populations may decrease slightly, increase slightly, or remain unaltered (Dührsen et al., 1988).

In mice and humans, the injection of G-CSF increases the proportion of early granulocytes in cell cycle (Lord et al., 1989, 1991), with an associated acceleration of maturation and release of mature cells from the bone marrow. This combination of changes could enable the production of sufficient additional mature neutrophils to account for the increased number of cells in the peripheral blood.

Based on changes in marrow alone, it could be concluded that the CSFs were inducing an increased production of maturing granulocytes and monocytes, often at the expense of depleting the marrow of stem cells and committed progenitor cells. However, changes in marrow offer an incomplete view of total body hemopoiesis because, to a large degree, these deficits are compensated for by corresponding increases in hemopoiesis in the spleen.

### *Spleen changes*

The changes in spleen induced by CSF injections have been well documented in mice, and although they have not been monitored in humans, similar changes almost certainly occur because of the frequent development of slight but clinically detected spleen enlargement.

In mice, the administration of each CSF for 6 days induces an increase in spleen size and cellularity, the effects being the greatest for G-CSF (up to 3-fold) and then, in sequence, Multi-CSF, GM-CSF, and M-CSF. In mice injected for 5 days with G-CSF, GM-CSF, or Multi-CSF, the increased cellularity is accompanied by an increase in the percentage of granulocytes and macrophage cells at various maturation stages and a 4- to 140-fold increase in the total number of stem and progenitor cells of all lineages (Metcalf et al., 1986a, 1987b; Pojda et al., 1990; Roberts and Metcalf, in press). In this regard, the changes in hemopoietic precursor cells in the spleen parallel those in peripheral blood, and the cell populations in both locations may well be in a certain equilibrium.

A striking change, seen with the injection of GM-CSF and Multi-CSF but most prominently with G-CSF, is an increase in the percentage of nucleated erythroid cells from a normal level of 1–5% to more than 60%. Calculations show that this increase essentially balances the decrease in marrow erythroid populations and allows red cell production to be maintained at nearly normal levels (Molineux et al., 1990a; de Haan et al., 1992). No mechanism has been advanced to account for the dramatic relocation of erythroid populations from the marrow to the spleen. However, it is a phenomenon seen in mice in a number of situations where granulopoiesis becomes excessive in the marrow, such as during infections, after the injection of endotoxin, and in certain transgenic mice or mice repopulated by CSF-producing cells. The population switch may be based either

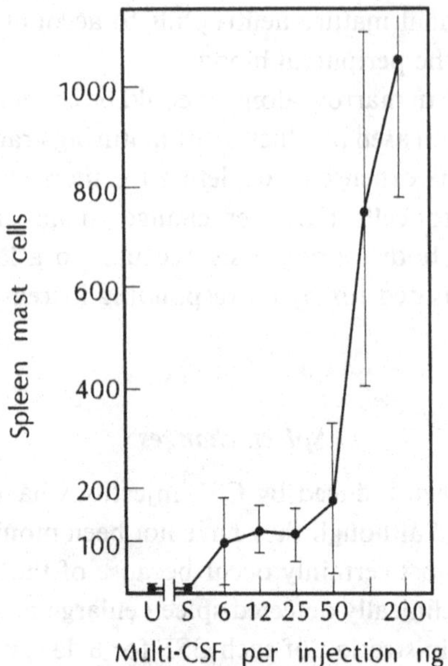


Figure 9.6. Increase in mast cells in the spleen of C57BL mice injected intraperitoneally three times daily for 6 days with various doses of Multi-CSF. U denotes uninjected; S, saline-injected. (Reproduced with permission from Metcalf et al., 1987a.)

on changes that result in the stroma no longer supporting erythropoiesis or on some mutual antagonism between these two hemopoietic populations.

In mice injected with Multi-CSF, the spleen exhibits a characteristic increase in small, incompletely granulated mast cells in the red pulp (Metcalf et al., 1986a). This population is quantitatively the most responsive of any in the body to stimulation by Multi-CSF, and rises in total spleen mast cells can be more than a hundredfold (Metcalf et al., 1987a) (Figure 9.6). An increase in the spleen content of megakaryocytes has also been noted in mice injected with GM-CSF or Multi-CSF (Metcalf et al., 1986a, 1987b).

### *Liver changes*

Changes in the liver parallel to a minor degree those in the spleen. During the height of a CSF-induced response, additional granulocytes can be present in the sinusoids, and most frequently in mice injected with Multi-CSF, small hemopoietic foci of granulocytes, monocytes, eosinophil cells, erythroid cells, and megakaryocytes can develop (Metcalf et al., 1986a).

In mice stimulated by GM-CSF or Multi-CSF, there is also an increase in the number of resident macrophages (Kupffer cells) in the liver (Metcalf et al., 1986a, 1987b).

### *Peritoneal cell population changes*

When CSF is injected intraperitoneally in mice, a pronounced increase occurs in the total number of peritoneal cells. In terms of absolute effect, GM-CSF is the most active of the CSFs, followed in order by Multi-CSF, G-CSF, and M-CSF (Metcalf, 1991a) (Figure 9.7). In mice injected with GM-CSF, the major cells involved are macrophages, which can increase 20-fold, but increases of lesser magnitude also occur with eosinophils and neutrophils. In the initial phase of a GM-CSF-induced response, there is a clear dose-related rise in mitotic activity of peritoneal macrophages, strongly suggesting that most of the increase in cell numbers occurs from local mitotic activity (Metcalf et al., 1987b). This cannot be the basis for changes in the number of eosinophils or granulocytes, since the cells appearing in the peritoneal cavity are exclusively postmitotic in type. Systemic injection of GM-CSF can also elevate peritoneal macrophage levels, but not to such high levels as are achieved by local intraperitoneal injection.

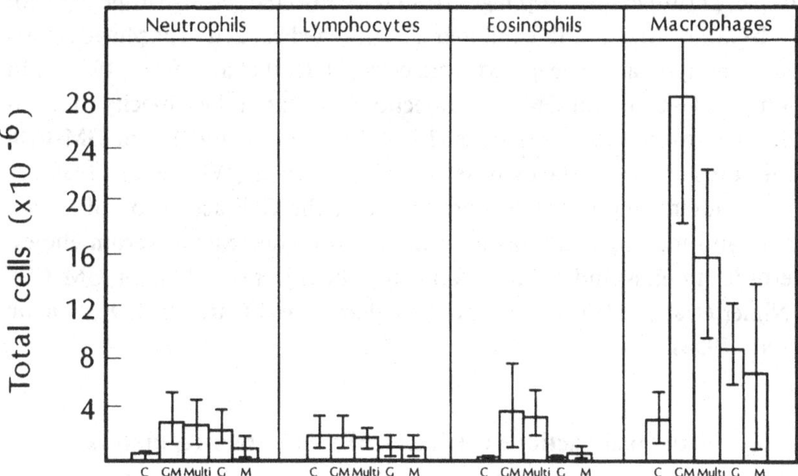


Figure 9.7. Comparative analysis of the capacity of various CSFs injected intraperitoneally three times daily for 6 days to elevate the number of cells in the peritoneal cavity of mice. Mice were injected with carrier solution (C) or 100 ng GM-CSF (GM), Multi-CSF (Multi), G-CSF (G), or M-CSF (M). (Reproduced with permission from Metcalf, 1991a.)

### *Changes in other organs*

Few changes have been noted in nonhemopoietic organs following the injection of CSF into normal animals other than minor increases in granulocytes and macrophages in various tissues such as the lung and the hilar regions of lymph nodes and, in the case of Multi-CSF, a two- to fourfold rise in mast cells in various tissues (Metcalf et al., 1986a, 1987b; Pojda et al., 1990).

One study of mice injected for 7 days with Multi-CSF revealed an increase in mitotic activity in epithelial crypt cells from the small and large intestine (Saxena et al., 1993), suggesting some direct or indirect action of Multi-CSF on these cells.

It is notable that regardless of the dose used, CSF-induced stimulation of hemopoiesis does not result in the development of hemopoietic tissue or the gross accumulation of mature blood cells in nonhemopoietic tissues, or in any obvious organ pathology.

### *Activation of mature cells*

In both mice and humans, the injection of CSF induces a measurable activation of various functions of mature granulocytes or monocytes. For example, peritoneal macrophages from mice injected intraperitoneally with GM-CSF or Multi-CSF exhibited a heightened capacity for phagocytosis of antibody-coated sheep erythroid cells (Metcalf et al., 1986a, 1987b). In humans, G-CSF and GM-CSF injections increased the capacity of granulocytes to produce superoxide (Lindemann et al., 1989), and GM-CSF injections increased the cytotoxicity of monocytes (Wing et al., 1989).

One interesting possible consequence of the CSF activation of monocytes and macrophages has been the reported decrease in serum cholesterol in humans and animals following the injection of either GM-CSF (Nimer et al., 1988a) or M-CSF (Stoudemire and Garnick, 1991; Schaub et al., 1994).

## Synergistic actions between CSFs and other regulators

It is evident in the mouse that each CSF induces a quite distinct pattern of hemopoietic responses, the two extremes being the selective increase of blood granulocytes induced by G-CSF and the rise in peritoneal macrophages induced by GM-CSF. In mice injected with a combination of G-CSF and GM-CSF, both responses are retained and some synergy is

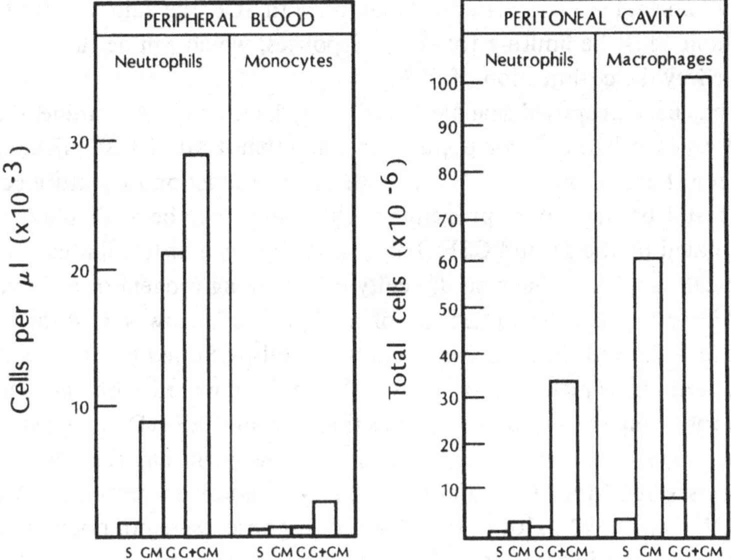


Figure 9.8. A potentiated response in blood or peritoneal cells occurs in mice injected with 100 ng G-CSF combined with 100 ng GM-CSF. Note the elevated cell numbers compared with those in mice injected with saline (S) or with GM-CSF (GM) or G-CSF (G) alone.

evident (D. Metcalf, unpublished data) (Figure 9.8). This parallels the phenomena documented in vitro, but extensive studies have not been performed in vivo on various possible CSF combinations.

As noted earlier, G-CSF, GM-CSF, or Multi-CSF can greatly amplify the production of progenitor cells from stem cells in vitro if acting in collaboration with SCF and/or IL-12. A characteristic of this process is the generation of a broad range of progenitor cells even as a consequence of the SCF–G-CSF interaction. This broad type of response may be the reason why none of the CSFs, on injection in vivo, induces a significant perturbation in the relative proportions of various progenitor cells in marrow populations.

The elevation of spleen and blood progenitor cells by injected G-CSF may well require a significant interaction with SCF. In studies using $W^v$ mice that lack SCF receptors and Sl mice lacking the capacity to produce SCF, the injection of G-CSF produced only a reduced granulocytic response (Cynshi et al., 1991). Conversely, the combination of SCF with G-CSF enhances the resulting increase in blood granulocytes and progenitor cells (Briddell et al., 1993). This suggests that even if G-CSF responses in vivo normally involve some interaction with SCF, the amounts of SCF available must be limiting for these responses, which can be further enhanced by the co-injection of SCF.

It has been proposed that Multi-CSF may have its most prominent actions on early hemopoietic populations, and that if Multi-CSF injections precede those of another CSF, an enhanced production of mature cells will result because more progenitor cells would then be available to be stimulated by the second CSF. This proposition is a little dubious, since stem cells appear to have no difficulty in sustaining progenitor cell numbers in response to the injection of a single CSF. However, studies in monkeys showed that the preinjection of Multi-CSF led to significantly enhanced subsequent responses to GM-CSF compared with responses seen following the simultaneous injection of both CSFs (Donahue et al., 1988; Mayer et al., 1989), and a similar enhancement has been noted in humans when Multi-CSF and GM-CSF were administered sequentially (Frisch et al., 1992). However, enhanced responses were not noted in another such trial in primates following radiation-induced marrow aplasia (Farese et al., 1993).

In general, such sequential administration of the CSFs seems of dubious value in leukopenic states because the greatest risk of infection occurs during the initial nadir of the leukopenia, and it would matter little whether a delayed enhancement of leukocyte levels could be achieved by such sequential administration of CSFs.

## Comment

The history of tissue culture contains many examples of phenomena detected in vitro that proved not to be demonstrable in vivo because they were based on various unrecognized in vitro artifacts. During the 20-year period when all studies on the CSFs were, of necessity, in vitro, there was the ever-present possibility that the phenomena being observed, although highly reproducible, were nonetheless in vitro artifacts not addressing the true regulatory biology of the populations in vivo.

It is remarkable how accurately the in vitro studies predicted the actions of the CSFs in vivo, although obviously certain responses such as the release of cells from the marrow or redistribution of populations between different organs could not be analyzed in vitro. Where discrepancies exist between in vitro and subsequent in vivo data, these are mainly quantitative, such as the unanticipated strength of the action of G-CSF on granulopoiesis in vivo.

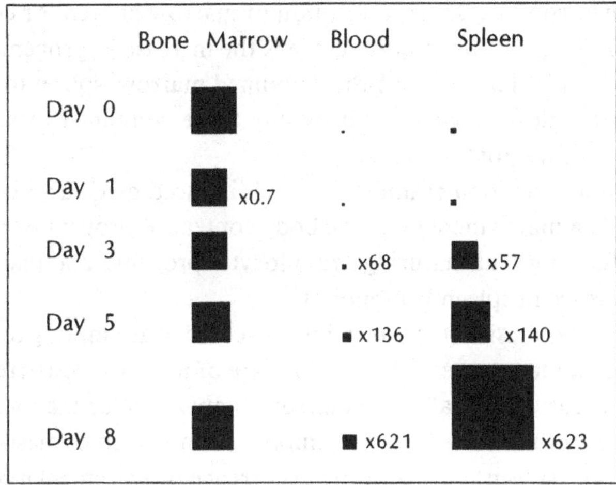


Figure 9.9. Scale drawing indicating the calculated total granulocyte-macrophage progenitor cells in the marrow, blood, and spleen in mice at intervals after the daily injection in two divided doses of 5 $\mu$g G-CSF. For each organ, the numbers indicate the fold elevation of the population compared with that in uninjected (day 0) mice. For example, by day 3, the spleen content of progenitor cells was 57 times that of uninjected mice.

The actions of the CSFs on cell proliferation and functional activation have been confirmed in vivo, as has the likely action of the CSFs on maturation induction. Differentiation commitment is a complex process that may not be capable of analysis in vivo. The in vitro action of the CSFs on cell viability remains the one aspect of CSF action yet to be established in vivo.

The overall proliferative effects of CSF injection on granulocyte-macrophage populations can best be appreciated from studies in mice, but this requires a consideration of all the relevant hemopoietic organs (Roberts and Metcalf, in press). Figure 9.9 is a scale drawing representing the total number of granulocyte-macrophage progenitor cells in marrow, blood, and spleen of mice responding to the injection of 5 $\mu$g G-CSF per day. Figures for the liver content of progenitor cells should be added to these data – for example, an additional 15% to the day 5 data shown. An essentially similar figure could be plotted for the total number of immature or mature granulocytes.

What the figure reveals is that most progenitor cells normally reside in the marrow and that the initial effect of G-CSF is to deplete the number of these cells, in part at least by accelerating the production and release of mature neutrophils. Some restoration of marrow progenitor cells subsequently occurs, but the major change is the increase in progenitor cells in the spleen such that by day 5 the combined marrow–spleen total is almost twice the normal value, and by day 8 the combined total greatly exceeds the normal total number.

Thus, the rise in blood granulocyte levels induced by G-CSF is eventually based on a major increase in the body content of progenitor cells and their proliferating and maturing granulocytic progeny, due mainly to a massive increase in spleen hemopoiesis.

This figure emphasizes the limitations involved in attempting to analyze responses in humans, where observations are of necessity restricted to the blood and occasional qualitative marrow analyses. Mice may well differ from humans in the magnitude of amplification of hemopoiesis elicited by CSFs in the spleen, but from the occurrence of spleen enlargement it is likely that the spleen does play an important role in human responses, even if much of that response involves an increase in the extensiveness of marrow hemopoiesis.

The overall conclusion from these observations is that when eliciting rises in the number of mature cells in the blood, the CSFs do not merely accelerate the maturation of existing marrow populations; they also induce major increases in the number of precursor and immature cells in the body.

# 10

# Role of the colony-stimulating factors in basal hemopoiesis

As noted in Chapter 8, early studies on the colony-stimulating factors documented that they are present in detectable amounts in the tissues and that their levels can rise dramatically in situations requiring an increased number of white cells. Subsequent work using the injection of recombinant CSFs in vivo certified their capacity to increase white cell production and function. While these data establish that the CSFs *can* regulate white cell production and function in vivo, they do not prove that the CSFs *do* function as important regulators of the basal production of these cells. The objection has been raised that levels of CSF in the serum or tissues of normal individuals are very low and become readily detectable only during infections. The argument has been advanced, therefore, that the CSFs might merely be "emergency" molecules, serving to enhance white cell production during infections, and that the production of basal levels of white cells in normal health is achieved by some other regulatory system.

Such criticisms can be countered in part by the fact that the CSFs are the strongest and most active stimuli for the formation of granulocytes and macrophages in vitro and by the data indicating that even when stromal cells support hemopoiesis, this process is associated with the production of CSFs by the stromal cells. Nevertheless, to prove formally that the CSFs are involved in the basal regulation of granulocyte and macrophage production, studies are required in which existing CSFs have been neutralized by the administration of antibodies or in which the various CSF genes have been inactivated. Such suppression studies might also provide important information on the consequences of CSF suppression on resistance to infections.

## In vivo effects of CSF suppression

While the data on the consequences of CSF suppression remain incomplete, there is already sufficient evidence to support the conclusion that the CSFs are required for the basal production of granulocytes and/or macrophages.

### *G-CSF*

Hammond et al. (1991) noted that dogs injected with human G-CSF developed neutralizing antibodies to the human G-CSF that cross-neutralized canine G-CSF. Following the development of such antibodies, the dogs developed neutropenia, and comparable neutropenia could be induced in other dogs by the injection of antibody-containing serum. The conclusion from these studies is that G-CSF is necessary to maintain the production of normal levels of neutrophils.

A similar conclusion has been reached in studies in progress with mice developed from embryonic stem cells in which the G-CSF gene had been inactivated by homologous recombination (G. Lieschke and D. Metcalf, unpublished data). Mice with a homozygous inactivation of the G-CSF gene exhibit normal fertility and growth, but their tissues have no capacity to produce G-CSF. In young adult mice, circulating neutrophil levels were only 10% of normal, and in the bone marrow there was a 50% reduction of granulocyte-macrophage progenitor cells as well as immature and mature granulocytes. These studies also indicate that G-CSF must be a major regulator of neutrophil production in normal animals. However, because neutrophil production continued to occur, albeit at a reduced level, there must be other mechanisms that stimulate granulocyte formation.

### *GM-CSF*

Studies on comparable mice with homozygous inactivation of the GM-CSF gene have revealed a more subtle series of changes (Dranoff et al., 1994; Stanley et al., 1994). Litter size and growth rates were normal, and the mice developed as apparently healthy young adult animals. Although the tissues failed to produce GM-CSF, the mice showed normal white cell levels and normal cellularity and progenitor cell content in the bone marrow, spleen, and peritoneal cavity. However, these mice exhibited an increased susceptibility to subclinical lung infections of bacterial or fungal type associated with the accumulation of surfactant lipids and proteinaceous fluid, as well as abnormal macrophages in the alveoli, with foci of B- and T-lymphocytes around the bronchi and major lung vessels. The lung lesions closely resemble those of the human disease alveolar proteinosis and appear to be due to inadequate functional activity of the alveolar macrophages. These observations also indicate that GM-CSF is required for normal resistance to lung infections in mice when there is exposure to suitable microorganisms. The consistent abnormalities noted in the lungs of mice with inactivation of the GM-CSF gene, despite the presence of macrophages in this tissue, suggests that normally GM-CSF is required to maintain macrophages in an adequate functional state. Further analysis of such mice has shown that they sometimes exhibit a significant reduction in dendritic cells in the lymph nodes and spleen (K. Shortman, D. Metcalf, and G. Lieschke, unpublished data). The possible defect in dendritic cells is in accord with the special role noted for GM-CSF in generating dendritic cells from marrow precursors in vitro and may provide a second basis for the defective resistance to infections exhibited in these mice. Since thymic dendritic cells appeared normal in mice with GM-CSF gene inactivation, it is evident that differing subsets of dendritic cells exist, but those of the lymph nodes and spleen may depend on GM-CSF stimulation in normal life.

## *M-CSF*

The necessary role played by M-CSF has been documented from studies on mice with the congenital defect of osteopetrosis (op/op), a disease state in which there is a defect in some macrophage populations, in particular in osteoclasts, cells of macrophage derivation. The defect in monocyte-macrophages is selective, being severe in the blood, peritoneal cavity, and marginal sinuses of the spleen and lymph nodes with a much less evident defect in the thymus, spleen red pulp, lymph node medulla, liver, lung, and brain (Witmer-Pack et al., 1993). The mice exhibit a failure of teeth eruption and an overgrowth of bone formation, leading to loss of hemopoietic cells from the marrow. There is a compensatory rise in granulocyte-macrophage progenitor cells in the spleen but still a threefold reduction in the total number of progenitor cells and a more severe lack of stem cells (Wiktor-Jedrzejczak et al., 1992).

The op/op gene responsible for this defect was localized to chromosome 3 in the region subsequently recognized to contain the M-CSF gene. Sequencing of the M-CSF gene in op/op mice revealed the presence of an additional thymidine nucleotide in the sequence, leading to an inactivating frameshift in the remaining sequence with an inability to transcribe M-CSF mRNA and an inability of op/op cells to produce M-CSF (Yoshida et al., 1990). The injection of M-CSF into op/op mice cured the defects in macrophage and osteoclast populations, stimulated teeth eruption, and reversed the osteopetrotic bone structure (Felix et al., 1990; Kodama et al., 1991; Wiktor-Jedrzejczak et al., 1991). From this evidence, it can be concluded that M-CSF is mandatory for the formation of osteoclasts and some macrophages. Again, since such mice are not totally devoid of monocytes or macrophages, it is evident that the formation of some subsets of these cells must be regulated by other means. The distribution and phenotype of dendritic cells appears normal in op/op mice, confirming studies indicating that GM-CSF, but not M-CSF, is involved in their regulation (Takahashi et al., 1993).

In line with the evidence linking M-CSF with trophoblastic cell function, homozygous op/op matings were consistently infertile. Male op/op mice exhibited nearly normal fertility, so the defect appears to be maternal. However, the studies showed that fetus-derived M-CSF or male seminal fluid M-CSF can partially compensate for the absence of maternal M-CSF (Pollard et al., 1991).

Studies on mice in which both the GM-CSF and M-CSF genes have been inactivated indicate that they exhibit both the lung abnormalities of GM-CSF-inactivated mice and the bone abnormalities of M-CSF-inactivated mice. However, the lung lesions are more severe, all mice showing patchy or complete consolidation by pneumonia that causes premature death (Lieschke et al., 1994). This indicates that M-CSF is also necessary to regulate the functional activity of macrophages in lung tissue. Although macrophage levels are reduced, they are still present in the blood and liver, with a large number being present in the lung lesions. This raises an unresolved problem. If, as seems possible, Multi-CSF is not present in normal tissues, some other regulator that can stimulate macrophage formation must exist but has yet to be characterized, apart from O-CSF reported by Lee et al. (1991).

A curious feature of op/op mice is that, in at least one colony, the disease has proved to be self-limiting in later life (Begg et al., 1993). This implies that, with time, other regulators take over the control of osteoclast and macrophage formation. This might have been anticipated from the overlapping actions of the CSFs, but the curious aspect of the natural history of the disease in these mice is that this compensatory process required months to develop, rather than hours or days.

### *Multi-CSF*

No information is available at present on the consequences of depressing Multi-CSF levels or of inactivating the Multi-CSF gene.

## Relative importance of the CSFs as regulators of granulocytes and macrophages

The experience in mice with inactivation of the M-CSF, GM-CSF, or G-CSF genes emphasizes the difficulty of using the gene inactivation approach to establish the consequences of deleting a particular regulator. The changes that occur following gene inactivation may eventually be corrected by some compensatory regulator, requiring some luck in choosing the optimal time for performing analyses. Alternatively, the defects may be of a quite subtle nature not readily apparent in animals maintained in the abnormally favorable environment of specific pathogen-free quarters.

The depletion data, at least for three of the CSFs, have shown that despite the fact that the CSFs have some actions in common, each has unique functions in the normal body that cannot be compensated for by the action of other CSFs or other regulatory systems. This supports the conclusion that the CSFs do function in normal health as significant regulators of granulocyte-macrophage populations, each CSF playing a special role in this complex process. However, it is also apparent that no individual CSF is wholly responsible for regulating the production of granulocytes or macrophages, confirming the in vitro data indicating that the CSFs must exhibit a certain level of redundancy.

Do the deletion data support the conclusion that the CSFs are the only, or the major, regulators of granulocyte and monocyte-macrophage formation? In the earlier discussion on the in vitro actions of the CSFs, it was pointed out that the CSFs were certainly more effective stimuli for granulocyte formation in vitro than other known agents. While some factors can enhance CSF-stimulated granulocyte formation, only SCF, IL-6, IL-11, and the flk-2 ligand have the capacity to stimulate granulocyte proliferation, and the concentrations of these factors that are required are much higher than those of the CSFs. Despite this, it is possible that membrane-displayed SCF is a more efficient stimulus than the secreted form of SCF usually used in such studies (Tokoz et al., 1992) and, furthermore, that SCF and IL-6 might be present in high concentrations in the marrow. It cannot be denied, therefore, that these or other agents yet to be detected may also play some role in stimulating granulopoiesis.

There are in fact some puzzling aspects of the relatively weak actions of SCF and IL-6 in elevating neutrophil levels in vivo. When used alone, SCF has only a weak action in elevating blood leukocyte levels (Briddell et al., 1993), although this action can be increased by combination with G-CSF. Similarly, the injection of IL-6 elicits very little response in peripheral blood leukocyte levels (Ishibashi et al., 1989a), although in mice with very high IL-6 levels, a neutrophil leukocytosis was observed (Hawley et al., 1992). This relative inactivity of IL-6 is curious, since in vitro, albeit at higher concentrations, its action in stimulating granulocytic colony formation is quite similar to that of G-CSF (Metcalf, 1989). Furthermore, as noted earlier, combination of IL-6 with SCF in vitro results in a major enhancement of colony formation, essentially similar to that observed when combining G-CSF with SCF (Metcalf, 1993a).

Whatever the underlying reasons, the present data suggest that SCF and IL-6 seem not to play a major role in regulating basal levels of granulocyte formation and that G-CSF is the major regulator of these cells.

Somewhat similar comments can be made regarding the role of the CSFs in the control of macrophage formation. Elimination of GM-CSF and M-CSF certainly depresses macrophage formation or function. Nevertheless, some macrophage formation continues, and it must be presumed that other factors exist with some action on this process.

Despite these unresolved issues, the combination of in vitro data with the gene inactivation data indicates that much of the granulocyte and macrophage formation and function in normal health is regulated by the CSFs. Further information on this question might be obtained by an analysis of mice with a combined inactivation of all CSF genes, but a continuing search for other regulatory factors is also warranted.

# 11

# Actions of the colony-stimulating factors in resistance to infections

The principal clinical interest in the colony-stimulating factors is based on the general proposition that because leukopenia is well recognized to be associated with enhanced susceptibility to infections (Bodey et al., 1966), the use of CSFs to increase white cell levels and/or function might result in increased resistance to infections.

Evidence was reviewed in Chapter 8 that serum CSF levels are often elevated during acute infections and that the local production of CSF can increase greatly after a local tissue infection. Nevertheless, the serum levels do not approach those produced by injecting CSF, and the possible capacity of injected CSF to enhance resistance to infections is an important question that warrants experimental and clinical investigation.

To investigate the possible value of CSF administration to experimental models that duplicate to some degree the common clinical situations in which leukopenia is present requires pretreatment of the animals in order to damage bone marrow cells or to lower their resistance to infections. A number of studies have revealed the enhancing effects of CSF injections on resistance to infections in models based on these considerations.

Matsumoto et al. (1987) showed that if mice were pretreated with cyclophosphamide, they became highly susceptible to death following challenge injection of organisms such as *Pseudomonas, Staphylococcus aureus,* or *Candida albicans.* The preinjection of cyclophosphamide-treated mice with G-CSF before challenge with microorganisms led to a thousandfold increase in their resistance to challenge infections (Figure 11.1).

In mice with induced leukopenia and infections, the commencement of G-CSF treatment *after* the induction of experimental infections was not effective, but if this was combined with cephem antibiotics, survival rates were significantly improved, and a decreased number of viable bacteria were recovered (Wakiyama et al., 1993).

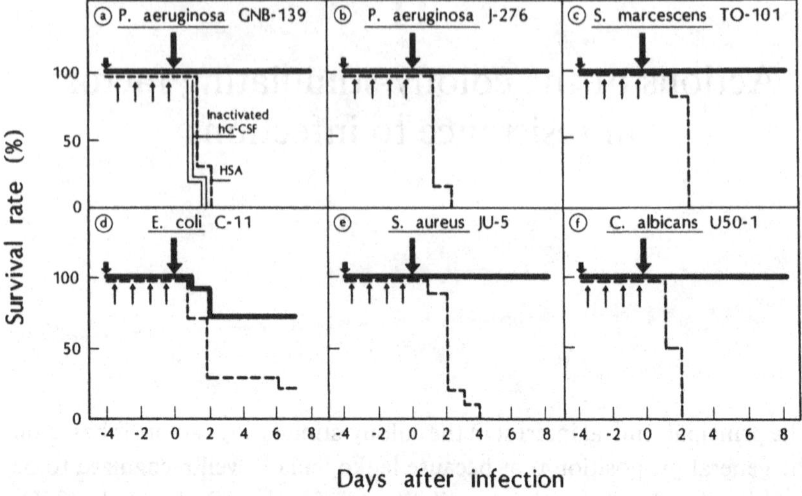


Figure 11.1. Mice preinjected with cyclophosphamide become highly susceptible to challenge with a variety of organisms (dashed lines). If mice are preinjected with G-CSF, resistance to these challenge infections is strongly enhanced (solid lines). HSA denotes human serum albumin. (Reproduced with permission from Matsumoto et al., 1987.)

In mice subjected to a burn injury followed by the local inoculation of *P. aeruginosa* to induce cellulitis, G-CSF treatment elevated neutrophil levels and improved survival rates when given with the antibiotic gentamicin (Silver et al., 1989). G-CSF also increased survival rates and decreased bacterial cell counts when given immediately following the intramuscular injection of *P. aeruginosa* (Yasuda et al., 1990). G-CSF alone had little effect in reducing mortality in newborn rats infected with streptococci, but improved survival was observed when G-CSF was combined with antibiotics (survival: G-CSF alone, 9%; antibiotics alone, 28%; antibiotics plus G-CSF, 91%; Cairo et al., 1990).

In splenectomized mice with *Streptococcus pneumoniae* infections, pretreatment with G-CSF enhanced survival (70 vs. 20%) and reduced the number of organisms recovered from the lungs (Hebert et al., 1990). Similarly, in ethanol-treated rats, pretreatment with G-CSF reduced the number of organisms recovered from the lungs following infection with *Klebsiella pneumoniae,* prevented bacteremia, and enhanced survival rates (Nelson et al., 1991). In a rat model involving ligation of the cecum and then a peritonitis induced by puncture of the cecum, G-CSF enhanced survival rates following the consequent infection (Toda et al., 1993).

Slightly more complex models employed mice given high doses of whole-body irradiation, a procedure commonly resulting in death from infections, presumably following the entry of organisms from the damaged gut. In such animals, the administration of either G-CSF or GM-CSF significantly reduced postirradiation mortality (Talmadge et al., 1989; Tanikawa et al., 1990).

The data from these animal models suggested the general principle that, if G-CSF was administered before challenge with microorganisms, protection resulted, whereas if infections were established before G-CSF treatment, improved survival rates usually required the combination of G-CSF treatment with antibiotics.

The injection of M-CSF into mice enhanced their resistance to challenge infection with *Listeria monocytogenes* (Kayashima et al., 1991) and reduced bacterial numbers in the spleen but not the liver in mice injected with *Brucella abortus* (Doyle et al., 1992). With infections in which the microorganism is a facultative parasite of macrophages, CSF action may be complex, and in one study of GM-CSF transgenic mice with *L. monocytogenes* infection, enhanced phagocytosis was noted but not enhanced killing of organisms, an outcome that emphasizes the selectivity of functional stimulation that can result from CSF action (Tran et al., 1990).

Injections of Multi-CSF into mice induced resistance against orally administered *Strongyloides ratti* worms but was not effective against tissue-migrating larvae. Analysis suggested that the protective effect was mediated by mast cell activation (Abe et al., 1993).

Clinical results have also documented the effectiveness of CSFs in at least some situations. The clearest evidence of enhanced resistance to infections or the resolution of existing infections has been obtained with the use of G-CSF in patients with cyclic or congenital neutropenia in whom daily injections of G-CSF result in a significant reduction in the occurrence of bacterial or fungal infections, antibiotic use, and hospitalization (Hammond et al., 1989; Welte et al., 1990; Dale et al., 1993). Patients with congenital neutropenia have proved hyporesponsive to the stimulation of white cell formation by G-CSF and require the use of higher doses than usual to maintain neutrophil levels.

In the least-favorable situation of patients with preexisting neutropenia and infections, the use of G-CSF only marginally reduced days of fever and antibiotic requirements (D. Maher, personal communication).

A somewhat intermediate situation has been noted in patients receiving marrow transplants or intensive chemotherapy. In neither situation are infections a major cause of death, but most studies have reported that the use of G-CSF or GM-CSF achieved a reduction in mucositis, days of fever, or antibiotic use. These observations were extended in a double-blind placebo-controlled study of patients subjected to chemotherapy for small-cell lung cancer. G-CSF decreased the frequency of febrile neutropenia, culture-confirmed infections, and days of treatment with intravenous antibiotics (Crawford et al., 1991). Treatment using M-CSF in marrow transplant patients with invasive fungal disease was reported to increase survival compared with historical control patients (Nemunaitis et al., 1993).

No clinical studies have yet been reported on the use of CSFs to enhance the functional activity of mature cells in infected patients with nearly normal hemopoietic populations. Such studies are difficult to design because of the heterogeniety of this patient group but would address a question of considerable practical consequence. There is also the possibility that the local injection of an agent such as GM-CSF around the site of chronically infected skin ulcers or wounds might enhance macrophage and granulocyte function and help resolve the infection, permitting healing.

# 12
# Role of the colony-stimulating factors in other disease states

The possibility must be considered that abnormally high or low levels of CSF, either systemic or at a local level, produce or contribute to disease development. Information on this issue remains somewhat limited because of the technical difficulty of estimating local-tissue CSF concentrations. The special question of the relation of the CSFs to myeloid leukemia development will be discussed in Chapter 13.

## Consequences of sustained excess levels of CSFs

Several models have been used to examine the consequences in mice of the sustained elevation of CSF levels. These have involved the production of GM-CSF transgenic mice with the inserted transgene under a viral long terminal repeat promoter (Lang et al., 1987) or the repopulation of irradiated mice by hemopoietic cells in which a retrovirus had been used to insert a CSF cDNA, again under the control of a strong viral promoter (Johnson et al., 1989; Chang et al., 1989a,b). Both maneuvers have achieved in mice the sustained elevation of circulating CSF levels (100-fold in the transgenic model and up to 10,000-fold for the repopulation models). However, in both types of model, the situation is artificial in terms of the cell types producing the additional CSF. In the case of the GM-CSF transgenic mice, expression of the transgene appeared to be restricted to macrophages, while, inevitably in the repopulation models, the cells expressing the inserted genes were entirely of hemopoietic type. Therefore, neither type of model duplicates the precise pattern of CSF-producing cells in the normal animal, and some of the abnormal consequences observed may well have been influenced by this aberrant tissue distribution of CSF-producing cells.

GM-CSF transgenic mice exhibit elevated serum GM-CSF levels from birth and maintain levels at least a hundredfold higher than normal throughout life (Lang et al., 1987; Metcalf, 1988b). In one transgenic line, comparable GM-CSF levels were observed in the urine of male mice but not in that of female mice. In the other transgenic line, no GM-CSF was detected in the urine of either sex. This curious sex difference remains unexplained. Mice of both sexes cleared injected native GM-CSF to the urine approximately equally, and while male transgenic bladder tissue produced two to four times more GM-CSF in vitro than did the corresponding female tissue, this difference does not satisfactorily account for the all-or-none sex difference observed.

GM-CSF transgenic mice exhibit normal fertility; litter sizes are normal, and apparently healthy young adult mice develop, with one notable exception. All transgenic mice are readily identifiable by the abnormally small size of their eyes and the opaque appearance of the cornea. This abnormal appearance is based on infiltration of both eye chambers by macrophages, destruction of the photoreceptor layer of the retina, and various degrees of iritis, corneal infiltration, and cataract-like lesions of the lens. These abnormalities are fully developed by the time of eyelid opening.

Curiously, the hemopoietic tissues of GM-CSF transgenic mice are essentially normal. White cell levels are normal, as are total marrow cell counts, spleen weights, and the cellular composition and content of progenitor cells in these tissues. GM progenitor cells from transgenic mice form colonies of normal size and cellular composition as well as exhibit normal dependency on, and quantitative responsiveness to, CSF stimulation. In older animals, abnormalities commonly develop in the spleen – some exhibiting enlargement by hemopoietic populations that are mostly erythroid in nature – while in other mice the spleen becomes aplastic for both lymphoid and hemopoietic elements. Where insertion of the transgene is on an unidentified autosomal chromosome, chronic bleeding into the peritoneal cavity is a common event, most likely from microhemorrhages in the gut, and this may have initiated the splenic erythroid hyperplasia evident in many of these mice.

The most striking feature of all GM-CSF transgenic mice is the hundredfold increase in the cellularity of the peritoneal and pleural cavities. Although elevated levels of eosinophils were common in these locations, the dominant population involved (>80%) was macrophages (Figure 12.1). Subsequent analysis has shown that 10% of these "macrophages" are in fact dendritic cells (K. Shortman and D. Metcalf, unpublished data), so

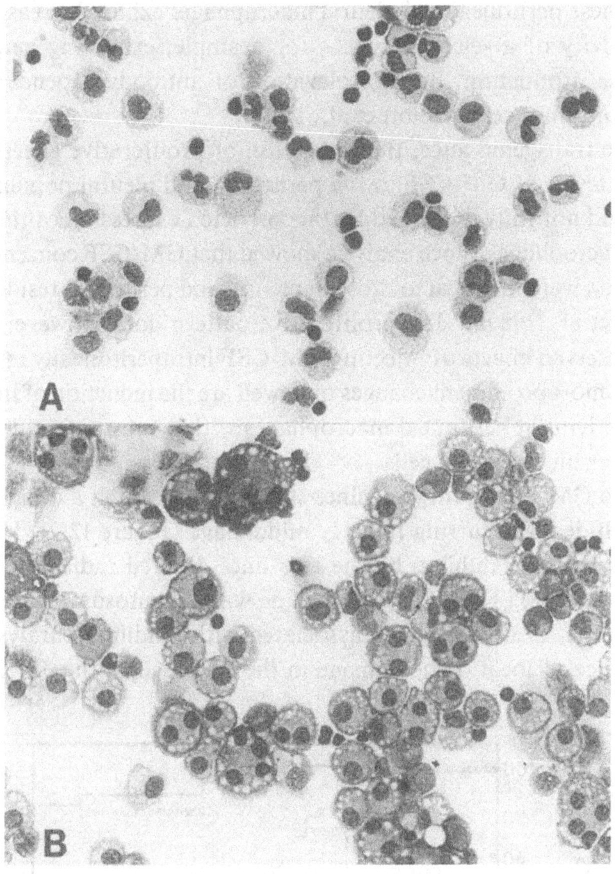


Figure 12.1. Peritoneal cell populations from normal (A) and GM-CSF transgenic (B) mice. Note the increased frequency of macrophages in the transgenic populations, their enlarged size, and the development of multinucleate cells.

this subset of dendritic cells is also elevated more than a hundredfold in GM-CSF transgenic mice. Macrophage cell levels commence rising from birth and achieve peak levels by 4–6 weeks of age, with some decline thereafter. Analysis showed that in these transgenic mice with normal marrow, spleen, and blood, the excess production of macrophages occurs locally in the peritoneal and pleural cavities due to the abnormal proliferative activity of a subset of local macrophage precursors (Metcalf et al., 1992a). This activity ceases when the mice reach 6–8 weeks of age, and thereafter the macrophages remain as a static population that exhibits a progressive tendency to form binucleate and multinucleate cells by cell fusion. These peritoneal and pleural macrophages exhibit increased functional activity of a selective type – for example, exhibiting heightened superoxide production, but not elevation of antibody-dependent cytotoxicity for tumor cells (Elliott et al., 1991).

In these transgenic mice, the restriction of proliferative effects of the increased levels of GM-CSF to the peritoneal and pleural populations is curious and not fully explained by the restricted expression of this transgene to macrophages, since analysis showed that GM-CSF concentrations in the blood were identical to those in pleural and peritoneal resident fluid (Gearing et al., 1989a). The proliferative pattern does, however, resemble the observed effects of injecting GM-CSF intraperitoneally into mice, where the most prominent changes observed are the induction of increased mitotic activity in peritoneal macrophages with a substantial increase in the number of peritoneal cells.

The two GM-CSF transgenic lines studied both exhibit a decreased life span, with death occurring in early middle age (Figure 12.2). However, the tissue lesions exhibited by the two lines differed radically (Metcalf and Moore, 1988) (Table 12.1). In the line with an autosomal insertion of the transgene, death was often associated with hindlimb paralysis without evidence of local tissue damage in the spinal cord, the development

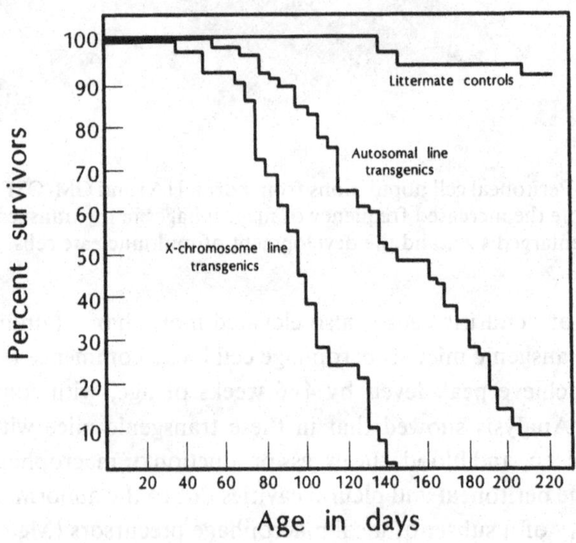


Figure 12.2. GM-CSF transgenic mice die prematurely, death occurring earlier in the line when the transgene was inserted on the X-chromosome. (Reproduced with permission from Metcalf, 1991c.)

Table 12.1. *Differing pattern of disease development in two GM-CSF transgenic mouse lines*

| Parameter | Autosomal line | X-Chromosomal line |
|---|---|---|
| Median survival (days) | 145 | 95 |
| Peritoneal macrophages ($\times 10^6$) | 100–200 | 25–50 |
| Peritoneal nodules (%) | 50–70 | 0 |
| Diffuse muscle lesions (%) | 3 | 57 |
| Bowel congestion (%) | 10 | 34 |
| Spleen atrophy (%) | 42 | 66 |
| Spleen hyperplasia (%) | 27 | 7 |

*Source:* Data from Metcalf and Moore (1988).

of inflammatory nodules in the peritoneal and pleural cavities, and intraperitoneal bleeding. In contrast, in the line where the transgene was inserted on the X-chromosome, the mice typically died with a wasting disease associated with extensive granulomatous lesions in skeletal muscle (Figure 12.3). The most likely basis for this miscellany of chronic inflammatory lesions and tissue damage is GM-CSF-stimulated production of toxic products by the increased number of macrophages. To date, studies have documented an increased production by the macrophages in these lesions of IL-1, TNF$\alpha$, and $\beta$-fibroblast growth factor, but other potentially toxic products may also be produced (Cuthbertson et al., 1990; Lang et al., 1992).

It is notable that no myeloid or myelomonocytic leukemias have developed in these transgenic mice, several thousand of which have been monitored in detail.

The development of distinctly different disease patterns in these two transgenic lines with similar elevations of GM-CSF levels indicates the need for some caution in ascribing all such changes simply to the effects of elevated GM-CSF levels. It is clear that the insertion site of the transgene significantly modified the disease pattern emerging, possibly indicating an action of the inserted transgene on some relevant adjacent genes in the macrophages presumably responsible for the tissue injury.

Irradiated mice repopulated by CSF-producing hemopoietic cells proved to be extreme models in which the circulating CSF levels achieved were very highly elevated. In mice repopulated by cells producing G-CSF, GM-CSF, or Multi-CSF, extreme hyperplasia was induced in granulocyte-

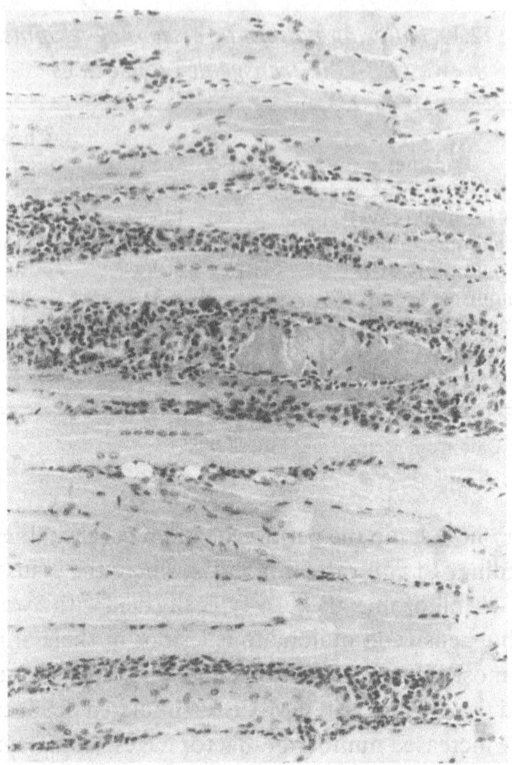

Figure 12.3. Granulomatous lesions in the skeletal muscle of GM-CSF transgenic mice. The major cells present in the foci are activated macrophages, and commonly there is destruction of adjacent muscle cells.

macrophage populations in the blood, spleen, and marrow, with parallel increases of progenitor cells.

Mice with excess G-CSF levels did not exhibit a reduced life span or evident disease other than the extreme hyperplasia of granulocyte populations and an increased number of mature granulocytes in organs such as the lung and kidney (Chang et al., 1989a).

In contrast, mice repopulated by GM-CSF- or Multi-CSF-producing cells died prematurely. In mice repopulated by GM-CSF-producing cells, the same inflammatory lesions were noted in muscle tissue as occur in GM-CSF transgenic mice, but in addition the liver and lung were extensively infiltrated by massive collections of proliferating granulocytic, macrophage, and eosinophil cells (Johnson et al., 1989). These lesions had the morphology of leukemic tissue, but transplantation tests show that the cells were nonleukemic. Mice repopulated by Multi-CSF-producing cells exhibited massive accumulations of mast cells in the marrow, spleen, skin, and other organs. This was associated with severe itching and skin ulceration following scratching (Chang et al., 1989b).

The conclusions from these studies on excess CSF models are that chronic excess stimulation by CSFs in general reproduces in exaggerated form the responses observed following the injection of CSF. While the models have the limitation of a reduced life span, no evidence was obtained to suggest that simple overstimulation of granulocyte-macrophage tissues by CSF leads to leukemic transformation. The benign nature of the tissue changes in mice with excess G-CSF levels supports the clinical data on the lack of serious adverse responses to G-CSF. Conversely, the shortened life span of mice with excess GM-CSF levels is again in line with clinical data indicating that high doses of GM-CSF can produce adverse responses, probably ascribable to stimulation of macrophages to produce tissue-damaging products.

## Actions of CSFs in immune responses and inflammatory states

Granulocytes and macrophages are regarded as having no capacity to exhibit selective proliferative responses to specific antigens but can respond in a broad manner if the antigens concerned can induce increased CSF production. Thus, the bacterial antigen flagellin is a highly effective elevator of CSF levels (Metcalf, 1971) and, via this mechanism, would be expected to induce both the general proliferation and activation of granulocyte-macrophage populations. In line with this expectation, levels of granulocyte-macrophage progenitor cells were elevated in the blood and spleen following the injection of flagellin (Metcalf and Stevens, 1972; Metcalf, 1974b). For comparable antigens or antigen mixtures of microbial origin, similar types of response have been documented. Foreign antigens of mammalian cell origin (proteins or carbohydrates) appear to be less effective in eliciting CSF responses unless T-cell activation results, in which case, from in vitro studies, the induction of CSF synthesis could be anticipated.

There are, however, major differences between the responses of lymphoid versus granulocyte-macrophage cells to foreign antigens. The hallmark of antigenic stimulation of lymphoid cells is that accelerated and heightened responses occur on second challenge. This feature has not been noted in CSF responses to the repeated injection of antigens (Metcalf,

1974b). Furthermore, repeated stimulation of T-lymphocytes by agents such as concanavalin A and antireceptor sera tend to lead to the development of an anergic state (Kelso and Metcalf, 1990). When microbial antigens or endotoxin enters the body, although lymphoid cells may respond, these are not the exclusive source of the CSF induced. Indeed, lymphocytes are likely to be a minor component of the CSF-producing population compared with endothelial cells, stromal cells, or fibroblasts. Thus, athymic or irradiated mice exhibit nearly normal CSF responses to injected microbial products (Metcalf, 1971). However, in one situation, hemopoietic cells seem either to be the major responding population or to be necessary for normal responses to occur. Thus, endotoxin-unresponsive C3H/HeJ mice cannot produce CSF following challenge by endotoxin but do so if repopulated by marrow cells from responsive syngeneic C3H/GSF mice (Hultner et al., 1982).

The elevated CSF levels in animals and humans with acute or chronic infections appear to be examples of responses to microbial antigens of the preceding type, and to a degree the CSF and consequent granulocyte-macrophage responses may be regarded as components of the broad immune response. Slightly more complex responses are observed in graft-versus-host disease developing after allogeneic marrow transplantation. The severity of the graft-versus-host response in mice and humans is paralleled by the degree of elevation of serum CSF levels (Hara et al., 1974; Singer et al., 1977). Of some interest has been the failure so far to document elevated serum CSF levels in a wide range of autoimmune diseases, again suggesting that mammalian antigens do not appear to provide effective inductive signals for elevating CSF production.

The role of granulocytes and macrophages in infected or inflammatory lesions has usually been regarded as merely being the relatively unsophisticated breakdown and removal of microorganisms and damaged cells. Macrophages may have additional roles, because of their capacity to produce a range of active signaling molecules potentially influencing revascularization or tissue repair processes (see Chapter 7).

In this context, there have been some intriguing anecdotal reports of the capacity of locally injected GM-CSF to facilitate the resolution of chronic ulcers and to induce regression of local Kaposi's sarcoma lesions. Such observations must be verified by more extensive studies but may indicate that CSF-activated macrophages and dendritic cells play an active role not only in local responses to microorganisms but also in local immune responses.

Levels of CSFs, along with many other cytokines, can be elevated at sites of chronic inflammation. It remains unclear in such situations (e.g., the joint fluid in acute arthritis; Williamson et al., 1988), what role is being played by the CSFs. Has CSF production been triggered locally to initiate removal of damaged tissue, or is it part of the abnormal process initiating tissue damage and inflammation? Here, the inflammatory lesions occurring in GM-CSF transgenic mice suggest that the CSF can actually initiate inflammatory tissue damage rather than serving as a repair mechanism. These questions require clarification by more extensive studies on human and experimental inflammatory states to establish the exact role being played by the CSFs. In experimental-induced cerebral malaria, in which release of the tumor necrosis factor by activated macrophages is believed to play a central role in disease development, administration of antibodies to both Multi-CSF and GM-CSF sharply reduced the development of the neurological syndrome (Grau et al., 1988), suggesting, at least in this model, that the CSF was involved in the pathogenesis of the lesions.

The human disease malignant histiocytosis exhibits many histological features in common with GM-CSF transgenic mice, and this disease and others such as polymyositis require careful analysis to establish whether CSF is similarly involved in the development of the granulomatous inflammatory lesions.

In a quite different category is the potential role played by GM-CSF in initiating immune responses that depend on the presentation of antigens by dendritic cells to reactive T-lymphocytes. In vitro studies have suggested that GM-CSF has a unique capacity to stimulate the formation of dendritic cells from marrow precursors (Inaba et al., 1992a). As noted earlier, in the spleen, lymph node, and peritoneal populations of GM-CSF transgenic mice, dendritic cells are abnormally numerous, and conversely, the number of these cells can be low in mice in which the GM-CSF gene has been inactivated. While there is evidence that not all dendritic cells have a common origin or regulatory system, for those that are GM-CSF-dependent, this regulation can be presumed to have a crucial role in the ability to develop effective T-lymphocyte responses to relevant antigens. In this context, the studies of Dranoff et al. (1993) are of particular interest. They used a variety of transplanted tumor models to determine which cytokines were relevant in promoting rejection of transplanted tumors. The procedure used was to insert cDNA for the test cytokine into tumor cells, irradiate the cells to prevent further cell division, then inject the cells into animals before subsequent challenge with viable tumor cells of the same type. Although some activity has been reported in such models for the lymphocyte-active cytokines IL-2, IL-4, and IL-6, the studies of Dranoff et al. (1993) showed that GM-CSF was outstanding in its capacity to induce tumor rejection.

Studies of this type need confirmation and extension but suggest that the capacity of GM-CSF to generate dendritic cells may give this regulator a crucial role in relevant T-lymphocyte immune responses. If so, GM-CSF could have a broader role as a highly effective adjuvant in potentiating a wide variety of immune responses involving or requiring initial antigen presentation by dendritic cells to achieve T-cell activation. In this context, GM-CSF has been noted to increase major histocompatibility complex, class II expression and augment antigen presentation by marrow-derived macrophages (Fischer et al., 1988) and, when fused to specific idiotypes, to elicit potent immune responses against B-cell lymphomas (Tao and Levy, 1993). Both observations suggest a useful role of GM-CSF as an adjuvant in eliciting immune responses.

The growing awareness of the importance of dendritic cells in the immune responses and the regulatory role played by GM-CSF in dendritic cell formation and/or function is providing experimental evidence of an unexpected link between lymphoid and granulocyte-macrophage populations. Such a link has been reinforced by the documentation that certain progenitor cells can generate both macrophage and B-lymphocyte progeny (Cumano et al., 1992).

Thus, the familiar co-involvement of both lymphoid and granulocyte-macrophage populations in naturally occurring inflammatory responses may be based on links in both the origin of the responding cells and the need for regulator-mediated functional interactions between these two general classes of white cells.

## Disease states associated with abnormal CSF levels

Surveys of human disease states have revealed consistent increases, particularly of G-CSF and M-CSF, and less often of GM-CSF, in acute infections. The reasons for this have just been discussed, as have the elevations noted in acute graft-versus-host disease.

With the exception of the increased levels of M-CSF in pregnant mice, to date the only noninfective and noninflammatory states in which serum CSF levels have been observed to be elevated are in occasional cancer patients exhibiting an associated leukocytosis. Most often the CSF involved has been G-CSF, and analysis has shown that the tumor cells concerned have acquired the capacity to produce CSF. Resection of the tumor led to a return to normal levels of CSF and white cells. In no case has this phenomenon been seen with all cancers of a particular histological type, and the cancers involved appear to represent exceptional examples of aberrant protein production by cancer cells.

While excess GM-CSF levels can lead to cachexia in mice, no evidence has so far been presented that excess GM-CSF levels are present in cachectic states in humans. Similarly, there are no data indicating elevated CSF levels in generalized inflammatory diseases. It should be commented that the biology of CSF production allows the possibility of excess local production of CSF without evidence of such activity in the peripheral blood. Because of this, the true situation in most human diseases involving local inflammatory lesions has yet to be established and requires some technique such as in situ hybridization to monitor CSF transcription in local tissue sites.

The situation in human myeloid leukemia is a special case that will be dealt with in Chapter 13, but there are no known diseases involving granulocyte or macrophage hyperplasia corresponding to secondary polycythemia with its link to elevated erythropoietin levels.

Naturally occurring neutropenia or monocyte defects are rare in humans. In severe congenital neutropenia (Kostmann's syndrome), serum levels of G-CSF are usually elevated rather than depressed (Mempel et al., 1991), and analysis has indicated that the disease is associated with a maturation block in granulopoiesis with an abnormally low responsiveness of the granulocytes to stimulation by G-CSF (Kobayashi et al., 1990). In one case this has been shown to be associated with defective G-CSF receptors present on the membrane of granulocytes (Dong et al., 1994).

In cyclic neutropenia, there is some evidence for the occurrence of cyclic fluctuations of CSF levels in the circulation (Moore et al., 1974a; Yujiri et al., 1992), and this may be a possible candidate for a disease based on recurrent abnormally low CSF levels. However, the disease can potentially involve hemopoietic cells in other lineages, so it probably cannot simply be regarded as the consequence of abnormally low CSF levels. Furthermore, hyporesponsiveness to stimulation by G-CSF or GM-CSF has been noted in granulocyte-macrophage progenitor cells from such patients (Hammond et al., 1992).

No examples have been observed of humans whose cells lack the capacity to produce CSF, nor have patient subgroups been identified that are capable of only subnormal CSF responses. However, this remains possible, and the question is in need of further exploration in, for example, elderly subjects or in U.S. blacks known to exhibit relative neutropenia.

In human osteopetrosis, no patients have been found with an inability to produce M-CSF corresponding to that of osteopetrotic mice (Orchard et al., 1992).

This largely negative information suggests that if aberrant CSF production is involved in the development of some disease states, the link will most likely be difficult to document, partly because of the existence of multiple regulators with potentially overlapping actions and partly because local dysfunction in CSF production is technically difficult to analyze in human subjects.

# 13

# The colony-stimulating factors and myeloid leukemia

Acute and chronic myeloid leukemias are clonal neoplasms in which granulocyte-macrophage populations are dominant members of the leukemic clone. However, in chronic leukemia and many cases of acute myeloid leukemia, it is evident that the originating clonogenic cell is multipotential and that cells in at least some other hemopoietic lineages are members of the neoplastic clone.

It could be argued that the CSFs are unlikely to be involved in a dominant manner in these diseases because of the involvement of multipotential cells in initiating the clone and because of the presence of other lineages in the neoplastic population. This reservation has some validity, and it will require a more complete knowledge of the regulatory biology of stem cells to establish with certainty whether novel regulator abnormalities are required for the transformation and emergence of myeloid leukemic clones. Nevertheless, it must be kept in mind that the CSFs do have obvious actions on multipotential stem cells and actions embracing eosinophil, erythroid, and megakaryocytic cells, the cell populations that can be present as additional members of the leukemic clone.

From the earliest phases of work on the CSFs, several questions were repeatedly raised with regard to the possible involvement of CSFs in the development of myeloid leukemia. Do myeloid leukemic cells continue to exhibit dependency on, or responsiveness to, proliferative stimulation by the CSFs? Is aberrant CSF stimulation involved in the emergence of myeloid leukemic clones? Do the CSFs have a capacity to restrict proliferation of leukemic clones because of their differentiation- and maturation-inducing actions?

Myeloid leukemia is not a particularly common disease in mice; nevertheless, two of the earliest studies on differing aspects of the biology of myeloid leukemia involved work on two murine myelomonocytic leukemias. The WEHI-3B leukemia was shown to be responsive to proliferative stimulation by CSF, and the leukemic cells themselves were shown to produce CSF (Metcalf et al., 1969). This was later documented to be Multi-CSF and to be aberrantly produced because of the insertion of an intracisternal A particle upstream of the Multi-CSF gene (Ymer et al., 1985). In concurrent studies, the M1 myelomonocytic leukemia was shown to respond in vitro to stimulation by various tissue-conditioned media by exhibiting pronounced maturation to granulocytes and monocyte-macrophages (Ichikawa, 1969, 1970). Subsequent analysis showed that several cytokines were likely to have been responsible for this type of phenomenon with murine leukemic cell lines - G-CSF, GM-CSF, IL-6, and LIF (Hilton et al., 1988; Lotem et al., 1989). These early observations set the stage for two distinct avenues of study on the CSFs and myeloid leukemia - their role as mandatory growth factors in the development of myeloid leukemia and their potential for the suppression of myeloid leukemia.

## Growth of myeloid leukemic cells in vitro

Using cells from patients with chronic myeloid leukemia (CML), it proved easy in semisolid cultures to grow granulocytic, macrophage, or eosinophil colonies the cells of which could be documented by karyotypic analysis to be Philadelphia-positive and derived from the clonal leukemic population (Moore et al., 1973a; Metcalf, 1984). In marrow populations, the frequency of such clonogenic cells was higher than normal, and in the blood, the frequency was many-fold higher than in normal blood, the frequency of clonogenic cells often equalling that in the marrow. The colonies grown were strikingly normal in general appearance and content of maturing cells, although the clonogenic cells did exhibit some abnormalities in cycling status, buoyant density, and responsiveness to agents such as prostaglandin E (Metcalf, 1984).

In contrast, results from the culture of cells from patients with acute myeloid leukemia (AML) proved highly variable - cells from a minor subset of patients failed to proliferate, and those from most patients produced small clones over a wide range of frequency (Moore et al., 1974b). The cells involved could be shown karyotypically to be members of the leukemic clone, but the clones commonly were of extremely small size and usually exhibited little capacity for cellular maturation. Subsequent improvement in culture techniques has resulted in some increase in clone size, often achieving the arbitrary limits of colony size, but primary AML cells continue to exhibit a strikingly abnormal proliferative capacity in vitro.

In AML there commonly is complete suppression of preexisting normal granulocyte-macrophage progenitor cells (Metcalf, 1984). In contrast, in CML normal progenitors coexist in normal numbers with leukemia-derived progenitor cells, although the latter cells greatly outnumber the normal progenitor cells (Eaves and Eaves, 1987).

When the potentially confounding effects of CSF production by accessory cells in marrow or blood cultures were appreciated (CML monocytes have the same capacity to produce CSF in vitro as normal monocytes; Moore et al., 1973b), a remarkably uniform picture emerged from studies on the dependency of myeloid leukemic cells on CSF. Without exception, the proliferation of CML colonies in vitro was shown to be dependent on stimulation by extrinsic CSF, and the concentrations required were essentially the same as those required for corresponding normal cells (Figure 13.1). All four CSFs exhibited proliferative actions, although there was some patient-to-patient variation in quantitative responsiveness to individual CSFs (Löwenberg and Touw, 1993).

The situation with AML cells was somewhat more varied and published data differ, probably due in large part to the selection of specimens from selected subsets of patients. As a generalization, it can be said that cells from the majority of patients are dependent on stimulation by extrinsic CSF, again with patient-to-patient variation concerning the most effective CSF and quite large variations in their quantitative responsiveness to stimulation (Francis et al., 1979; Metcalf, 1984; Begley et al., 1987; Löwenberg and Touw, 1993). However, it must be remembered that AML populations are clonal and that quantitative responsiveness to CSF stimulation is to some degree a heritable trait. Thus, the range of quantitative responsiveness observed with different AML populations does not exceed the range of responsiveness of normal progenitor cells.

There is clearly a subset of AML cells that exhibit an unambiguous capacity for proliferation in unstimulated in vitro cultures. In different studies the proportion of such patients has varied from 3 to 30%. Even where AML cells exhibit a capacity for autonomous proliferation in vitro, it is not uncommon to observe that the addition of CSF to the cultures produces an enhancement of clonal proliferation (Young and Griffin, 1986; Young et al., 1987; Löwenberg et al., 1993).

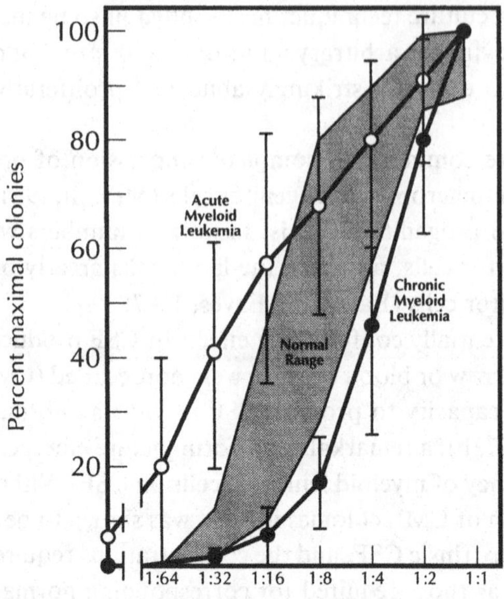


Figure 13.1. Clonogenic leukemic cells from patients with CML or AML exhibit continuing dependency on proliferative stimulation by CSF when cultured in vitro. In general, their quantitative responsiveness to stimulation is similar to that of normal cells. The data with AML cells include some samples where the cells exhibited some capacity for autonomous proliferation. (Reproduced with permission from Metcalf, 1977.)

What was unanticipated from model studies using long-established leukemic cell lines, where the clonogenic cells exhibit a high capacity for self-renewal, was that most clones of leukemic cells grown from CML or AML patients do not contain clonogenic cells capable of further clone or colony formation when recultured in secondary cultures. This is not the expected behavior of genuine stem cells in a leukemic clone and has led many investigators to conclude that the clonogenic cells detected in such cultures are not the true clonogenic cells of the leukemic population. Modification of the culture technique has documented the existence of less numerous clonogenic cells that can form blast colonies containing cells with some capacity for further clonogenic proliferation (Buick et al., 1979; Griffin and Löwenberg, 1986). Such cells are also dependent for proliferation on CSF stimulation but are not wholly convincing representatives of the true clonogenic cells in these leukemic populations.

Two quite different interpretations of the existing data are possible. First, true clonogenic cells have yet to be grown clonally in vitro and their regulation remains unknown. Second, true clonogenic cells have been grown, but the culture conditions have resulted in a truncation of their proliferative potential, possibly because the growth factors used to stimulate proliferation also induced differentiation commitment, with or without maturation induction.

In this context, the frequency of clonogenic cells in AML populations, as defined by a capacity to generate a transplanted leukemia in SCID mice, was estimated to be only 1 in 250,000 cells (Lapidot et al., 1994). If "true" clonogenic cells are of such low frequency, in vitro studies to date have not addressed their properties or response to regulatory factors.

This unresolved question does leave some continuing doubts regarding the relevance of what has been observed in in vitro studies, and the biology revealed may merely relate to the major components of the leukemic population, not necessarily to the originating clonogenic cells.

However, in vitro observations do allow one fairly secure conclusion to be drawn. The expansion of a myeloid leukemic clone to attain clinically recognizable size is likely to be dependent on CSF stimulation, and at a minimum, therefore, CSF stimulation is a mandatory cofactor in the emergence of myeloid leukemic clones (Metcalf, 1994).

## CSF levels in leukemia

The dependency of myeloid leukemia cells on stimulation by CSF immediately raises the question of whether CSF levels are abnormally high before or during myeloid leukemia development and the related question of whether myeloid leukemic cells produce CSF in an autocrine manner. Neither question can be answered in a wholly satisfactory manner because of the unresolved problems relating to the biology of CSF production and distribution discussed earlier – the difficulties in determining local versus systemic levels of CSF and in establishing the precise status of CSF-producing cells in vivo.

Much of the early work on CSF levels in serum and urine of leukemic patients was undertaken before it was possible to distinguish between the four CSFs, and subsequent specific radioimmunoassays have not been particularly extensive. It can certainly be concluded from published data that serum CSF levels are not uniformly elevated in either AML or CML but can be elevated if the patient is suffering from an associated infection and in some other situations. Individual sets of data are quite variable on these questions (Watari et al., 1989; Sallerfors and Olofsson, 1991; Janowska-Wieczorek et al., 1991; Omori et al., 1992; Verhoef et al., 1992).

There have been a number of studies on the apparent ability of myeloid leukemic cells to produce CSF in vitro, but the data are difficult to translate into the possible situation in vivo because of the transcriptional activation of CSF in cultured cells. Most studies have shown unequivocally that leukemic monocytes from patients with CML or chronic myelomonocytic leukemia have a readily detected capacity to produce CSF in vitro. However, the levels produced are comparable to those produced by normal monocytes in vitro, and in both cases the actual functional activity of these cells in vivo is undocumented. Monocytes from patients with AML are often subnormal in their capacity to produce CSF in vitro, except those from patients with monocytic or myelomonocytic leukemias (Metcalf, 1984; Metcalf and Nicola, 1985a).

The possible capacity of clonogenic leukemic blast cells to produce CSF is of particular interest for reasons to be discussed later. More recent studies have shown that a high proportion of AML blast cells have the capacity to transcribe one or another CSF (Young and Griffin, 1986; Oster et al., 1988; Murohashi et al., 1989) in a process that is highly inducible by IL-1 (Delwel et al., 1989). This raises the possibility that many such blast cell populations have an autocrine capacity to produce CSF – a property that most researchers do not believe is exhibited by corresponding normal progenitor cells. The data are potentially important but must be assessed with caution, since handling such cells can induce CSF production that is not apparent in unmanipulated cells.

## Autocrine production of CSF in myeloid leukemia

The data raise the tantalizing possibility that myeloid leukemia is a disease state associated with, and possibly consequent upon, acquisition by cells of an autocrine capacity to produce their own growth factors. It is necessary, therefore, with the use of animal models to assess whether such an event can be an important part of the pathogenic process in myeloid leukemia development.

As discussed earlier, prolonged overstimulation of otherwise normal granulocyte-macrophage populations by excessive levels of CSF leads to extreme hyperplasia of these populations, but not to leukemic transformation.

The failure of an acquired capacity for autocrine production of CSF to transform normal hemopoietic cells is in sharp contrast to the results of similar experiments performed using continuous CSF-dependent cell lines such as the FDC-P1. Such cell lines are dependent for all proliferation on CSF stimulation but are immortalized, with a highly abnormal capacity for self-renewal of the clonogenic cells in the population (80–90% of all cells). These immortalized cell lines are not, however, transformed and cannot produce leukemia when transplanted into syngeneic recipients.

The insertion of a retrovirus containing GM-CSF cDNA into FDC-P1 cells led to the rapid transformation of the cells to grow autonomously in cultures lacking added CSF, and assays on such autonomous cells showed that the cells now behaved as transplantable leukemic cells (Lang et al., 1985; Laker et al., 1987). Although transformation was dependent on the autocrine production of GM-CSF, the key GM-CSF involved was cell-associated, even though the cells usually also exhibited a capacity to secrete GM-CSF.

A more subtle outcome was observed when Multi-CSF cDNA was inserted into FDC-P1 cells. While the cells again transformed to leukemic cells and again produced cell-associated and -secreted Multi-CSF, the transformed cells did not necessarily behave autonomously in vitro (Metcalf, 1988a). In some instances, the cells remained wholly dependent on added extrinsic CSF for continued proliferation – the behavior of typical human myeloid leukemic cells in vitro.

A somewhat comparable outcome was observed when FDC-P1 cells were injected into irradiated syngeneic recipient mice. Such recipients reproducibly developed myeloid leukemia after a delay of 2–4 months, and the leukemias were demonstrated to have arisen from the injected FDC-P1 cells (Dührsen and Metcalf, 1988, 1989). While these leukemic cells could now be readily transplanted into normal recipients, they again did not always behave as autonomous cells in vitro and in some cases remained wholly dependent on added extrinsic CSF for proliferation. An analysis of this engraftment model showed that a frequent feature of the transformed cells was an acquired capacity to produce either GM-CSF or Multi-CSF, based on the insertion of an intracisternal A particle upstream of the relevant gene (Dührsen et al., 1990).

In a further model involving the use of FDC-P1 cells, transformation of the cells was accomplished by infection with the Moloney leukemia virus. The majority of the transformed cell lines had acquired an autocrine capacity to produce either GM-CSF or Multi-CSF, with rearrangement of one or another gene presumably consequent upon adjacent insertion of the Moloney virus (J. Rasko, unpublished data).

These various models indicated that acquisition of an autocrine capacity to produce CSF is a transforming event if it occurs in cells already exhibiting an abnormal capacity for self-renewal.

An important experiment linking the two disparate sets of observations on normal versus immortalized cells followed the recognition that in WEHI-3B leukemic cells, there are activating intracisternal A particle insertions upstream not only of the Multi-CSF gene, but also of the homeobox gene *Hox* 2.4 (Blatt et al., 1988; Kongsuwan et al., 1989). This prompted an experiment in which normal marrow cells were infected with a retrovirus containing the cDNAs both for Multi-CSF and *Hox* 2.4, with the resulting overexpression of both genes. When irradiated mice were engrafted with such cells, they rapidly developed donor-derived leukemias resembling WEHI-3B leukemias (Perkins et al., 1990). Subsequent experiments showed that the induced overexpression of *Hox* 2.4 by normal cells results in these cells acquiring an abnormal capacity for CSF-dependent self-renewal (Perkins and Cory, 1993).

These experiments identified a combination of two intrinsic changes as being necessary for myeloid leukemia development in mice - acquisition of an abnormal capacity for self-renewal divisions and acquisition of an autocrine capacity to produce a relevant CSF. This formula for leukemic transformation should be viewed as merely documenting two basic abnormalities that a hemopoietic cell must acquire for neoplastic transformation. It should be emphasized that there are other mechanisms for achieving both abnormal states (Metcalf, 1994).

First, aberrant self-renewal can probably be induced by a variety of other genes encoding nuclear transcription factors that influence the genetic events controlling self-renewal versus differentiation commitment. From various studies, it is likely that v-*erb* A can also achieve this outcome, as can v-*myb*, possibly v-*myc*, and various other genes in the homeobox, helix–loop–helix, and zinc finger group of genes encoding nuclear transcription factors.

Second, autocrine stimulation need not necessarily involve acquisition of a capacity to produce a relevant growth factor. A similar outcome could result from production of an oncogene product such as that of the *raf*, *lck*, *ras*, *abl* and *bcr/abl* oncogenes that either is part of or can enter the mitotic signaling pathway normally activated by the binding of a growth factor to its receptor. Alternatively, a mutation leading to the constitutive activation of a growth factor receptor such as occurs with v-*fms* or v-*erb* B can produce a surrogate system for continuous cell stimulation (Metcalf, 1994). In the latter context, an analysis of GM-CSF receptors in AML cells has failed to reveal rearrangements of the receptor genes that might lead to constitutive activation of the receptors (Brown et al., 1993).

Although autocrine production of CSF in appropriate abnormal cells can lead to myeloid leukemic transformation, it is obvious that this is only one possible method for achieving transformation. Nevertheless, the fact that many human myeloid leukemias appear to exhibit some capacity for autocrine CSF production is potentially relevant to the transformation. Studies on FDC-P1 cells have revealed that such CSF production need not be quantitatively large; nor is it necessary for the cells to secrete CSF, because cell-related CSF appears to be particularly effective in mediating transformation. Attempts to detect the CSF production by leukemic cells using assays on medium conditioned by the cells can be difficult if the cells actively consume the CSF by receptor-mediated endocytosis (Metcalf and Rasko, 1993). Under conditions where the transforming CSF is present in very low concentrations, and possibly detectable only in concentrates of cell extracts, it becomes very difficult to certify that such CSF is not being produced and equally difficult to determine whether there is some critical concentration threshold that must be exceeded if the CSF is to function as a co-transforming agent.

At present, the exact situation remains unclear with human myeloid leukemic cells, but autocrine production of CSFs seems likely to be involved in the initiation of many of these acute leukemias.

It could be questioned why autocrine production of CSF should be a necessary situation. What would happen if a suitably abnormal cell was exposed to excess (or even normal) concentrations of extrinsic CSF derived from some other tissue? Would this also tend to result in leukemic transformation?

This possibility was investigated by comparing the fate of FDC-P1 cells engrafted into normal recipients with that of cells engrafted into transgenic GM-CSF mice with excess circulating levels of GM-CSF. A striking difference was observed in that leukemic transformation of the injected FDC-P1 cells occurred in all transgenic recipients within 3 months, whereas no transformation occurred in normal recipients during a 6-month observation period (Metcalf and Rasko, 1993) (Figure 13.2). It is intriguing that the majority of the leukemias developing in transgenic recipients also had acquired an autocrine capacity to produce either GM-CSF or

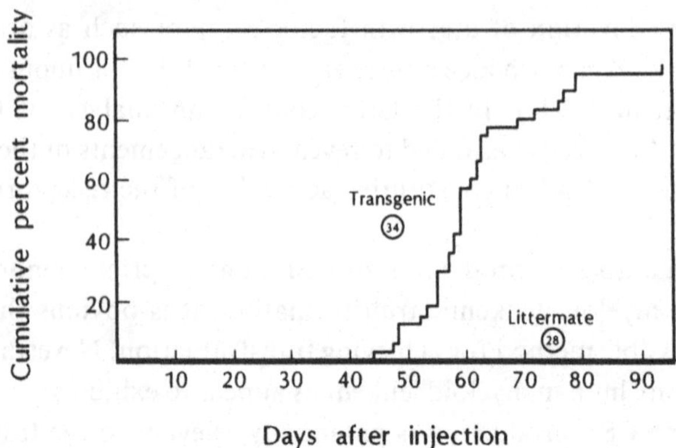


Figure 13.2. When nonleukemic FDC-P1 cells are injected into histocompatible GM-CSF transgenic mice, all recipients develop leukemia due to the transformation of the injected FDC-P1 cells, an event not occurring in similarly injected littermate control mice. (Reproduced with permission from Metcalf and Rasko, 1993.)

Multi-CSF, despite the fact that in the presence of the excess levels of extrinsic CSF, there would have been no obvious selective advantage for such autocrine-producing cells. The results did indicate, however, that the excessive stimulation by extrinsic CSF greatly accelerates the leukemic transformation process, perhaps merely by expanding the size of the population of FDC-P1 cells at risk of transformation.

To the degree that FDC-P1 cells might resemble the abnormal granulocyte-macrophage populations in patients with myelodysplasia, these data suggest that the prolonged administration of CSF might entail some risk of increasing the possibility of transformation to AML in these patients.

A possibly related set of observations was made on mice developing myeloid leukemia following whole-body irradiation plus the administration of dexamethasone. A short course of injections of M-CSF soon after irradiation increased the frequency of myeloid leukemia but had no effect if administered 4 months after irradiation. Conversely, the injection of GM-CSF early after irradiation was without effect but, if administered 4 months after irradiation, increased the frequency of myeloid leukemia (Haran-Ghera et al., 1992).

In principle, the CSFs could play an indirect, quite different role in myeloid leukemia development. At least in vitro, the CSFs sustain cell viability and delay death from apoptosis. Studies have shown an association between prolonged lymphocyte survival induced by activation of *bcl*-2 and a predisposition to develop follicular lymphomas (Tsujimoto et al., 1984). Conversely, the tumor-suppressive action of p53 has been linked with its capacity to enforce death by apoptosis (Yonish-Rouach et al., 1991), a process that would result in elimination of both normal cells and cells exhibiting preneoplastic changes. If CSF can exhibit a significant capacity in vivo to extend the life span of abnormal granulocyte-macrophage cells, it might allow such cells to develop further abnormalities leading to leukemic transformation. This possibility is highly speculative and constitutes a much less likely link between CSF action and myeloid leukemia development than the studies described earlier in which CSF has a more active transforming role.

These studies indicate that the CSFs are likely to be mandatory cofactors in the emergence of human myeloid leukemic clones and in many instances may play a direct role in the transformation process. While the models discussed have implicated GM-CSF and Multi-CSF, other models have shown that M-CSF can play a similar role (Wheeler et al., 1986). It is unclear whether G-CSF can play an active role in transformation, mainly because no G-CSF-dependent models have been analyzed. It remains an intriguing possibility, however, that G-CSF may not be involved in such events because of its prominent capacity to initiate differentiation commitment and maturation - processes that would abort the emergence of a transformed clone.

## Suppression of myeloid leukemias by CSFs

The polyfunctional actions of the CSFs allow these agents potentially to play a quite opposite role in the biology of myeloid leukemia development. If the capacity of CSFs to influence differentiation commitment and initiate maturation extends also to comparable actions on myeloid leukemia cells, these could result in suppression of a leukemic population by a combination of the suppression of leukemic stem cell self-generation and enforced differentiation and maturation either to postmitotic cells or to cells with a finite proliferative capacity.

Studies using the WEHI-3B myelomonocytic leukemic cell line documented that GM-CSF had a minor capacity to suppress colony formation by these cells (Metcalf, 1979). However, G-CSF had a much more marked capacity to induce differentiation in such colonies, and recloning studies showed that this was associated with an obvious reduction of stem cell self-renewal, with the asymmetrical generation of cells with irreversible changes involving loss of clonogenicity, death of the affected cells, or retention of some capacity to proliferate, but only to form differentiating progeny (Metcalf, 1982a; Nicola et al., 1983). Following treatment in vitro with G-CSF, WEHI-3B cells exhibited a reduced capacity to produce transplanted leukemias in syngeneic recipients (Metcalf, 1982b).

In parallel studies using a comparable mouse leukemic cell line, the injection of G-CSF in animals bearing transplanted leukemias derived from this cell line prolonged survival in the mice with, in some cases, complete suppression of the transplanted leukemias (Tamura et al., 1989).

While these actions on appropriate cell lines could be impressive, the suppressive effects were slow and incremental. Complete suppression of a leukemic population in vitro required multiple reculture cycles in the presence of G-CSF and sometimes led to the emergence of resistant subclones. Furthermore, studies on other leukemic cell lines resulted in the complete failure to suppress cell growth or induce maturation. In some instances, the cells lacked receptors for G-CSF, and in other cases presumably there was a failure of the cells to respond effectively to CSF-initiated signals. It is likely that most often these cellular defects are based on abnormal genetic programming of the type needed to achieve abnormal self-renewal during the initiation of the leukemia, the failures then indicating that these abnormalities could not have been corrected by CSF signaling (Sachs, 1987; Metcalf, 1994).

More recent evidence on the separate locations of mitotic signaling and differentiation-inducing domains in the G-CSF receptor support the additional possibility that in some leukemic cells the receptors may have a mutation that prevents initiation of differentiation-inducing signals.

Parallel studies on human myeloid leukemic cell lines have documented a situation somewhat similar to that noted for murine leukemic lines. Some human leukemic cell lines exhibit some reduction in the self-renewal of clonogenic cells with or without evidence of maturation induction when cultured repeatedly in the presence of CSF (Maekawa and Metcalf, 1989). Thus, U937 cells can be significantly suppressed by GM-CSF, and HL60 cells exhibit partial responses to G-CSF.

It has also been observed that combinations of CSFs, or CSFs in combination with regulators such as IL-6 or LIF, can enhance the suppression process (Maekawa et al., 1990) (Figure 13.3), a phenomenon also noted with murine cell lines (Metcalf, 1989).

As in the case of murine cell lines, many human leukemic cell lines are refractory to suppression by CSFs. As noted earlier, primary AML cells in culture usually exhibit little or no capacity for maturation in the presence of CSF, although a careful analysis of self-renewal characteristics has revealed some influence of the CSFs, particularly M-CSF, in partially

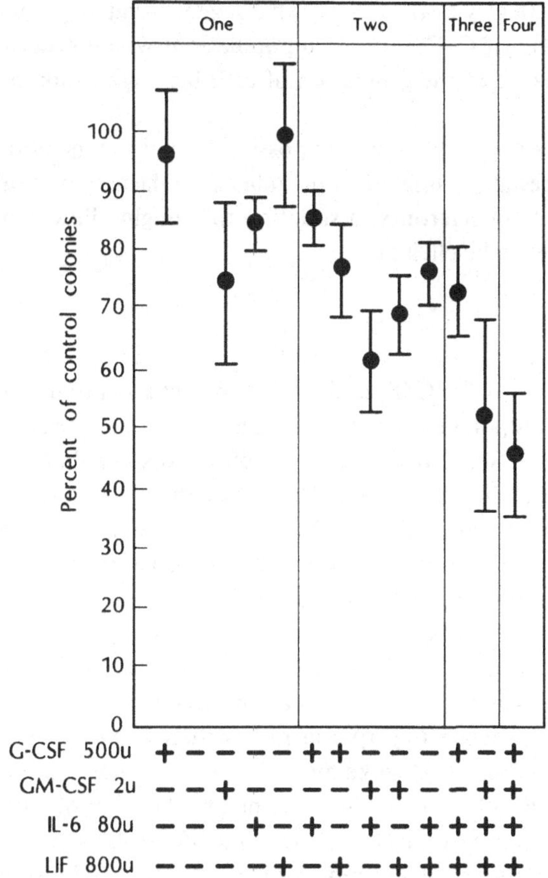


Figure 13.3. The clonogenicity of human leukemic U937 cells in culture can be suppressed by the action of G-CSF, GM-CSF, IL-6, or LIF. This suppression is enhanced by combining two or more of these regulators. Plus signs denote factors used in each case. (Reproduced with permission from Maekawa et al., 1990.)

suppressing the self-renewal of clonogenic cells (Miyauchi et al., 1988a,b). Indeed, as commented earlier, the absence of clonogenic cells from most colonies or clones grown from primary human myeloid leukemic cells may possibly result from a differentiation-inducing action of the CSFs used to stimulate cell proliferation.

One study on cells from patients with AML or CML showed that G-CSF receptors were often present on leukemic cells, as expected from the capacity of G-CSF to stimulate the proliferation of such cells. However, in most cases a subset of the leukemic blast cells was present that exhibited no receptors (Begley et al., 1987b). This suggests that any differentiation-inducing action of G-CSF on such populations would necessarily be incomplete because of the generation of cells lacking membrane receptors for G-CSF.

Few studies have addressed the possibility that the membrane expression of CSF receptors might be upregulated by the action of other agents such as IL-1 or interferon $\gamma$, a situation that might allow more effective CSF responses to be elicited.

## Comment

The role played by the CSFs in the development and progression of myeloid leukemia is potentially highly complex because of the polyfunctional actions of the CSFs. From in vitro studies and some data from clinical trials, it is clear that the CSFs can stimulate the proliferation of myeloid leukemic cells at concentrations similar to those active on corresponding normal cells. It seems inescapable that this action of the CSFs has a major influence on the clonal expansion of the leukemic clone.

Patients with preleukemic syndromes or myeloid leukemia have not so far been documented to have unusually high levels of CSF either in local hemopoietic tissues or in the circulation, and simple elevations of CSF levels merely provoke hyperplasia rather than leukemia. Given the responsiveness of myeloid leukemic cells, even normal concentrations of CSF would be sufficient to stimulate the proliferation of leukemic cells, and the progressive expansion of the population is likely to be the consequence of an abnormal self-renewal capacity of the clonogenic cells in the population rather than of excess stimulation.

It must be presumed that there are significant concentrations of CSF in the environment of normal hemopoietic cells, in which case it is difficult to explain why an acquired capacity to produce CSF should give myeloid leukemic cells any proliferative advantage over normal hemopoietic cells, the more so since leukemic cycle times are longer than those of normal cells. When the leukemic cells have left the hemopoietic tissues, the situation may differ, and the restricted availability of CSF may become limiting. In this circumstance, the autocrine capacity to produce CSF may well represent a significant advantage. Certainly in the FDC-P1 model system, the acquisition of an autocrine capacity to produce CSF is a key step in leukemogenesis and occurs even in animals already possessing excess CSF levels. It remains difficult to establish what percentage of AML populations in humans exhibit autocrine CSF production, but it is significant.

Given the multiplicity of gene rearrangements associated with myeloid leukemia development, none of which involve CSF genes, it is a little surprising that autocrine CSF production should be as common as it appears to be. There are many alternative ways in which a cell might acquire independence of growth factor stimulation, and animal models have documented successful leukemic transformation by these alternative methods for activating the mitotic signaling pathway. Future studies may produce more convincing evidence of these alternative methods in human leukemias; the most promising candidate at present is the possible proliferative stimulation by the *bcr–abl* fusion protein in CML. Even with this fusion protein, which, after induced expression, leads to sustained hyperplasia and, eventually, leukemic transformation (Daley and Baltimore, 1988), one study suggested that its action might be indirect by inducing CSF production (Hariharan et al., 1988).

Whatever the method used by leukemic cells to achieve autocrine stimulation, it remains puzzling that the affected cells usually exhibit absolute dependency in vitro on proliferative stimulation by *extrinsic* CSF. Models in which transformation was triggered by acquisition of an autocrine capacity to produce CSF verified this curious anomalous behavior of apparent autonomy in vivo and dependency in vitro.

Complicating the whole question of the role played by the CSFs in myeloid leukemia is the fact that the same CSFs can actually suppress myeloid leukemia populations by reducing stem cell self-generation and inducing differentiation commitment. While this is a highly reproducible phenomenon with suitable cell lines, it must be emphasized that many leukemic populations are quite refractory to these actions of the CSFs, often presumably because of severe derangement of the gene program controlling self-generation.

The present knowledge of the role played by the CSFs in the biology of myeloid leukemia is seriously incomplete and full of unexplained paradoxes. Clinicians are probably justifiably wary about using the CSFs in the management of myeloid leukemia until some of these paradoxes are resolved. It may well be, however, that an analysis of CSF action on various myeloid leukemias will offer the best prospects for determining the mechanisms controlling self-renewal versus differentiation commitment and the role played by CSF signaling in this process.

# 14

# Clinical uses of the colony-stimulating factors

The first clinical trials involving the colony-stimulating factors were undertaken using GM-CSF in AIDS patients (Groopman et al., 1987), and these were followed by studies using G-CSF in patients with lymphoma and cancer (Gabrilove et al., 1988; Morstyn et al., 1988). In both series of studies the administration of CSF elicited a dose-related increase in granulocytes and, in the case of GM-CSF, an increase in monocytes and eosinophils.

The following obscure and confusing generic names have been assigned to recombinant G-CSF and GM-CSF for clinical use:

| | | |
|---|---|---|
| G-CSF: | Filgrastim | (*E. coli*, nonglycosylated) |
| | Lenograstim | (CHO cells, glycosylated) |
| GM-CSF: | Molgramostim | (*E. coli*, nonglycosylated) |
| | Sargramostim | (yeast, glycosylated) |
| | Regramostim | (CHO cells, glycosylated) |

While these generic names are beginning to appear in publications on the clinical use of the CSFs, they will not be used in this chapter, because we feel it is more important to maintain the uniformity of presentation of information on the CSFs throughout the book.

## Adverse responses

As dose escalation studies were extended, no significant dose-limiting toxicity was encountered with G-CSF in doses up to 60 $\mu$g/kg per day. The only regularly observed side effect was bone pain in approximately 20% of the patients, and this was often mild. The data from an analysis of adverse events in phase III trials of G-CSF in cancer patients (Decoster et al., 1994) are shown in Table 14.1 and indicate the overall very low frequency of side effects that might be ascribed to G-CSF.

Table 14.1. *Adverse events in Phase III cancer patients administered G-SCF or placebo*

| System | G-SCF patients (237) | | | | | Placebo patients (171) | | | | |
|---|---|---|---|---|---|---|---|---|---|---|
| | Total patients | Percent | Mild | Moderate | Severe | Total patients | Percent | Mild | Moderate | Severe |
| Musculoskeletal | 46 | 19 | 13 | 20 | 13 | 8 | 5 | 2 | 5 | 1 |
| Skin reactions | 20 | 8 | 7 | 11 | 2 | 8 | 5 | 4 | 4 | 0 |
| General disorders | 17 | 8 | 1 | 13 | 3 | 4 | 2 | 2 | 2 | 0 |
| Gastrointestinal | 13 | 5 | 4 | 3 | 6 | 6 | 4 | 5 | 1 | 0 |
| Application site | 6 | 3 | 6 | 0 | 0 | 0 | 0 | 0 | 0 | 0 |

*Source:* Modified from Decoster et al. (1994).

Table 14.2. *Adverse events following GM-CSF treatment (less than 10 μg/kg per day) in Phase I/II trials*

| Route of injection | Patients | First dose reaction | Fever | Bone pain | Thrombosis | Pericarditis | Systemic symptoms |
|---|---|---|---|---|---|---|---|
| Subcutaneous | 34 | 1 | 18 | 12 | 0 | 0 | 10 |
| Intravenous bolus or short infusion | 136 | 2 | 23 | 16 | 0 | 0 | 27 |
| Continuous intravenous | 125 | ?4[a] | 23 | 16 | 0 | 0 | 44 |
| Total events | 295 | 3 + ?4[a] (2%) | 64 (22%) | 44 (14%) | 0 | 0 | 81 (27%) |
| WHO Grade III/IV | 295 | 3 + ?4[a] | 0 | 5 | 0 | 0 | 4 |

[a] Question mark denotes reactions of an uncertain nature.
*Source:* Data from Scarffe (1991).

Table 14.3. *Adverse responses following treatment with Multi-CSF (IL-3)*

| | IL-3 (μg/kg per day) | | |
|---|---|---|---|
| | 1–4 | 8 | 15 |
| Assessable patients | 10 | 4 | 5 |
| Fever (WHO grade 2) | 2 (20) | 3 (75) | 5 (100) |
| Influenza-like symptoms | 2 (20) | 3 (75) | 4 (80) |
| Headache | 0 | 2 (50) | 4 (80)[a] |
| Local erythema | 4 (40) | 0 | 0 |
| Facial flushing | 1 (10) | 0 | 0 |
| Rash | 0 | 1 (25) | 1 (20) |
| Nausea | 0 | 0 | 1 (20) |

*Note:* Figures represent number of patients; those in parentheses are percentages.
[a] No adequate control with acetaminophen in two patients.
*Source:* Data from Postmus et al. (1992).

In the case of GM-CSF, adverse responses have been observed in patients receiving relatively high daily doses (15–64 μg/kg). These have included pericarditis (resolving after cessation of treatment) and possibly thromboembolism. A syndrome of transient hypoxia and hypotension has been observed in some patients, characteristically restricted to the period following the first dose of GM-CSF (Lieschke et al., 1989) and being more common in patients receiving high doses of GM-CSF. In patients receiving less than 10 μg/kg per day (the usual therapeutic dosage), less severe side effects have been noted that include fever, bone pain, myalgia, lethargy, skin rashes, and dyspnea (Scarffe, 1991). As shown in Table 14.2, few of these reached World Health Organization (WHO) grade III or IV, and resolution occurred following cessation of therapy.

Dose escalation studies using Multi-CSF (IL-3) in patients with lung cancer encountered frequent adverse responses with daily doses of 8 μg/kg and higher. The most frequent of these were fever, influenza-like symptoms, and headache (Postmus et al., 1992) (Table 14.3).

The experience with M-CSF has been less extensive, but in one study the maximum tolerated dose was established as 100 μg/kg per day, with adverse responses including thrombocytopenia, ocular inflammation, and retinal hemorrhages (Cole et al., 1994). Another study also revealed a range of ophthalmological side effects in addition to malaise, headache, and nausea (Sanda et al., 1992).

Because significant hemopoietic responses can be stimulated in most patients with daily doses below 10 μg/kg, the CSFs as a group have proved relatively nontoxic. In reviewing the current clinical use of the CSFs, it is more convenient to discuss their use in particular disease situations.

## Cancer patients receiving chemotherapy

Many of the cytotoxic agents used in cancer chemotherapy are myelotoxic and cause various degrees of marrow aplasia with a consequent fall in neutrophil levels below 500–1,000 per microliter. Often platelet levels also fall to dangerously low levels in such patients. Progenitor cell levels are subnormal, but unless these patients have had extensive previous treatment, they possess a sufficient number of stem cells to initiate hemopoietic regeneration eventually. This process is slow, however, and results in extended hospitalization with antibiotic use; it often leads to interruption or abandonment of planned further courses of chemotherapy.

As noted earlier, such patients often have elevated plasma levels of G-CSF and less often of GM-CSF or M-CSF. From animal studies discussed earlier, one would surmise that these probably represent responses to microbial invasion rather than to leukopenia. Much higher CSF levels can be achieved by the administration of CSF. In principle, therefore, such patients can be regarded as capable of responding to the consequences of induced aplasia but do so in a suboptimal manner that can be accelerated by the administration of growth factors.

The earliest clinical trials on G-CSF and GM-CSF made it evident that the administration of CSF after chemotherapy could accelerate recovery of neutrophil levels in such patients. CSF administration did not prevent the occurrence of an initial neutropenic nadir but did reduce the time to recovery of neutrophil levels above 500 or 1,000 per microliter (Bronchud et al., 1987, 1989; Gabrilove et al., 1988; Morstyn et al., 1988; Neidhart et al., 1989). There was also an associated reduction in the frequency and severity of the accompanying debilitating mucositis and a reduction in antibiotic use.

These initial results were extended with three placebo-controlled studies using G-CSF in small-cell lung cancer patients receiving chemotherapy (Crawford et al., 1991; Green et al., 1991; Trillet-Lenoir et al., 1993b). All three studies showed that G-CSF reduced by approximately twofold the incidence of febrile neutropenia, antibiotic use, and days of hospitalization.

The administration of GM-CSF to cancer patients following chemotherapy showed that GM-CSF induced a dose-related increase in neutrophils, eosinophils, and monocytes (Antman et al., 1988; Leischke et al., 1990) with no significant effects on reticulocyte or platelet levels. A number of studies have been made on the effects of GM-CSF treatment subsequent to a single cycle of cytotoxic therapy in patients with a variety of cancers. These revealed an accelerated recovery from neutropenia (Antman et al., 1988; Gianni et al., 1990; Herrmann et al., 1990; Logothetis et al., 1990; Morstyn et al., 1990; Steward et al., 1990; Gerhartz et al., 1993) with, in some cases, a reduction in febrile days, a reduction in days on antibiotics, or a reduction in infections. In some patients, an accelerated recovery of platelets was observed with a reduction in the need for platelet transfusions, but the latter response was variable. In one study of patients with small-cell lung cancer, GM-CSF treatment reduced neutropenia, but when chemotherapy was used simultaneously with GM-CSF, increased thrombocytopenia and neutropenia were observed (Havemann et al., 1991). The occurrence of fever in some patients as a response to injected GM-CSF can make it difficult to distinguish this pharmacological response from infection-related fevers.

The useful responses elicited by G-CSF and GM-CSF in cancer patients given single courses of chemotherapy have been extended to studies designed to determine whether CSF treatment can permit multiple courses of chemotherapy to be completed on schedule. Studies using both G-CSF and GM-CSF have shown that this is achievable in the majority of patients (Trillet-Lenoir et al., 1993a).

These trials form the basis for the most frequent current clinical use of G-CSF and GM-CSF. Apart from achieving a useful reduction in antibiotic use and hospitalization for such patients, the ultimate value of CSF therapy in permitting more intensive or sustained chemotherapy can be assessed only with a long-term analysis of remission or survival rates in such patients – aspects that really relate to the question of whether more intensive chemotherapy can achieve higher cure rates than less intensive chemotherapy. This is a matter of particular relevance to patients with breast cancer, who tend to be younger and whose survival rates appear to be increased by chemotherapy. Such intensification of chemotherapy with the use of CSF therapy is now being linked to the use of peripheral blood stem cell autografts (as discussed later).

Administration of Multi-CSF (IL-3) following chemotherapy in lung cancer patients elevated the level of and reduced the time to recovery of leukocytes, which included neutrophils, monocytes, and eosinophils; no consistent effects were observed on platelet or hemoglobin levels (Postmus et al., 1992). Similar results were obtained with the use of Multi-CSF in patients with ovarian cancer receiving multiple courses of chemotherapy, and Multi-CSF markedly reduced the number of postponements in scheduled chemotherapy (Biesma et al., 1992). In another study, the administration of Multi-CSF to lung cancer patients following chemotherapy elicited a significant increase in platelet levels (D'Hondt et al., 1993).

## Chemotherapy plus bone marrow transplantation

For patients with lymphoid leukemia, lymphoma, or solid tumors, the combination of chemotherapy with marrow transplantation is similar in principle to treatment with chemotherapy alone, except that the chemotherapy is more intensive and, for patients with leukemia or lymphoma, is designed to ablate myeloid and lymphoid populations. It is not intended that the patients' hemopoietic cells survive such treatment, and hemopoietic regeneration therefore requires the use of an autologous or matched allogeneic marrow transplant to provide the needed stem and progenitor cells. Although somewhat elevated serum levels of G-CSF, and less frequently of GM-CSF, have been reported in such patients following transplantation (Sallerfors et al., 1991; Cairo et al., 1992; Baiocchi et al., 1993; Kawano et al., 1993b), such elevations are small as well as variable and do not provide the maximal stimulation of hemopoiesis. In such patients, recovery of neutrophil and platelet levels is slow, requiring extensive antibiotic and platelet therapy and prolonged hospitalization – sometimes with a fatal outcome because transplanted marrow cells fail to regenerate.

The administration of GM-CSF to such patients following transplantation, in some cases in randomized double-blind studies, has accelerated recovery of neutrophil levels to above 500 or 1,000 per microliter within 7–10 days (Brandt et al., 1988; Nemunaitis et al., 1988; De Witte et al., 1990; Link et al., 1990; Powles et al., 1990) with a reduction in the occurrence of infections (Link et al., 1990) and fewer febrile days (Nemunaitis et al., 1988; De Witte et al., 1990) but with inconsistent effects on platelet recovery.

Similarly, G-CSF treatment resulted in a reduced period of neutropenia following marrow transplantation with fewer febrile episodes, less severe mucositis, and reduced days in hospital (Sheridan et al., 1989; Taylor et al., 1989b; Takahashi et al., 1991) (Figure 14.1).

GM-CSF has also been reported (Klingemann et al., 1990; Nemunaitis et al., 1990; Thomas et al., 1990) to have been successful in triggering

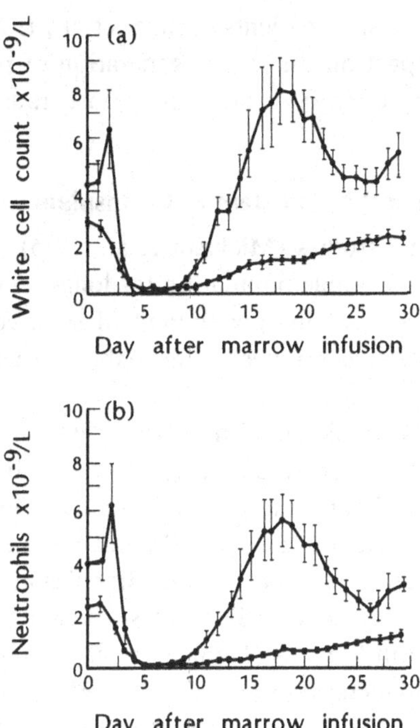


Figure 14.1. Accelerated recovery of neutrophil levels in cancer or lymphoma patients receiving autologous bone marrow transplants by the injection of G-CSF for up to 8 days following transplantation. The lower line in each panel represents leukocyte recovery in a historical series of transplant recipients. (Reproduced with permission from Sheridan et al., 1989.)

hemopoietic regeneration and enhancing survival in transplanted patients who were exhibiting a protracted failure of regeneration following autologous or allogeneic transplantation. The use of GM-CSF did not exacerbate the severity of graft-versus-host disease in such patients.

Pretreatment of marrow donors with GM-CSF combined with Multi-CSF augmented the repopulating capacity of the bone marrow (Mumcuoglu et al., 1990). In patients with invasive fungal infections following bone marrow transplantation, administration of M-CSF was reported to have increased survival to 27% compared with 5% in historical controls (Nemunaitis et al., 1993).

There are two deficiencies in these CSF-initiated responses. First, they fail to prevent the initial nadir of neutrophil levels following chemotherapy plus transplantation, and it is in these early days that infections are most likely to occur in such patients (Spitzer et al., 1994). Second, CSF therapy has little impact on the slow regeneration of platelets, a major reason for the need of intensive management post-transplantation.

## Peripheral blood stem cell transplantation

Based on early animal studies (Micklem et al., 1975), peripheral blood was not regarded as a suitable population for long-term repopulation of ablated subjects because of its low content of stem cells and evidence that blood-derived stem cells appeared incapable of successful long-term repopulation.

This situation must be distinguished from that with blood collected after the administration of cytotoxic drugs or CSFs. In the rebound period following cytotoxic drug administration, the stem and progenitor cell content of the blood rises sharply (Richman et al., 1976), and such cells are suitable for use in transplantation (Gianni et al., 1989). Similarly, the injection for 4–7 days of G-CSF increases stem and progenitor cells up to a hundredfold in humans (Dührsen et al., 1988), while GM-CSF causes a 10- to 20-fold increase (Socinski et al., 1988a; Villeval et al., 1990) and Multi-CSF a 2- to 4-fold increase (Ottman et al., 1990). The combination of cytotoxic drugs with G-CSF elicits even higher increases in the number of progenitor cells in the peripheral blood.

In the context of autologous transplantation, the frequencies of progenitor and presumably stem cells in the blood cell populations after CSF pretreatment approximate those in the bone marrow. Peripheral blood cells harvested by leukapheresis therefore become a realistic alternative source of cells for subsequent transplantation following either ablative or intensive chemotherapy. In initial studies, G-CSF-induced peripheral blood cells were supplemented with marrow cells in patients who then received G-CSF to stimulate hemopoietic regeneration. This procedure did not result in a further acceleration of the neutrophil recovery over that obtained by the use of G-CSF alone but did result in a remarkable acceleration of platelet recovery to 50,000 per microliter from 39 to 15 days (Figure 14.2) (Sheridan et al., 1992). Subsequent studies have confirmed this effect of peripheral blood stem cells in accelerating platelet recovery (Chao et al., 1993; Spitzer et al., 1994), and a comparable acceleration of platelet recovery was obtained using peripheral blood cells alone after elicitation either by G-CSF (Schmidt et al., 1992) or by chemotherapy plus G-CSF (Pettengell et al., 1992). In such procedures it is

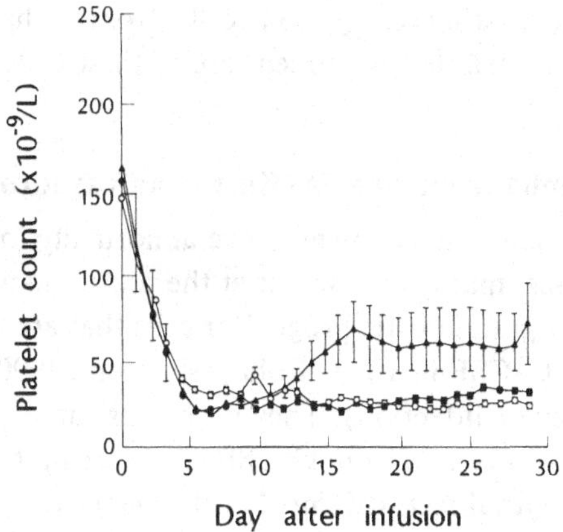


Figure 14.2. Accelerated recovery of platelet levels in patients receiving a combined transplant of marrow cells plus G-CSF-elicited peripheral blood stem cells. The lower two curves indicate platelet regeneration in control patients receiving marrow transplantation with or without G-CSF. (Reproduced with permission from Sheridan et al., 1992.)

becoming evident that treatment of the patient with G-CSF following peripheral blood transplantation does not further accelerate the recovery of either neutrophil or platelet levels.

A similar response pattern in patients undergoing chemotherapy has been observed using autografts of peripheral blood cells elicited by GM-CSF plus chemotherapy (Gianni et al., 1989). Again, there was acceleration of neutrophil recovery and a marked shortening of the recovery time for platelets.

The use of peripheral blood autografts following priming by CSF (Peters et al., 1993) or chemotherapy plus CSF (Elias et al., 1992) in patients receiving intensive chemotherapy is beginning to have a marked effect on current clinical chemotherapy because of its simplicity and capacity to reduce patient hospitalization and to permit the completion of chemotherapy courses. For such autologous grafts, the procedure raises one problem that must be resolved, namely, the possible presence of tumor cells in the reinfused peripheral blood. While this risk is probably lower than that following the use of corresponding autologous marrow transplants, the anticipated more extensive use of peripheral blood autografts increases the magnitude of the problem. Lowering this risk will require the development of effective methods for killing tumor cells in the harvested peripheral blood population or, alternatively, the use of methods for selectively recovering the repopulating cells ($CD34^+$ cells) from the harvested peripheral blood cells and then the subsequent use of these cells for grafting.

### Congenital neutropenia (Kostmann's syndrome)

Patients with congenital neutropenia have abnormally low levels of circulating neutrophils, maturation arrest at the promyelocytic stage in the bone marrow, and granulocytic progenitor cells that are hyporesponsive to stimulation by G-CSF in vitro (Kobayashi et al., 1990). The patients suffer recurring severe infections. They do possess an ability to produce G-CSF in vivo, and in fact serum G-CSF levels are up to 10-fold higher than those in normal subjects (Mempel et al., 1991). In at least one study, a heterozygous defect in the G-CSF receptor was found to allow proliferative but not maturation-inducing signaling (Dong et al., 1994); however, the disease is believed to be heterogeneous, and in studies on other patients no such defect in G-CSF receptors was noted (Sandoval et al., 1993).

The administration of GM-CSF was not successful in elevating neutrophil levels, although some eosinophil responses were noted (Vadhan-Raj et al., 1990; Welte et al., 1990). The administration of G-CSF has been successful in increasing and sustaining the number of neutrophils to normal levels in such patients, although the doses required are usually higher than those required in other patients (Figure 14.3) (Bonilla et al., 1989; Welte et al., 1990; Dale et al., 1993). This has resulted in a substantial reduction in the frequency of infections, resolution of preexisting infections, and reduced antibiotic use and hospitalization.

There is little doubt that G-CSF treatment can be a lifesaving procedure in these patients, but the maintenance of an adequate number of neutrophils requires continuing G-CSF treatment, and these patients are comparable to those with insulin-dependent diabetes in their daily need for injected G-CSF.

### Cyclic neutropenia

In cyclic neutropenia, patients exhibit 21-day cyclic fluctuations in the number of blood neutrophils, monocytes, eosinophils, lymphocytes, platelets, and reticulocytes. As a consequence, during recurring neutropenic periods they suffer from fevers, mucosal ulcers, and, less often, life-threatening infections. Some data suggest that in the disease, as in the

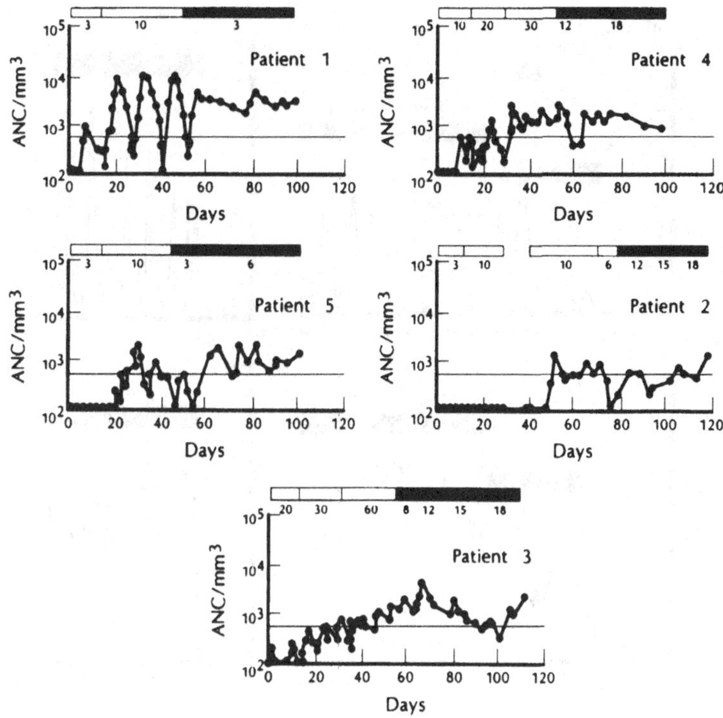


Figure 14.3. Peripheral blood neutrophil (ANC) responses in a group of patients with congenital agranulocytosis receiving various doses of G-CSF. (Reproduced with permission from Bonilla et al., 1989.)

corresponding disease in gray collie dogs, CSF levels may also fluctuate in a cyclical manner, although in dogs the disease can be cured by marrow transplantation. The neutropenia could be corrected in dogs by the administration of G-CSF (Lothrop et al., 1988; Hammond et al., 1990) or GM-CSF (Hammond et al., 1990), but not by Multi-CSF (Hammond et al., 1990), and on this basis G-CSF therapy was initiated in humans with cyclic neutropenia (Hammond et al., 1989).

The administration of G-CSF daily did not correct the cyclical fluctuations in neutrophil levels; indeed, cycling occurred with a shortened periodicity of 14 days (Figure 14.4). However, the nadirs of the neutropenia were significantly elevated, and in such patients it has proved possible to maintain neutrophil levels above 1,000 per microliter. Such patients have maintained responses of this type throughout 3–5 years of G-CSF treatment without developing antibodies to the G-CSF, becoming refractory

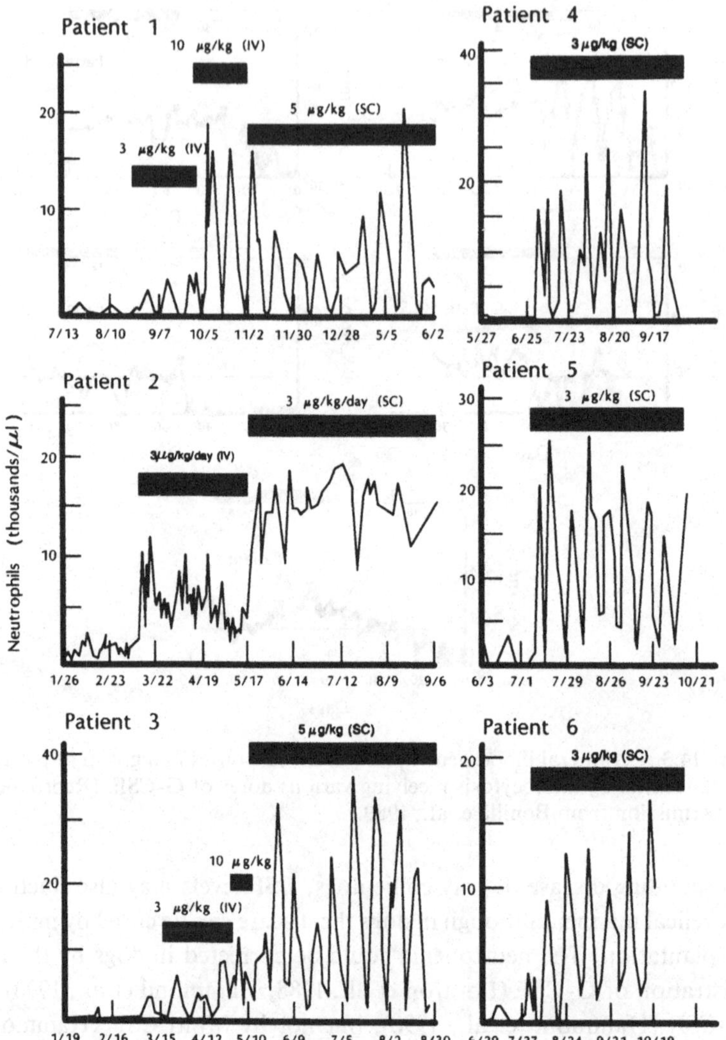


Figure 14.4. Peripheral blood neutrophil responses in a group of patients with cyclic neutropenia after treatment with various doses of G-CSF. IV denotes intravenous; SC, subcutaneous. The horizontal scale is month/day. (Reproduced with permission from Hammond et al., 1989.)

to stimulation, or developing anemia or thrombocytopenia. These patients have exhibited significant changes in their pattern of infectious disease development with reduced frequencies of infections, antibiotic use, and hospitalization (Dale et al., 1993).

## Myelodysplasia

This is a heterogeneous group of myeloproliferative disorders, often clonal in nature, with a subset displaying a predisposition to terminate in the development of AML. The patients commonly exhibit anemia, neutropenia, and thrombocytopenia. Elevated levels of CSF have been noted in some patients but not others. Potentially, these patients might be responsive to growth factor stimulation, and of the CSFs, the broader-acting GM-CSF and Multi-CSF might appear to be the more promising. The use of such stimulating factors carries the potential risk of stimulating the proliferation of any cells already transformed to leukemic cells or, as discussed earlier, of possibly making transformation a more frequent occurrence.

Clinical experience with the use of CSF therapy has been variable and somewhat disappointing, no doubt due to a heterogeneity of the disease state and the abnormal nature of the cells available for stimulation.

The administration of GM-CSF resulted in increased neutrophil and eosinophil levels (Vadhan-Raj et al., 1987; Antin et al., 1988; Ganser et al., 1989; Gerhartz et al., 1989; Nagler et al., 1990; Willemze et al., 1993), and the best responses were observed in those patients with no karyotypic abnormalities (Willemze et al., 1993). In some patients with refractory anemia and an excess of blast cells, an increase in blast cells was observed following GM-CSF treatment (Esty et al., 1991), but other studies suggested no significant stimulation of clonal blast cell proliferation (Nagler et al., 1990). In some patients, a rise in hematocrit levels was observed with a reduced dependency on transfusions (Vadhan-Raj et al., 1987).

Administration of G-CSF also increased neutrophil levels in the peripheral blood (Kobayashi et al., 1989; Negrin et al., 1989, 1990; Nagler et al., 1990; Yoshida et al., 1991), sometimes with the loss of chromosomally abnormal cells in the marrow. The cessation of therapy led to a fall in neutrophil levels and a return of cytogenetic abnormalities. Again, some patients have progressed to AML during the G-CSF therapy.

The administration of Multi-CSF also increased neutrophil, eosinophil, lymphocyte, basophil, and monocyte levels in all patients, but only in some patients were transient hematocrit or platelet responses observed (Ganser et al., 1990b).

The combination of G-CSF with erythropoietin has been noted to elevate both neutrophil and hematocrit levels and to reduce transfusion requirements in myelodysplastic patients treated for prolonged periods (Negrin et al., 1993).

It appears that the use of CSFs has some value in the management of myelodysplasia, but whether sustained responses can be achieved with a significantly increased resistance to infections and whether there is no significantly increased risk of leukemic transformation have yet to be established.

## Aplastic anemia

In aplastic anemia there is a profound aplasia of precursor and mature cells, and the situation is unfavorable for the use of growth factors because of the virtual absence of target cells available for stimulation.

Some improvement in white cell levels with reduced infections was reported following the use of GM-CSF (Vadhan-Raj et al., 1988), although in another study the results were quite variable (Antin et al., 1988). The combination of GM-CSF treatment with antithymocyte globulin has also been reported to increase the frequency of complete remissions (Gordon-Smith et al., 1991). GM-CSF did not achieve a significant reduction in the need for red cell or platelet transfusions, although both GM-CSF and Multi-CSF improved erythropoiesis in some patients with Diamond-Blackfan anemia (Dunbar et al., 1990). Some lymphocyte responses have also been observed in aplastic anemic patients following the administration of GM-CSF (Faisal et al., 1990).

## Myeloid leukemia

In myeloid leukemia, leukemic cells from the majority of patients respond to proliferative stimulation by the CSFs, and the administration of CSF would be expected to increase the size of the leukemic clone and so worsen the disease state. No clinical studies have been reported on the use of CSFs in CML.

The cell-cycle-activating properties of the CSFs in vivo have been verified in patients injected with GM-CSF (Aglietta et al., 1989). In principle, this action of the CSFs should render concomitant chemotherapy more effective when the drugs used include S-phase-specific agents because many leukemic blast cells appear either to be noncycling or to have extended $G_1$ periods. This has been tested clinically in trials combining chemotherapy and GM-CSF treatment, with the successful induction of remissions (Estey et al., 1990; Bettelheim et al., 1991).

A similar study on patients with refractory AML combined intensive chemotherapy with G-CSF to enhance subsequent hemopoietic regeneration.

This resulted in accelerated neutrophil recovery and a reduced incidence of infections (Ohno et al., 1990). In a subsequent study, G-CSF was used following the induction of remissions if life-threatening infections developed during the subsequent period of neutropenia. A tendency was noted in these patients for a subsequently longer disease-free survival (Ohno et al., 1993).

None of these studies has provided definitive indications for the use of CSFs during treatment of AML, but their cautious use may be possible in special circumstances.

## AIDS

In addition to the well-documented T-lymphocyte deficiency in AIDS, there are hemopoietic defects, including abnormally low levels of monocytes and neutrophils, the latter possibly based on an immune response to viral antigens displayed on the surface of these cells. Furthermore, zidovudine (AZT) used in the therapy of the viral infection is myelotoxic and can cause profound cytopenias.

The initial clinical trial of GM-CSF was in AIDS patients (Groopman et al., 1987) and documented that GM-CSF increased both peripheral white cell levels and bone marrow cellularity. Subsequent studies showed that GM-CSF can correct AZT-induced cytotoxic effects (Bhalla et al., 1989) and the neutropenia associated with the use of gancyclovir (Grossberg and Bonnem, 1989).

The use of GM-CSF to treat AIDS was questioned on the grounds that GM-CSF increased HIV replication in an infected cell line and in monocytes (Folks et al., 1987; Koyanagi et al., 1988). However, when combined with AZT, GM-CSF enhances the inhibitory action of AZT (Perno et al., 1989; Hammer et al., 1990). The clinical use of GM-CSF and AZT in an alternating regimen has helped some AIDS patients tolerate AZT therapy (Pluda et al., 1990).

G-CSF has no action on HIV replication in monocytes (Koyanagi et al., 1988) and, in principle, should be a useful agent for restoring neutrophil levels and enhancing resistance to some of the secondary infections in AIDS patients. The administration of G-CSF improved neutropenia in patients with AIDS (Kimura et al., 1990) and also increased neutrophil counts during antiviral therapy. The combination of G-CSF with erythropoietin to correct anemia was successful in elevating neutrophil levels during long-term treatment and also achieved increases in hemoglobin levels (Miles et al., 1991).

In the absence so far of clear evidence for a reduction in infections in AIDS patients, a role for the CSFs in the management of these patients has yet to be firmly established.

## Use of the CSFs in radiation accidents

Studies in animals indicated that the use of G-CSF or GM-CSF accelerates regeneration of hemopoietic populations following whole-body irradiation and reduces mortality, presumably by increasing resistance to secondary infections. In principle, the same effects should be observed in humans, but to date experience has been restricted to the use of GM-CSF in eight of the people exposed to the Brazil radiation accident (Butturini et al., 1988). Although neutrophil recovery occurred during GM-CSF treatment in seven evaluable patients, there were four deaths from radiation toxicity or sepsis, and it was not possible to establish whether the use of GM-CSF had been beneficial.

Since the data from animal studies are so unambiguous, it would seem prudent to maintain stocks of G-CSF and GM-CSF for use in possible future accidents.

## Comment

The responses to the administration of G-CSF or GM-CSF in cancer patients with cytotoxic drug-induced leukopenia indicate that although such patients undoubtedly have depleted populations of stem and progenitor cells, those remaining are capable of being stimulated to regenerate mature hemopoietic populations more rapidly than if left untreated. This establishes the principle that while sensor systems may exist to detect and respond to leukopenia, these "natural" regulator responses cannot elicit maximal regeneration. This conclusion is supported by the relatively low and variable levels of relevant regulators in the circulation of such patients.

The data therefore indicate the desirability of administering hemopoietic regulators to such patients, not only on the grounds of reducing the complexity and expense of hospitalization, but also to minimize the risks of disabling infections or hemorrhage. To date, most clinical use has involved the administration of a single hemopoietic regulator. While this may have resulted from the regulatory requirement to demonstrate the efficacy of individual agents, the use of single regulators must be replaced by regulator combinations for a variety of reasons alluded to earlier: (a) It is more efficient to use regulator combinations to generate mature cells in any one lineage. The consequent capacity to use lower doses of individual agents reduces the likelihood of adverse responses and should eventually prove less expensive. (b) Regulator combinations are needed to stimulate efficient progenitor cell formation by stem cells and to stimulate many progenitor cells. (c) The use of regulator combinations broadens the range of hemopoietic cells responding and can result in more effective responses in certain locations.

In this latter context, it is unclear what types of white cell are needed to constitute the ideal response to any infectious agent. However, from the pathology of infected tissues, there are no infections where only a single lineage of hemopoietic cells is involved. It makes little biological sense, therefore, to rely on the use of a single agent such as G-CSF, which can essentially elicit only a neutrophil response. Although G-CSF, used alone, can be surprisingly effective, a combined response involving neutrophils, monocyte-macrophages, eosinophils, and possibly other cell types should provide a more versatile and effective cellular response, particularly for many fungal and bacterial infections where monocytes play a prominent role in tissue responses.

Indeed, as discussed earlier, it is probable that G-CSF-elicited responses do depend on interactions with other regulators already present in the body, particularly with SCF. As already commented, it cannot be assumed that the body is capable of producing optimal concentrations of any regulator during emergencies – hence the need to modify current therapy by employing regulator combinations.

There are certain combinations that it would seem logical to test – particularly that of a granulocyte-active and a macrophage-active regulator – either G-CSF plus GM-CSF or G-CSF plus M-CSF. One or two trials have combined Multi-CSF with GM-CSF on the grounds of combining an early-acting with a late-acting agent. However, as noted earlier, the CSFs cannot be clearly categorized as early- or late-acting, and some other basis must be established to justify the use of such combinations.

The use of G-CSF in congenital neutropenia may closely approximate substitution therapy akin to the use of insulin in insulin-dependent diabetics, but there are diseases based on defective macrophage function where the use of a macrophage-active CSF may prove of similar value.

The results so far of the use of CSFs in the management of AIDS have been relatively disappointing, but the clinical state of these patients is highly complex, combining obvious hemopoietic cell defects with complex simultaneous infections. From general principles, the use of CSF combinations should be more efficacious than the use of single CSFs.

To date, all clinical studies on the CSFs have been on patients with spontaneous or induced leukopenia where CSFs have primarily been used to increase hemopoietic cell numbers. However, the CSFs are strong enhancers of the functional activity of mature neutrophils, monocytes, and eosinophils, and it would seem logical to extend the clinical use of the CSFs to the many patients with, or at risk of, infections, where hemopoiesis appears normal. Many such patients do not respond to the use of antibiotics, and there is some prospect that enhancement of cellular function might achieve resolution or prevention of such infections. The possible use of CSFs could therefore be considered in a variety of chronic infections, wound infections, and recurrent lung or urinary tract infections in addition to situations where infections are likely to occur, such as in patients with burns, skin grafts, or severe trauma or patients undergoing complex abdominal surgery.

Improved protocols must be designed for patients undergoing chemotherapy, because the use of CSFs following chemotherapy does not prevent the initial fall in leukocyte levels with its attendant risk of infections. There has been a reluctance to use CSF treatment before chemotherapy for reasons that are difficult to comprehend. It may be that the use of CSF-primed peripheral blood autografts will somewhat improve the situation by providing a population of hemopoietic cells that can initiate regeneration more rapidly. Possibly, the preliminary amplification of such harvested cells by in vitro culture with growth factors will provide an even more rapidly regenerating population also containing some maturing cells to be reinfused.

The major hemopoietic problems attending chemotherapy are neutropenia and thrombocytopenia. To a degree, CSF therapy has partially solved the problem of neutropenia, and the use of CSF-elicited peripheral blood autografts has diminished the problem of the slow regeneration of platelets. However, there is clearly a need to combine CSF treatment with the use of a regulatory factor stimulating platelet formation. There are four available agents with some capacity to stimulate platelet formation – IL-6, LIF, IL-11, and Multi-CSF – but none of these has a particularly strong action in vivo and all involve a considerable delay before platelet levels rise. The recent cloning of cDNA for thrombopoietin and the demonstration of its powerful effects in elevating platelet levels may well provide the therapeutic agent needed to solve the clinical problem of thrombocytopenia (de Sauvage et al., 1994; Kaushansky et al., 1994; Lok et al., 1994).

Although the CSFs have been used in the treatment of myeloid leukemia, their use has been restricted either to increasing sensitivity to cycle-specific agents or to enhancing subsequent hemopoietic regeneration following therapy where all leukemic cells were believed to have been eliminated. So far, no attempt has been made to explore the differentiation-committing actions of the CSFs to help induce remissions or to suppress residual leukemic cells during remission. While it is unlikely that all myeloid leukemias would respond positively to such treatment, some may, and since studies on leukemic cell lines have indicated the superiority of regulator combinations in achieving suppression, it is worth considering the use of combinations of CSFs or CSFs with active agents such as IL-6 or LIF in such an approach.

All studies to date have used injected recombinant CSFs, with the need for repeated injections, but this method of delivery can be improved. Given more complete information on the three-dimensional structure of CSF receptor complexes, it may be possible to develop low-molecular-weight, orally ingestible agonists that mimic the combining sites of the CSFs. Initial studies have suggested that it is feasible to inject cDNA intravenously in liposomes and then obtain extended expression of the cDNA by transfected endothelial and other cells (Zhu et al., 1993). If this approach could be extended to CSF cDNA, it might offer clear advantages for those patients currently facing a lifetime of CSF injections. A less speculative advance would be the development of new CSF formulations allowing depot injections of CSF with slow release to reduce the currently necessary daily or twice-daily injections.

This critical appraisal is not intended to diminish the success so far achieved by the clinical use of single CSFs. The shortcomings discussed are well recognized by the clinicians involved. The present phase of clinical CSF use should be viewed as a transient one, preceding the use of more effective and sophisticated treatment regimens based on principles already established from in vitro studies and work with experimental animals. Even if none of the proposed new regimens proves superior, the CSFs have still firmly established themselves as useful therapeutic agents in a wide variety of disease states.

# 15
# Conclusions

The discovery and characterization of the CSFs occurred at a time when the only previously known hemopoietic regulator, erythropoietin, appeared to be highly specific in its action, to have a single organ source, and to be unique in its actions on late-stage erythropoiesis. Subsequent studies have shown erythropoietin not to be entirely lineage-specific, not to have a single organ source, and not usually to be involved solely in the development of diseases of erythroid populations. Even so, erythropoietin remains the "gold standard" model for a regulatory system in which individual single-function regulators might control specific aspects of the biology of hemopoietic populations.

Present concepts of the control of hemopoiesis differ radically from such a simple model in that they have had to take into account the following data: (a) Multiple regulators have major overlapping of functions (if not entirely redundant actions), (b) regulators are typically polyfunctional, (c) regulators usually originate from a multiplicity of cell types, and (d) estimates of circulating levels of these regulators can give a very misleading impression of their likely importance or action.

The CSFs display all the features now recognized to be characteristic of the complex biology of hemopoietic regulators but, in hindsight, are intermediate in position between the largely single-function erythropoietin and newer regulators (typified by LIF, IL-6, IL-11, and oncostatin-M), which reach extraordinary levels of polyfunctionality involving a wide range of nonhemopoietic tissues.

Despite exhibiting certain actions on nonhemopoietic cells, it seems broadly valid to continue to regard the CSFs as hemopoietic regulators. This view is based on the present knowledge of their most obvious actions in vitro, their actions in vivo when administered clinically, and the consequences of artificially inducing elevations or depletion of CSF levels.

The evolution of our understanding of the regulatory control of various tissues does suggest, however, the wisdom of retaining some reservations about the ability to identify any regulator with a single tissue system. Future discoveries may well force some revision of the view that the CSFs are essentially hemopoietic regulators.

The hemopoietic populations most clearly influenced by CSF action are cells of the numerically large granulocyte-macrophage system. There is a temptation to oversimplify the CSFs by referring to them as a family of related regulators that control granulocyte-macrophage populations. The evidence that they are a related family comes from their overlapping range of actions, the close physical linkage of two of the genes - for GM-CSF and Multi-CSF - and their receptors, as well as the structural homology evident between the CSFs themselves and between the receptors for G-CSF, GM-CSF, and Multi-CSF. This notion of the CSF "family" probably should not be pressed too hard. In particular, M-CSF differs significantly in its biology because of its relatively high concentrations in the body, the obvious fluctuations in its levels during pregnancy, and the quite different nature of the M-CSF receptor. On this last basis, it could be argued that M-CSF might be more appropriately linked with other regulators, such as SCF, which have more closely related receptors.

The concept that the CSFs can simply be described as granulocyte-macrophage regulators is probably valid enough if based on a restricted view of their actions on these two prominent white cell lineages. The description is most valid for G-CSF and M-CSF and may be appropriate enough for GM-CSF if low concentrations are involved. Such a simple concept, however, ignores the prominent action of the CSFs on stem cells with the generation of committed progenitor cells in multiple lineages and the obvious actions of GM-CSF on dendritic cells and of Multi-CSF on mast cells, erythroid cells, and megakaryocytes.

It is perhaps better to refer to the CSFs as being major regulators involved in the control of granulocyte-macrophage populations - a subtle change in the preceding generalization, but one less prone to arousing misconceptions regarding the broad biological role of these regulators.

As discussed earlier, the CSFs can probably be regarded as the *major* regulators of granulocyte-macrophage populations, although it must be accepted that other regulators are potentially involved. Included in this category are SCF and IL-6, with some actions on granulocytic cells, and O-CSF, with actions on at least some macrophage populations. The failure of a homozygous inactivation of the G-CSF, GM-CSF, and M-CSF genes to suppress completely the formation either of granulocytic or macrophage cells suggests that other regulators of these populations may exist and are yet to be discovered.

One of the general principles emerging from the work on the CSFs is that although the tissues can rapidly alter their levels of CFS production in response to emergency situations, the CSF-producing system cannot be relied on to achieve the very high CSF levels necessary to stimulate maximal granulocyte-macrophage responses. In all situations so far analyzed, the administration of additional CSF achieves more rapid and greater hemopoietic responses than can be initiated either by infections or complete aplasia of the hemopoietic population. In the case of infections, it can be assumed that if a host cellular response is rapid, it can usually adequately eliminate the initial microorganisms with no tissue damage in a process requiring only moderate CSF concentrations. Disease development is the exceptional outcome in which the microorganisms escape early elimination and the usual CSF responses become inadequate to marshal the vastly increased granulocyte-macrophage responses then needed. This general principle appears similar to that applying to hormones such as the corticosteroids, where once a major inflammatory state has developed, normally achievable corticosteroid levels are inadequate and the administration of extra corticosteroids elicits dramatic responses. This principle probably also applies to regulatory systems for other tissues where similar limitations result in suboptimal responses. For example, it could be anticipated that the regulatory system controlling epithelial and mesenchymal cells probably does not achieve optimal rates of healing for major wounds and that, once developed, the administration of appropriate regulators would accelerate these processes.

From in vitro analyses and more limited studies in vivo, it seems that multiple regulatory factors control granulocyte-macrophage formation and function with some functional overlap, but not complete redundancy. The studies indicate that superior granulocyte-macrophage formation can be achieved using combinations of these regulators rather than by increasing the concentration of a single regulator. This arrangement probably places a lower demand on CSF-producing tissues and has the likely benefit of improving the precise localization of responding cells to affected tissues and the involvement of a broader range of responding cells. The optimal clinical use of CSFs must make use of this regulator design feature, but there are obvious practical problems. There are 15 possible combinations of the four CSFs using a single dosage schedule and route of administration. If it proves advantageous to combine CSFs with other regulators, then with the 20 regulators now available, there are more than a million such combinations. It is evident that extensive studies in vitro and with animal models will be needed to identify advantageous combinations for particular disease situations.

Studies designed to establish the physiology of the CSFs seem to have less appeal now that these agents are in clinical use. However, it is a questionable medical practice to use CSFs in the continuing absence of precise information on which cells produce CSF, and at what levels and under what circumstances. Similarly, there is a need to establish much more clearly the usual fate of these molecules. Is it target cell consumption, or degradation and clearance? If the latter, what are the cell types involved and what cellular processes achieve this? These questions must be resolved not only for the tissues in normal health, but also in the wide variety of disease situations in which local or systemic CSF may be involved in initiating the disease. As a consequence of these deficiencies, knowledge of the role played by the CSFs in disease development, whether for good or bad, remains rudimentary. An involvement of the CSFs is already evident for diseases such as chronic inflammatory states and myeloid leukemia but may also be the case for a much wider range of disease states.

Despite the major limitations in our understanding of the physiology of the CSFs, there appears to be a certain elegance about the design system of these regulators in the context of a multicellular organism in which the special functions permitting resistance to invading microorganisms have been delegated to the specialized granulocyte-macrophage population. Many, if not all, of the cells of the organism have a readily inducible set of CSF genes allowing these cells to produce CSF for either local or systemic use. This CSF can marshal the services of the protective granulocyte-macrophage population by localizing and functionally activating existing cells and then, if need be, by stimulating the production of additional cells. When demand ceases with the elimination of the microorganisms, the system returns promptly to basal levels of activity due to the short half-lives of both the mRNAs involved and the CSFs in circulation with the possibility that the additional CSF produced is actually consumed by the responding granulocyte-macrophage cells during their functional stimulation.

It should be possible to make use of the known actions of the CSFs to establish more precisely which hemopoietic cells are required under various abnormal circumstances and for what purposes. The logic of this approach is based on the assumption that the diverse actions exhibited by the CSFs are not side effects or retained vestigial functions, but are purposeful. It then becomes important to establish precisely under what circumstances each CSF is produced. For example, when is GM-CSF produced in unusual amounts? The capacity of GM-CSF to stimulate not only granulocyte and macrophage populations but also eosinophils can be taken as an indication that eosinophils play an important role in that particular abnormal circumstance. This logic can probably be fruitfully exploited not only for the CSFs, but also for those regulators with seemingly bizarre sets of unrelated responding cells. It may be that regulator molecules do possess purposeless side actions, but until this becomes clear, it is more prudent to accept that the various tissues do interact efficiently and, where polyfunctionality seems at odds with established notions of organ biology, to explore very carefully radically different possibilities that might link apparently disparate tissues in integrated biosystems.

There are now more than 20 defined hemopoietic regulators, but most researchers expect that the discovery process may have achieved only the halfway mark, with an equal number of hemopoietic regulators still to be identified. The search for these regulators preoccupies the attention and ambitions of most of the investigators in this field, their hope being to discover yet another hemopoietic regulator with the broad clinical applications and lucrative commercial potential of G-CSF. It could be questioned whether a new granulocyte-stimulating factor, if discovered, would ever find clinical use, given the availability of G-CSF. The cost of bringing a new factor to the clinic is about 200 million dollars, and few pharmaceutical companies now contemplate with equanimity the prospect of developing a competitor regulator whose actions might overlap those of an existing regulator. To a degree, the G-CSF example may prove to be exceptional because of the very large number of patients who could be treated with it – the one-fifth of the population destined to develop cancer and probably to have chemotherapy, as well as those with a wide variety of infections. Should a newly discovered regulator prove to have useful actions on a minor subset of hemopoietic cells of value in far less numerous disease states, it is doubtful whether such a regulator could ever be developed for clinical use because of the costs involved in the present methods of development and licensing.

These considerations may be overly pessimistic because the cost of producing clinical-quality recombinant regulators can certainly be greatly reduced, and there may be far less expensive ways of licensing agents for clinical use than the present cumbersome methods. From the biological viewpoint, it seems premature to discount the possibility that an agent acting on a currently obscure hemopoietic subpopulation will necessarily have little relevance in clinical medicine. The information beginning to emerge - for example, regarding dendritic cells, which were formerly an obscure population, and the action of GM-CSF on these cells - serves as a warning. Dendritic cell function may prove to be crucial for adequate T-cell responses to infections and cancer, and an agent with the capacity to amplify this function would clearly have broad potential clinical applications. The constant delight of experimental biology is the emergence of the unexpected to confound the model builders and prognosticators.

While the hemopoietic system admittedly consists of highly complex tissue, some of whose features, such as the need for continuous new cell formation, set it apart from many other tissues, it is becoming evident that most tissues, either in their developmental or mature phase, must solve the same general regulatory problems. It can be anticipated that, in time, the hemopoietic regulatory factors will be matched by an equally complex array of regulatory factors for other tissues. Given the development of adequate selective tissue culture systems for these other cell types, the technology exists to discover and apply these tissue regulators. We are indeed fortunate to be living in such an exciting time of discovery where opportunities abound for major advances in understanding the biology of multicellular organisms and for improving the management of disease.

# References

Abe, T., Sugaya, H., Ishida, K., Khan, W. I., Tasdemir, I., and Yoshimura, K. (1993). Intestinal protection against *Strongyloides rattii* and mastocytosis induced by administration of interleukin-3 in mice. *Immunology* **80:** 116–121.

Aglietta, M., Piacibello, W., Sanavio, F., Stacchini, A., Apra, F., Schena, M., Mosetti, C., Carnino, F., Caligaris-Cappio, F., and Gavosto, F. (1989). Kinetics of human hemopoietic cells after *in vivo* administration of granulocyte-macrophage colony-stimulating factor. *Journal of Clinical Investigation* **83:** 551–557.

Aharon, T., and Schneider, R. J. (1993). Selective destabilization of short-lived mRNAs with the granulocyte-macrophage colony-stimulating factor AU-rich 3′ noncoding region is mediated by a cotranslational mechanism. *Molecular and Cellular Biology* **13:** 1971–1980.

Aihara, T., Misago, M., Hanamura, T., Kikuchi, M., Toshimitsu, H., Ootani, H., Chiba, S., and Eto, S. (1993). Within-day and day-to-day variations of serum M-CSF levels in healthy volunteers. *Rinsho Byori* **41:** 268–272.

Altmann, S. W., Johnson, G. D., and Prystowsky, M. B. (1991). Single proline substitutions in predicted alpha-helices of murine granulocyte-macrophage colony-stimulating factor result in a loss of bioactivity and altered glycosylation. *Journal of Biological Chemistry* **266:** 5333–5341.

Antin, J. H., Smith, B. R., Holmes, W., and Rosenthal, D. S. (1988). Phase I/II study of recombinant human granulocyte-macrophage colony-stimulating factor in aplastic anemia and myelodysplastic syndrome. *Blood* **72:** 705–713.

Antman, K. S., Griffin, J. D., Elias, A. Socinski, M. A., Ryan, L., Cannistra, S. A., Oette, D., Whitley, M., Frei, E., and Schnipper, L. E. (1988). Effect of recombinant human granulocyte-macrophage colony-stimulating factor on chemotherapy-induced myelosuppression. *New England Journal of Medicine* **319:** 593–598.

Arai, K. I., Lee, F., Miyajima, A., Miyatake, S., Arai, N., and Yokota, T. (1990). Cytokines: Coordinators of immune and inflammatory responses. *Annual Review of Biochemistry* **59:** 783–836.

Arai, N., Naito, Y., Watanabe, M., Masuda, E. S., Yamaguchi-Iwai, Y., Tsuboi, A., Heike, T., Matsuda, I., Yokota, K., Koyano-Nakagawa, N., Li, H. J., Muramatsu, M., Yokota, T., and Arai, K. I. (1992). Activation of lymphokine genes in T cells: Role of cis-acting DNA elements that respond to T cell activation signals. *Pharmacology and Therapeutics* **55:** 303–318.

Arceci, R. J., Shanahan, F., Stanley, E. R., and Pollard, J. W. (1989). Temporal expression and location of colony-stimulating factor 1 (CSF-1) and its receptor in the female reproductive tract are consistent with CSF-1-regulated placental development. *Proceedings of the National Academy of Sciences, U.S.A.* **86:** 8818–8822.

Asano, M., and Nagata, S. (1992). Constitutive and inducible factors bind to regulatory element 3 in the promoter of the gene encoding mouse granulocyte colony-stimulating factor. *Gene* **121:** 371–375.

Asano, S., Sato, N., Mori, M., Ohsawa, W., Kosaka, K., and Ueyama, Y. (1980). Detection and assessment of human tumors producing granulocyte-macrophage colony-stimulating factor (GM-CSF) by heterotransplantation into nude mice. *British Journal of Cancer* **41:** 689–694.

Ashworth, A., and Kraft, A. (1990). Cloning of a potentially soluble receptor for human GM-CSF. *Nucleic Acids Research* **18:** 7178.

Athanassakis, I., Bleackley, C. R., Paetkau, V., Guilbert, L., Barr, P. J., and Wegmann, T. G. (1987). The immunostimulatory effect of T cells and T cell lymphokines on murine fetally derived placental cells. *Journal of Immunology* **138:** 37–44.

Azuma, J., Kurimoto, T., and Awata, S., et al. (1989). Phase I study of KRN 8601 (rhG-CSF) in normal volunteers: Safety and pharmacokinetics in single subcutaneous administration. *Rinsho Iyaku* **5:** 2231–2252.

Baccarini, M., Dello, S. P., Buscher, D., Bartocci, A., and Stanley, E. R. (1992). IFN-gamma/lipopolysaccharide activation of macrophages is associated with protein kinase C-dependent down-modulation of the colony-stimulating factor-1 receptor. *Journal of Immunology* **149:** 2656–2661.

Baccarini, M., and Stanley, E. R. (1990). Colony stimulating factor-1. In A. Habenicht (ed.), *Growth Factors, Differentiation Factors, and Cytokines, 1990,* pp. 189–200. Berlin: Springer-Verlag.

Bagby, G. C., McCall, E. A., Bergstrom, K. A., and Burger, D. (1983). A monokine regulates colony-stimulating activity production by vascular endothelial cells. *Blood* **62:** 663–668.

Baiocchi, G., Scambia, G., Benedetti, P., Menichella, G., Testa, U., Pierelli, L., Martucci, R., Foddai, M. L., Bizzi, B., Mancuso, S., and Peschle, C. (1993). Autologous stem cell transplantation: Sequential production of hematopoietic cytokines underlying granulocytic recovery. *Cancer Research* **53:** 1297–1303.

Baldwin, G. C., Benveniste, E. N., Chung, G. Y., Gasson, J. C., and Golde, D. W. (1993). Identification and characterization of a high-affinity granulocyte-macrophage colony-stimulating factor receptor on primary rat oligodendrocytes. *Blood* **82:** 3279–3282.

Baldwin, G. C., Gasson, J. C., Kaufman, S. E., Quan, S. G., Williams, R. E., Avalos, B. R., Gazdar, A. F., Golde, D. W., and DiPersio, J. F. (1989). Nonhematopoietic tumor cells express functional GM-CSF receptors. *Blood* **73:** 1033–1037.

Balkwill, F. R., and Burke, F. (1989). The cytokine network. *Immunology Today* **10:** 299–304.

Barlow, D. P., Bucan, M., Lehrach, H., Hogan, B. L., and Gough, N. M. (1987). Close genetic and physical linkage between the murine haemopoietic growth factor genes GM-CSF and Multi-CSF (IL-3). *EMBO Journal* **6:** 617–623.

Bartocci, A., Mastrogiannis, D. S., Migliorati, G., Stockert, R. J., Wolkoff, A. W., and Stanley, E. R. (1987). Macrophages specifically regulate the concentration of their own growth factor in the circulation. *Proceedings of the National Academy of Sciences, U.S.A.* **84:** 6179–6183.

Bartocci, A., Pollard, J. W., and Stanley, E. R. (1986). Regulation of colony-stimulating factor 1 during pregnancy. *Journal of Experimental Medicine* **164:** 956–961.

Bazan, J. F. (1990a). Haemopoietic receptors and helical cytokines. *Immunology Today* **11:** 350–354.

Bazan, J. F. (1990b). Structural design and molecular evolution of a cytokine receptor superfamily. *Proceedings of the National Academy of Sciences, U.S.A.* **87:** 6934–6938.

Bazan, J. F. (1991a). Genetic and structural homology of stem cell factor and macrophage colony-stimulating factor [letter]. *Cell* **65:** 9–10.

Bazan, J. F. (1991b). Neuropoietic cytokines in the hematopoietic fold. *Neuron* **7:** 197–208.

Bazill, G. W., Haynes, M., Garland, J., and Dexter, T. M. (1983). Characterization and partial purification of a haemopoietic growth factor in WEHI-3 conditioned medium. *Biochemical Journal* **210:** 747–759.

Begg, S. K., Radley, J. M., Pollard, J. W., Chisholm, O. T., Stanley, E. R., and Bertoncello, I. (1993). Delayed hematopoietic development in osteopetrotic (*op/op*) mice. *Journal of Experimental Medicine* 177: 237–242.

Begley, C. G., Lopez, A. F., Nicola, N. A., Warren, D. J., Vadas, M. A., Sanderson, C. J., and Metcalf, D. (1986). Purified colony stimulating factors enhance the survival of human neutrophils and eosinophils *in vitro*: A rapid and sensitive microassay for colony stimulating factors. *Blood* **68:** 162–166.

Begley, C. G., Metcalf, D., Lopez, A. F., and Nicola, N. A. (1985). Fractionated populations of normal human marrow cells respond to both human colony-stimulating factors with granulocyte-macrophage activity. *Experimental Hematology* **13:** 956–962.

Begley, C. G., Metcalf, D., and Nicola, N. A. (1987). Primary human myeloid leukemia cells: Comparative responsiveness to proliferative stimulation by GM-CSF or G-CSF and membrane expression of CSF receptors. *Leukemia* **1:** 1–8.

Begley, C. G., Nicola, N. A., and Metcalf, D. (1988). Proliferation of normal human promyelocytes and myelocytes after a single pulse stimulation by purified GM-CSF or G-CSF. *Blood* **71:** 640–645.

Berdel, W. E., Danhauser-Riedl, S., Steinhauser, G., and Rastetter, J. (1990). Stimulation of clonal growth of human colorectal tumor cells by IL-3 and GM-CSF. Modulation of 5-FU cytotoxicity by GM-CSF. *Onkologie* **13:** 437–443.

Bettelheim, P., Valent, P., Andreeff, M., Tafuri, A., Haimi, J., Gorischek, C., Muhm, M., Sillaber, C., Haas, O., Vieder, L., Maurer, D., Schultz, G., Speiser, W., Geissler, K., Kier, P., Hinterberger, W., and Lechner, K. (1991). Recombinant human granulocyte-macrophage colony-stimulating factor in combination with standard induction chemotherapy in *de novo* acute myeloid leukemia. *Blood* **77:** 700–711.

Bhalla, K., Birkhofer, M., Grand, S., and Graham, G. (1989). The effect of recombinant human granulocyte-macrophage colony-stimulating factor (rGM-CSF) on 3′-Azido-3′-deoxythymidine (AZT)-mediated biochemical and cytotoxic effects on normal human myeloid progenitor cells. *Experimental Hematology* **17:** 17–20.

Biesma, B., Pokorny, R., Kovarik, J. M., Duffy, F. A., Willemse, P. H. B., Mulder, N. H., and de Vries, E. G. E. (1993). Pharmacokinetics of recombinant human interleukin 3 administered subcutaneously and by continuous intravenous infusion in patients after chemotherapy for ovarian cancer. *Cancer Research* **53:** 5915–5919.

Biesma, B., Willemse, P. H. B., Mulder, N. H., Sleijfer, D. Th., Gietema, J. A., Mull, R., Limburg, P. C., Bouma, J., Vellenga, E., and de Vries, E. G. E. (1992). Effects of interleukin-3 after chemotherapy for advanced ovarian cancer. *Blood* **80:** 1141–1148.

Blatt, C., Aberdam, D., Schwartz, R., and Sachs, L. (1988). DNA rearrangement of a homeobox gene in myeloid leukaemic cells. *EMBO Journal* **7:** 4283–4290.

Bocchietto, E., Guglielmetti, A., Silvagno, F., Taraboletti, G., Pescarmona, G. P., Mantovani, A., and Bussolino, F. (1993). Proliferative and migratory responses of murine microvascular endothelial cells to granulocyte-colony-stimulating factor. *Journal of Cellular Physiology* **155:** 89–95.

Bodey, G. P., Buckley, M., Sathe, Y. S., and Freireich, E. J. (1966). Quantitative relationships between circulating leukocytes and infections in patients with acute leukemia. *Annals of Internal Medicine* **64:** 328–340.

Bonilla, M. A., Gillio, A. P., Ruggeiro, M., Kernan, N. A., Brochstein, J. A., Abboud, M., Fumagalli, L., Vincent, M., Gabrilove, J. L., Welte, K., Souza, L. M., and O'Reilly, R. J. (1989). Effects of recombinant human granulocyte colony stimulating factor on neutropenia in patients with congenital agranulocytosis. *New England Journal of Medicine* **320:** 1574–1580.

Borzillo, G. V., and Sherr, C. J. (1989). Early pre-B-cell transformation induced by the v-fms oncogene in long-term mouse bone marrow cultures. *Molecular and Cellular Biology* **9:** 3973–3981.

Bot, F. J., Schipper, P., Broeders, L., Delwel, R., Kaushansky, K., and Löwenberg, B. (1990a). Interleukin 1-$\alpha$ also induces granulocyte-macrophage colony-stimulating factor in immature normal bone marrow cells. *Blood* **76:** 307–311.

Bot, F. J., van Eijk, L., Schipper, P., Backx, B., and Löwenberg, B. (1990b). Synergistic effects between GM-CSF and G-CSF or M-CSF on highly enriched human marrow progenitor cells. *Leukemia* **4:** 325–328.

Bot, F. J., van Eijk, L., Schipper, P., and Löwenberg, B. (1989). Human granulocyte-macrophage colony-stimulating factor (GM-CSF) stimulates immature marrow precursors but no CFU-GM, CFU-G or CFU-M. *Experimental Hematology* **17:** 292–295.

Boyd, A. W., and Metcalf, D. (1984). Induction of differentiation in HL60 leukemic cells: A cell cycle dependent all-or-none effect. *Leukemia Research* **8:** 27–43.

Brach, M. A., Arnold, C., Kiehntopf, M., Gruss, H. J., and Herrmann, F. (1993). Transcriptional activation of the macrophage colony-stimulating factor gene by IL-2 is associated with secretion of bioactive macrophage colony-stimulating factor protein by monocytes and involves activation of the transcription factor NF-kappa B. *Journal of Immunology* **150:** 5535–5543.

Bradley, T. R., Hodgson, G. S., and Bertoncello, I. (1980). Characterization of macrophage progenitor cells with high proliferative potential: Their relationships to cells with marrow repopulating ability in 5-fluorouracil treated mouse bone marrow. In S. J. Baum, G. D. Ledney, and D. W. Van Bekkum (eds.), *Experimental Hematology Today, 1980,* pp. 285–297. New York: Karger.

Bradley, T. R., and Metcalf, D. (1966). The growth of mouse bone marrow cells in vitro. *Australian Journal of Experimental Biology and Medical Science* **44:** 287–300.

Bradley, T. R., Metcalf, D., Sumner, M., and Stanley, R. (1969). Characteristics of *in vitro* colony formation by cells from haemopoietic tissues. In P. Farnes (ed.), *Hemic Cells In Vitro,* Vol. 4, pp. 22–35. Philadelphia: Williams & Wilkins.

Brandt, S. J., Peters, W. P., Atwater, S. K., Kurtzberg, J., Borowitz, M. J., Jones, R. B., Shpall, E. J., Bast, R. C., Jr., Gilbert, C. J., and Oette, D. H. (1988). Effect of recombinant granulocyte-macrophage colony-stimulating factor on hematopoietic reconstitution after high-dose chemotherapy and autologous bone marrow transplantation. *New England Journal of Medicine* **318:** 869–876.

Briddell, R. A., Hartley, C. A., Smith, K. A., and McNiece, I. K. (1993). Recombinant rat stem cell factor synergizes with recombinant human granulocyte colony-stimulating factor *in vivo* in mice to mobilize peripheral blood progenitor cells that have enhanced repopulating potential. *Blood* **82:** 1720–1723.

Bronchud, M. H., Howell, A., Crowther, D., Hopwood, P., Souza, L., and Dexter, T. M. (1989). The use of granulocyte colony-stimulating factor to increase the intensity of treatment with doxorubicin in patients with advanced breast and ovarian cancer. *British Journal of Cancer* **60:** 121–125.

Bronchud, M. H., Scarffe, J. H., Thatcher, N., Crowther, D., Souza, L. M., Alton, W. K., Testa, N. G., and Dexter, T. M. (1987). Phase I/II study of recombinant human granulocyte colony-stimulating factor in patients receiving intensive chemotherapy for small cell lung cancer. *British Journal of Cancer* **56:** 809–813.

Broudy, V. C., Kaushansky, K., Harlan, J. M., and Adamson, J. W. (1987). Interleukin 1 stimulates human endothelial cells to produce granulocyte-macrophage colony-stimulating factor and granulocyte colony-stimulating factor. *Journal of Immunology* **139:** 464–468.

Broudy, V. C., Kaushansky, K., Segal, G. M., Harlan, J. M., and Adamson, J. W. (1986a). Tumor necrosis factor type $\alpha$ stimulates human endothelial cells to produce granulocyte/macrophage colony stimulating factor. *Proceedings of the National Academy of Sciences, U.S.A.* **83:** 7467–7471.

Broudy, V. C., Zuckerman, K. S., Jetmalani, S., Fitchan, J. H., and Bagby, G. C., Jr. (1986b). Monocytes stimulate fibroblastoid bone marrow stromal cells to produce multilineage hematopoietic growth factors. *Blood* **68:** 530–534.

Brown, C. B., Hart, C. E., Curtis, D. M., Bailey, M. C., and Kaushansky, K. (1990). Two neutralizing monoclonal antibodies against human granulocyte-macrophage colony-stimulating factor recognize the receptor binding domain of the molecule. *Journal of Immunology* **144:** 2184–2189.

Brown, M. A., Gough, N. M., Willson, T. A., Rockman, S., and Begley, C. G. (1993). Structure and expression of the GM-CSF receptor $\alpha$ and $\beta$ chain genes in human leukemia. *Leukemia* **7:** 63–74.

Broxmeyer, H. E., Cooper, S., Lu, L., Miller, M. E., Langefeld, C. D., and Ralph, P. (1990). Enhanced stimulation of human bone marrow macrophage colony formation *in vitro* by recombinant human macrophage colony-stimulating factor in agarose medium and at low oxygen tension. *Blood* **76:** 323–329.

Buchberg, A. M., Bedigian, H. G., Taylor, B. A., Brownell, E., Ihle, J. N., Nagata, S., Jenkins, N. A., and Copeland, N. G. (1988). Localization of

Evi-2 to chromosome 11: Linkage to other proto-oncogene and growth factor loci using interspecific backcross mice. *Oncogene Research* **2:** 149–165.

Budel, L. M., Elbaz, O., Hoogerbrugge, H., Delwel, R., Mahmoud, L. A., Löwenberg, B., and Touw, I. P. (1990). Common binding structure for granulocyte macrophage colony-stimulating factor and interleukin-3 on human acute myeloid leukemia cells and monocytes. *Blood* **75:** 1439–1445.

Budel, L. M., Touw, I. P., Delwel, R., and Löwenberg, B. (1989). Granulocyte colony-stimulating factor receptors in human acute myelocytic leukemia. *Blood* **74:** 2668–2673.

Buick, R. N., Minden, M. D., and McCulloch, E. A. (1979). Self-renewal in culture of proliferative blast progenitor cells in acute myeloblastic leukemia. *Blood* **54:** 95–104.

Bungart, B., Loeffler, M., Goris, H., Dontje, B., Diehl, V., and Nijhof, W. (1990). Differential effects of recombinant human colony stimulating factor (rh G-CSF) on stem cells in marrow, spleen and peripheral blood in mice. *British Journal of Haematology* **76:** 174–179.

Burgess, A. W., Camakaris, J., and Metcalf, D. (1977). Purification and properties of colony-stimulating factor from mouse lung conditioned medium. *Journal of Biological Chemistry* **252:** 1998–2003.

Burgess, A. W., and Metcalf, D. (1977). Serum half-life and organ distribution of radiolabeled colony stimulating factor in mice. *Experimental Hematology* **5:** 456–464.

Burgess, A. W., and Metcalf, D. (1980). Characterization of a serum factor stimulating the differentiation of myelomonocytic leukemic cells. *International Journal of Cancer* **26:** 647–654.

Burgess, A. W., Metcalf, D., Russell, S. H. M., and Nicola, N. A. (1980). Granulocyte/macrophage-, megakaryocyte-, eosinophil- and erythroid-colony-stimulating factors produced by mouse spleen cells. *Biochemical Journal* **185:** 301–314.

Bussolino, F., Wang, J. M., Defilippi, P., Turrini, F., Sanavio, F., Edgell, C.-J. S., Aglietta, M., Arese, P., and Mantovani, A. (1989). Granulocyte- and granulocyte-macrophage colony stimulating factors induce endothelial cells to migrate and proliferate. *Nature (London)* **337:** 471–473.

Butturini, A., Gale, R. P., Lopes, D. M., Cunha, C. B., Ilo, W. G., Sanpai, J. M., De Souza, P. C., Cordiero, J. M., Neto, C., De Souza, C. E. P., Tabak, D. G., Burla, A., and the Navy Hospital Radiation Team. (1988). Use of recombinant granulocyte-macrophage colony stimulating factor in the Brazil radiation accident. *Lancet* **2:** 471–475.

Byrne, P. V., Guilbert, L. J., and Stanley, E. R. (1981). Distribution of cells bearing receptors for a colony-stimulating factor (CSF-1) in murine tissues. *Journal of Cellular Biology* **91:** 848–853.

Cairo, M. S., Mauss, D., Kommareddy, S., Norris, K., Van de Ven, C., and Modanlou, H. (1990). Prophylactic or simultaneous administration of recombinant human granulocyte colony stimulating factor in the treatment of group B streptococcal sepsis in neonatal rats. *Pediatric Research* **27:** 612–616.

Cairo, M. S., Suen, Y., Sender, L., Gillan, E. R., Ho, W., Plunkett, J. M., and Van de Ven, C. (1992). Circulating granulocyte colony-stimulating factor (G-CSF) levels after allogeneic and autologous bone marrow transplantation: Endogenous G-CSF production correlates with myeloid engraftment. *Blood* **79:** 1869–1873.

Campbell, H. D., Ymer, S., Fung, M. C., and Young, I. G. (1985). Cloning and nucleotide sequence of the murine interleukin-3 gene. *European Journal of Biochemistry* **150:** 297–304.

Cantrell, D. A., and Smith, K. A. (1984). The interleukin-2 T-cell system: A new cell growth model. *Science (Washington)* **224:** 1312–1316.

Cantrell, M. A., Anderson, D., Cerretti, D. P., Price, V., McKereghan, K., Tushinski, R. J., Mochizuki, D. Y., Larsen, A., Grabstein, K., Gillis, S., and Cosman, D. (1985). Cloning, sequence and expression of a human granulocyte/macrophage colony stimulating factor. *Proceedings of the National Academy of Sciences, U.S.A.* **82:** 6250–6254.

Caput, D., Beutler, B., Hartog, K., Thayer, R., Brown, S. S., and Cerami, A. (1986). Identification of a common nucleotide sequence in the 3′-untranslated region of mRNA molecules specifying inflammatory mediators. *Proceedings of the National Academy of Sciences, U.S.A.* **83:** 1670–1674.

Caracciolo, D., Shirsat, N., Wong, G. G., Lange, B., Clark, S., and Rovera, G. (1987). Recombinant human macrophage colony-stimulating factor (M-CSF) requires sublimal concentrations of granulocyte/macrophage (GM)-CSF for optimal stimulation of human macrophage colony formation *in vitro. Journal of Experimental Medicine* **166:** 1851–1860.

Carlberg, K., Tapley, P., Haystead, C., and Rohrschneider, L. (1991). The role of kinase activity and the kinase insert region in ligand-induced internalization and degradation of the c-fms protein. *EMBO Journal* **10:** 877–883.

Carnot, P., and Deflandre, G. (1906). Sur l'activité hemopoietique du serum au cours de la régeneration du sang. *Comptes Rendu Académie Science, Paris* **143:** 384–386.

Carrington, P. A., Hill, R. J., Stenberg, P. E., Levin, J., Corash, L., Schreurs, J., Baker, G., and Levin, F. C. (1991). Multiple *in vivo* effects of interleukin-3 and interleukin-6 on murine megakaryocytopoiesis. *Blood* **77:** 34–41.

Carrol, M. P., Clark-Lewis, I., Rapp, U. R., and May, W. S. (1990). Interleukin-3 and granulocyte-macrophage colony-stimulating factor mediate rapid phosphorylation and activation of cytosolic c-raf. *Journal of Biological Chemistry* **265:** 19812–19817.

Cebon, J. S., Bury, R. W. Lieschke, G. J., and Morstyn, G. (1990a). The effects of dose and route of administration on the pharmacokinetics of granulocyte-macrophage colony-stimulating factor. *European Journal of Cancer* **26:** 1064–1069.

Cebon, J., Layton, J. E., Maher, D., and Morstyn, G. (1994). Endogenous haemopoietic growth factors in neutropenia and infection. *British Journal of Haematology* **86:** 265–274.

Cebon, J., Nicola, N., Ward, M., Gardner, I., Dempsey, P., Layton, J., Dührsen, U., Burgess, A. W., Nice, E., and Morstyn, G. (1990b). Granulocyte-macrophage colony stimulating factor from human lymphocytes: The effect of glycosylation on receptor binding and biological activity. *Journal of Biological Chemistry* **268:** 4483–4491.

Cerretti, D. P., Wignall, J., Anderson, D., Tushinski, R. J., Gallis, B. M., Stya, M., Gillis, S., Urdal, D. L., and Cosman, D. (1988). Human macrophage-colony stimulating factor: Alternative RNA and protein processing from a single gene. *Molecular Immunology* **25:** 761–770.

Chan, J. Y., Slamon, D. J., Nimer, S. D., Golde, D. W., and Gasson, J. C. (1986). Regulation of expression of human granulocyte/macrophage colony-stimulating factor. *Proceedings of the National Academy of Sciences, U.S.A.* **83:** 8669–8673.

Chan, S. H. (1972). Bone marrow colony stimulating factor (CSF) and inhibitor levels in renal disease. *Revue Europeenne D'endes Cliniques et Biologiques* **17:** 686–690.

Chan, S. H., and Metcalf, D. (1972). Local production of colony-stimulating factor within the bone marrow: Role of nonhematopoietic cells. *Blood* **40:** 646–653.

Chang, J. M., Metcalf, D., Gonda, T. J., and Johnson, G. R. (1989a). Long-term exposure to retrovirally-expressed G-CSF induces a non-neoplastic granulocytic and progenitor cell hyperplasia without tissue damage in mice. *Journal of Laboratory Clinical Investigation* **84:** 1488–1496.

Chang, J. M., Metcalf, D., Lang, R. A., Gonda, T. J., and Johnson, G. R. (1989b). Non-neoplastic hematopoietic myeloproliferative syndrome induced by dysregulated Multi-CSF (IL-3) expression. *Blood* **73:** 1487–1497.

Chao, N. J., Schriber, J. R., Grimes, K., Long, G. D., Negrin, R. S., Raimondi, C. M., Horning, S. J., Brown, S. L., Miller, L., and Blume, K. G. (1993). Granulocyte colony-stimulating factor "mobilized" peripheral blood progenitor cells accelerate granulocyte and platelet recovery after high-dose chemotherapy. *Blood* **81:** 2031–2035.

Cheers, C., Haigh, A. M., Kelso, A., Metcalf, D., Stanley, E. R., and Young, A. M. (1988). Production of colony-stimulating factors (CSFs) during infection: Separate determinations of macrophage-, granulocyte-, granulocyte-macrophage and Multi-CSFs. *Infection and Immunity* **56:** 247–251.

Chen, A. R., and Rohrschneider, L. R. (1993). Mechanism of differential inhibition of factor-dependent cell proliferation by transforming growth factor $\beta$1: Selective uncoupling of FMS from MYC. *Blood* **81:** 2539–2546.

Chen, B. D. (1991). In vivo administration of recombinant human interleukin-1 and macrophage colony-stimulating factor (M-CSF) induce a rapid loss of M-CSF receptors in mouse bone marrow cells and peritoneal macrophages: Effect of administration route. *Blood* **77:** 1923–1928.

Chen, B. D., Chou, T. H., and Sensenbrenner. L. (1993). Downregulation of M-CSF receptors by lipopolysaccharide in murine peritoneal exudate macrophages is mediated through a phospholipase C dependent pathway. *Experimental Hematology* **21:** 623–628.

Chervenak, R., Dempsey, D., Soloff, R. S., and Smithson, G. (1992). *In vitro* growth of bone marrow-resident T cell precursors supported by mast cell growth factor and IL-3. *Journal of Immunology* **149:** 2851–2856.

Chikkappa, G., Broxmeyer, H. E., Cooper, S. Williams, D. E., Hangoc, G., Greenberg, M. L., Waheed, A., and Shadduck, R. K. (1989). Effect *in vivo* of multiple injections of purified murine and recombinant human macrophage colony-stimulating factor to mice. *Cancer Research* **49:** 3558–3561.

Claesson, M. H., Olsson, L., Martinsen, L., and Brix-Poulsen, P. (1982). Bone marrow derived diffuse colonies: Their cytotoxic potential, morphology and antigenic phenotype. *Experimental Hematology* **10:** 708–721.

Clark, D. I., Chaouat, G., Mogil, R., and Wegmann, T. G. (1994). Prevention of spontaneous abortion in DBA/2-mated CBA/J mice by GM-CSF involves $CD8^+$ T-cell dependent suppression of natural effector cell cytotoxicity against trophoblast target cells. *Cellular Immunology* **154:** 143–152.

Clark-Lewis, I., Aebersold, R., Ziltener, H., Schrader. J. W., Hood, L. E., and Kent, S. B. (1986). Automoted chemical synthesis of a protein growth factor for hemopoietic cells, interleukin-3. *Science (Washington)* **231:** 134–139.

Clark-Lewis, I., Hood, L. E., and Kent, S. B. (1988a). Role of disulfide bridges in determining the biological activity of interleukin 3. *Proceedings of the National Academy of Sciences, U.S.A.* **85:** 7897–7901.

Clark-Lewis, I., Kent, S. B. H., and Schrader, J. W. (1984). Purification to apparent homogeneity of a factor stimulating the growth of multiple lineages of hemopoietic cells. *Journal of Biological Chemistry* **259:** 7488–7494.

Clark-Lewis, I., Lopez, A. F., To, L. B., Vadas, M. A., Schrader, J. W., Hood, L. E., and Kent, S. B. (1988b). Structure-function studies of human granulocyte-macrophage colony-stimulating factor. Identification of residues required for activity. *Journal of Immunology* **141:** 881–889.

Clark-Lewis, I., and Schrader, J. W. (1988). Molecular structure and biological activities of P cell-stimulating factor (interleukin 3). *Lymphokines* **15:** 1–37.

Clayberger, C., Luna-Fineman, S., Lee, J. E., Pillai, A., Campbell, M., Levy, R., and Krensky, A. M. (1992). Interleukin 3 is a growth factor for human folicular B cell lymphoma. *Journal of Experimental Medicine* **175:** 371–376.

Cockerill, P. N., Shannon, M. F., Bert, A. G., Ryan, G. R., and Vadas, M. A. (1993). The granulocyte-macrophage colony-stimulating factor/interleukin 3 locus is regulated by an inducible cyclosporin A-sensitive enhancer. *Proceedings of the National Academy of Sciences, U.S.A.* **90:** 2466–2470.

Cole, D. J., Sanda, M. G., Yang, J. C., Schwartzentruber, D. J., Weber, J., Ettinghausen, S. E., Pockaj, B. A., Kim, H. I., Levin, R. D., Pogrebniak, H. W., Balkissoon, J., Fenton, R. M., DeBarge, L. R., Kaye, J., Rosenberg, S. A., and Parkinson, D. R. (1994). Phase I trial of recombinant human macrophage colony-stimulating factor administered by continuous intravenous infusion in patients with metastatic cancer. *Journal of the National Cancer Institute* **86:** 39–45.

Conlon, P. J., Luk, K. H., Park, L. S., March, C. J., Hopp, T. P., and Urdal, D. L. (1985). Generation of anti-peptide monoclonal antibodies which recognize mature CSF-2 alpha (IL3) protein. *Journal of Immunology* **135:** 328–332.

Courtneidge, S. A., Dhand, R., Pilat, D., Twamley, G. M., Waterfield, M. D., and Roussel, M. F. (1993). Activation of Src family kinases by colony stimulating factor-1, and their association with its receptor. *EMBO Journal* **12:** 943–950.

Coussens, L., Van Beveren, C., Smith, D., Chen, E., Mitchell, R. L., Isacke, C. M., Verma, I. M., and Ullrich, A. (1986). Structural alteration of viral homologue of receptor proto-oncogene fms at carboxyl terminus. *Nature (London)* **320:** 277–280.

Crawford, J., Ozer, H., Stoller, R., Johnson, D., Lyman, G., Tabbara, I., Kris, M., Grous, J., Picozzi, V., Rausch, G., Smith, R., Gradishar, W., Yahanda, A., Vincent, M., Stewart, M., and Glaspy, J. (1991). Reduction by granulocyte colony-stimulating factor of fever and neutropenia induced by chemotherapy in patients with small-cell lung cancer. *New England Journal of Medicine* **325:** 164–170.

Crosier, K. E., Wong, G. G., Mathey, P. B., Nathan, D. G., and Sieff, C. A. (1991). A functional isoform of the human granulocyte/macrophage colony-stimulating factor receptor has an unusual cytoplasmic domain. *Proceedings of the National Academy of Sciences, U.S.A.* **88:** 7744–7748.

Cumano, A., Paige, C. J., Iscove, N. N., and Brady, G. (1992). Bipotential precursors of B cells and macrophages in murine fetal liver. *Nature (London)* **356:** 612–615.

Cuthbertson, R. A., Lang, R. A., and Coghlan, J. P. (1990). Macrophage products IL-1 alpha, TNF alpha and bFGF may mediate multiple cytopathic effects in the developing eyes of GM-CSF transgenic mice. *Experimental Eye Research* **51:** 335–344.

Cutler, R. L., Metcalf, D., Nicola, N. A., and Johnson, G. R. (1985). Purification of a multipotential colony stimulating factor from pokeweed mitogen-stimulated mouse spleen cell conditioned medium. *Journal of Biological Chemistry* **260:** 6579–6587.

Cynshi, O., Satoh, K., Shimonaka, Y., Hattori, K., Nomura, H., Imai, N., and Hirashima, K. (1991). Reduced response to granulocyte colony-stimulating factor in $W/W^v$ and $Sl/Sl^d$ mice. *Leukemia* **5:** 75–77.

Dale, D. C., Bonilla, M. A., Davis, M. W., Nakanishi, A. M., Hammond, W. P., Kurtzberg, J., Wang, W., Jakubowski, A., Winton, E., Lalezari, P., Robinson, W., Glaspy, J. A., Emerson, S., Gabrilove, J., Vincent, M., and Boxer, L. A. (1993). Randomized controlled Phase III trial of recombinant human granulocyte colony-stimulating factor (Filgrastim) for treatment of severe chronic neutropenia. *Blood* **81:** 2496–2502.

Daley, G. Q., and Baltimore, D. (1988). Transformation of an interleukin 3-dependent hematopoietic cell line by the chronic myelogenous leukemia-specific $P210^{bcr/abl}$ protein. *Proceedings of the National Academy of Sciences, U.S.A.* **85:** 9312–9316.

Das, S. K., and Stanley, E. R. (1982). Structure-function studies of a colony stimulating factor (CSF-1). *Journal of Biological Chemistry* **257:** 13679–13684.

Davies, K., TePas, E. C., Nathan, D. G., and Mathey-Prevot, B. (1993). Interleukin-3 expression by activated T cells involves an inducible, T-cell specific factor and an octamer binding protein. *Blood* **81:** 928–934.

Decoster, G., Rich, W., and Brown, S. L. (1994). Safety profile of filgrastim (r-metHuG-CSF). In G. Morstyn and T. M. Dexter (eds.), *Filgrastim (r-metHuG-CSF) in Clinical Practice,* pp. 267–290. New York: Dekker.

Dedhar, S., Gaboury, L., Galloway, P., and Eaves, C. (1988). Human granulocyte-macrophage colony-stimulating factor is a growth factor active on a variety of cell types of nonhemopoietic origin. *Proceedings of the National Academy of Sciences, U.S.A.* **85:** 9253–9257.

de Haan, G., Loeffler, M., and Nijhof, W. (1992). Long-term recombinant human granulocyte colony-stimulating factor (rhG-CSF) treatment severely depresses murine marrow erythropoiesis without causing an anemia. *Experimental Hematology* **20:** 600–604.

DeLamarter, J. F., Hession, C., Semon, D., Gough, N. M., Rothenbuhler, R., and Mermod, J.-J. (1987). Nucleotide sequence of a cDNA encoding murine CSF-1 (macrophage-CSF). *Nucleic Acids Research* **15:** 2389–2390.

DeLamarter, J. F., Mermod, J.-J., Liang, C. M., Eliason, J. F., and Thatcher, D. R. (1985). Recombinant murine GM-CSF from *E. coli* has biological activity and is neutralized by a specific antiserum. *EMBO Journal* **4:** 2575–2581.

DeLuca, E., Sheridan, W. P., Watson, D., Szer, J., and Begley, C. G. (1992). Prior chemotherapy does not prevent effective mobilisation by G-CSF of peripheral blood progenitor cells. *British Journal of Cancer* **66:** 893–899.

Delwell, R., Van Buitenen, C., Salem, M., Bot, F., Gillis, S., Kaushansky, K., Altrock, B., and Löwenberg, R. (1989). Interleukin-1 stimulates proliferation of acute myeloblastic leukemia cells by induction of granulocyte-macrophage colony-stimulating factor release. *Blood* **74:** 586–593.

Demetri, G. D., Ernst, T. J., Pratt, E. S., II, Zenzie, B. W., Rheinwald, J. G., and Griffin, J. D. (1990). Expression of ras oncogenes in cultured human cells alters the transcriptional and posttranscriptional regulation of cytokine genes. *Journal of Clinical Investigation* **86:** 1261–1269.

Demetri, G. D., and Griffin, J. D. (1991). Granulocyte colony-stimulating factor and its receptor. *Blood* **78:** 2791–2808.

Demetri, G. D., Zenzie, B. W., Rheinwald, J. G., and Griffin, J. D. (1989). Expression of colony-stimulating factor genes by normal human mesothelial cells and human malignant mesothelioma cell ines *in vitro. Blood* **74:** 940–946.

de Sauvage, F. J., Hass, P. E., Spencer, S. D., Malloy, B. E., Gurney, A. L., Spencer, S. A., Darbonne, W. C., Henzel, W. J., Wong, S. C., Kuang, W.-J., Oes, K. J., Hultgren, B., Solberg, L. A., Jr., Goeddel, D. V., and Eaton, D. L. (1994). The c-mpl ligand, a novel cytokine that stimulates megakaryocytopoiesis and thrombopoiesis. *Nature (London)* **369:** 533–538.

de Vos, A. M., Ultsch, M., and Kossiakoff, A. A. (1992). Human growth hormone and extracellular domain of its receptor: Crystal structure of the complex. *Science (Washington)* **255:** 306–312.

de Vries, P., Brasel, K. A., Eisenman, J. R., Alpert, A. R., and Williams, D. E. (1991). The effect of recombinant mast cell growth factor on purified murine hematopoietic stem cells. *Journal of Experimental Medicine* **173:** 1205–1211.

Dexter, T. M., Spooncer, E., Simons, P., and Allen, T. D. (1984). Long-term marrow culture: An overview of techniques and experience. In D. G. Wright and J. S. Greenberger (eds.), *Long-Term Bone Marrow Culture,* pp. 57–96. New York: Liss.

De Witte, T., Gratwohl, A., Van Der Lely, N., Muus, P., Stern, A., Speck, B., Nissen, C., Marmont, A., Bacigalupo, A., Gluckman, E., and Zwann, F. (1990). A multicentre double blind randomized trial of recombinant human granulocyte-macrophage colony stimulating factor (rhGM-CSF) in recipients of allogenic T-cell depleted bone marrow. *Blood* **76:** suppl. 1, 139a.

D'Hondt, V., et al. (1993). Dose-dependent interleukin-3 stimulation of thrombopoiesis and neutropoiesis in patients with small-cell lung carcinoma before and following chemotherapy: A placebo-controlled randomized phase Ib study. *Journal of Clinical Oncology* **11:** 2063–2071.

Diederichs, K., Boone, T., and Karplus, P. A. (1991). Novel fold and putative receptor binding site of granulocyte-macrophage colony-stimulating factor. *Science (Washington)* **254:** 1779–1782.

Dieterlen-Lievre, F., and Martin, C. (1981). Diffuse intraembryonic hemopoiesis in normal and chimeric avian development. *Developmental Biology* **88:** 180–191.

Di Persio, J., Billing, P., Kaufman, S., Eghtesady, P., Williams, R. E., and Gasson, J. C. (1988). Characterization of the human granulocyte-macrophage colony-stimulating factor receptor. *Journal of Biological Chemistry* **263:** 1834–1841.

Disteche, C. M., Brannan, C. I., Larsen, A., Adler, D. A., Schorderet, D. G., Gearing, D., Copeland, N. G., Jenkins, N. A., and Park, L. S. (1992). The human pseudoautosomal GM-CSF receptor and subunit gene is autosomal in mouse. *Nature Genetics* **1:** 333–336.

Donahue, R. E., Seehra, J., Metzger, M., Lefebvre, D., Rock, B., Carbone, S., Nathan, D. G., Garnick, M., Sehgal, P. K., Laston, D., LaVallie, E., McCoy, J., Schendel, P. F., Norton, C., Turner, K., Yang, Y., and Clark, S. C. (1988). Human IL-3 and GM-CSF act synergistically in stimulating hematopoiesis in primates. *Science (Washington)* **241:** 1820–1823.

Dong, F., Hoefsloot, L. H., Schelen, A. M., Broeders, L. C. A. M., Meijer, Y., Veerman, A. J. P., Touw, I. P., and Löwenberg, B. (1994). Identification of nonsense mutation in the granulocyte-colony-stimulating factor receptor in severe congenital neutropenia. *Proceedings of the National Academy of Sciences, U.S.A.* **91:** 4480–4484.

Dong, F., Van Buitenen, C., Pouwels, K., Hoefsloot, L. H., Löwenberg, B., and Touw, I. P. (1993). Distinct cytoplasmic regions of the human granulocyte colony-stimulating factor receptor involved in induction of proliferation and maturation. *Molecular and Cellular Biology* **13:** 7774–7778.

Dorssers, L. C., Mostert, M. C., Burger, H., Janssen, C., Lemson, P. J., van Lambalgen, R., Wagemaker, G., and van Leen, R. W. (1991). Receptor and antibody interactions of human interleukin-3 characterized by mutational analysis. *Journal of Biological Chemistry* **266:** 21310–21317.

Downing, J. R., Roussel, M. F., and Sherr, C. J. (1989). Ligand and protein kinase C down-modulate the colony-stimulating factor 1 receptor by independent mechanisms. *Molecular and Cellular Biology* **9:** 2890–2896.

Doyle, A. G., Halliday, W. J., Barnett, C. J., Dunn, T. L., and Hume, D. A. (1992). Effect of recombinant human macrophage colony-stimulating factor on immunopathology of experimental brucellosis in mice. *Infection and Immunity* **60:** 1465–1472.

Dranoff, G., Crawford, A. D., Sadelain, M., Ream, B., Rashid, A., Bronson, R. T., Dickersin, G. R., Bachurski, C. J., Mark, E. L., Whitsett, J. A., and Mulligan, R. C. (1994). Involvement of granulocyte-macrophage colony-stimulating factor in pulmonary homeostasis. *Science (Washington)* **264:** 713–716.

Dranoff, G. Jaffe, E., Lazenby, A., Golumbek, P., Levitsky, H., Brose, K., Jackson, V., Hamada, H., Pardoll, D., and Mulligan, R. C. (1993). Vaccination with irradiated tumor cells engineered to secrete murine granulocyte-macrophage colony-stimulating factor stimulates potent, specific, and long-lasting anti-tumor immunity. *Proceedings of the National Academy of Sciences, U.S.A.* **90:** 3539–3543.

Dührsen, U., and Metcalf, D. (1988). A model system for leukemic transformation of immortalized hemopoeitic cells in irradiated recipient mice. *Leukemia* **2:** 329–333.

Dührsen, U., and Metcalf, D. (1989). Factors influencing the time and site of leukemic transformation of factor-dependent cells in irradiated recipient mice. *International Journal of Cancer* **44:** 1074–1081.

Dührsen, U., Stahl, J., and Gough, N. M. (1990). In vivo transformation of factor-dependent hemopoietic cells: Role of intracisternal A-particle transposition for growth factor gene activation. *EMBO Journal* **9:** 1087–1096.

Dührsen, U., Villeval, J.-L., Boyd, J., Kannourakis, G., Morstyn, G., and Metcalf, D. (1988). Effects of recombinant human granulocyte-colony stimulating factor on hemopoeitic progenitor cells in cancer patients. *Blood* **72:** 2074–2081.

Dunbar, C. E., Smith, D., Kimball, J., Garrison, L., Nienhuis, A. W., and Young, N. S. (1990). Hematopoietic growth factor treatment of Diamond-Blackfan anemia. (Abstract 554). *Blood* **76:** suppl., 141a.

Eaves, C. J., and Eaves, A. C. (1987). Cell culture studies in CML. In J. M. Goldman (ed.), *Baillière's Clinical Haematology, 1987,* Vol. 1, pp. 931–961. London: Baillière Tindall.

Eckmann, L., Freshney, M., Wright, E. G., Sproul, A., Wilkie, N., and Pragnell, I. B. (1988). A novel *in vitro* assay for murine haematopoietic stem cells. *British Journal of Cancer (Supplement)* **9:** 36–40.

Elbaz, O., Budel, L. M., Hoogerbrugge, H., Touw, I. P., Delwel, R., Mahmoud, L. A., and Löwenberg, B. (1991). Tumor necrosis factor downregulates granulocyte-colony-stimulating factor receptor expression on human acute myeloid leukemia cells and granulocytes. *Journal of Clinical Investigation* **87:** 838–841.

Elias, A. D., Ayash, L., Anderson, K. C., Hunt, M., Wheeler, C., Schwartz, G., Tepler, I., Mazanet, R., Lynch, C., Pap, S., Pelaez, J., Reich, E., Critchlow, J., Demetri, G., Bibbo, J., Schnipper, L., Griffin, J. D., Frei, E., III, and Antman, K. H. (1992). Mobilization of peripheral blood progenitor cells by chemotherapy and granulocyte-macrophage colony-stimulating factor for hematologic support after high-dose intensification for breast cancer. *Blood* **79:** 3036–3044.

Eliason, J. F. (1986). Granulocyte-macrophage colony formation in serum-free culture: Effects of purified colony stimulating factor and modulation by hydrocortisone. *Journal of Cellular Physiology* **128:** 231–238.

Elliott, M. J., Strasser, A., and Metcalf, D. (1991). Selective up-regulation of macrophage function in granulocyte-macrophage colony-stimulating factor transgenic mice. *Journal of Immunology* **147:** 2957–2963.

Elliott, M. J., Vadas, M. A., Eglinton, J. M., Park, L. S., To, L. B., Cleland, L. G., Clark, S. C., and Lopez, A. F. (1989). Recombinant human interleukin-3 and granulocyte-macrophage colony-stimulating factor show common biological effects and binding characteristics on human monocytes. *Blood* **74:** 2349–2359.

Ernst, T. J., Ritchie, A. R., Demetri, G. D., and Griffin, J. D. (1989). Regulation of granulocyte- and monocyte-colony stimulating factor mRNA levels in human blood monocytes is mediated primarily at a post-transcriptional level. *Journal of Biological Chemistry* **264:** 5700–5703.

Estey, E. H., Dixon, D., Kantarjian, H. M., Keating, M. J., McCredie, K., Bodey, G. P., Kuzrock, R., Talpaz, M., Freireich, E. J., Deisseroth, A. B., and Gutterman, J. U. (1990). Treatment of poor-prognosis, newly diagnosed acute myeloid leukemia with ara-C and recombinant human granulocyte-macrophage colony-stimulating factor. *Blood* **75:** 1766–1769.

Estey, E. H., Kurzrock, R., Talpaz, M., McCredie, K. B., O'Brien, S., Kantarjian, H. M., Keating, M. J., Deisseroth, A. B., and Gutterman, J. U. (1991). Effects of low doses of recombinant human granulocyte-macrophage colony stimulating factor (GM-CSF) in patients with myelodysplastic syndromes. *British Journal of Haematology* **77:** 291–295.

Fairbairn, L. J., Cowling, G. J., Reipert, B. M., and Dexter, T. M. (1993). Suppression of apoptosis allows differentiation and development of a multipotent haemopoietic stem cell line in the absence of added growth factors. *Cell* **74:** 823–832.

Faisal, M., Cumberland, W., Champlin, R., and Fahey, J. L. (1990). Effect of recombinant human granulocyte-macrophage colony-stimulating factor administration on the lymphocyte subsets of patients with refractory aplastic anemia. *Blood* **76:** 1580–1585.

Farese, A. M., Williams, D. E., Seiler, F. R., and MacVittie, T. J. (1993). Combination protocols of cytokine therapy with interleukin-3 and granulocyte-macrophage colony-stimulating factor in a primate model of radiation-induced marrow aplasia. *Blood* **82:** 3012–3018.

Felix, R., Cecchini, M. G., and Fleisch, H. (1990). Macrophage colony stimulating factor restores *in vivo* bone resorption in the op/op osteopetrotic mouse. *Endocrinology* **127:** 2592–2594.

Fibbe, W. E., Damme, J., Billiau, A., Goselink, H. M., Voogt, P. J., Eeden, G., Ralph, P., Altrock, B. W., and Falkenburg, J. H. F. (1988). Interleukin 1 induces human marrow stromal cells in long-term culture to produce granulocyte colony-stimulating factor and macrophage colony-stimulating factor. *Blood* **71:** 430–435.

Filderman, A. E., Bruckner, A., Kacinski, B. M., Deng, N., and Remold, H. G.

(1992). Macrophage colony-stimulating factor (CSF-1) enhances invasiveness in CSF-1 receptor-positive carcinoma cell lines. *Cancer Research* **52:** 3661–3666.

Fischer, H.-G., Frosch, S., Reske, K., and Reske-Kunz, A. B. (1988). Granulocyte-macrophage colony-stimulating factor activates macrophages derived from bone marrow cultures to synthesis of MHC class II molecules and to augmented antigen presentation function. *Journal of Immunology* **141:** 3882–3888.

Folks, T. M., Justement, J., Kinter, A., Dinarello, C. A., and Fauci, A. S. (1987). Cytokine-induced expression of HIV-1 in a chronically infected promonocyte cell line. *Science (Washington)* **238:** 800–802.

Foster, R., Metcalf, D., and Kirchmyer, R. (1968a). Induction of bone marrow colony stimulating activity by a filterable agent in leukemic and normal mouse serum. *Journal of Experimental Medicine* **127:** 853–866.

Foster, R., Metcalf, D., Robinson, W. A., and Bradley, T. R. (1968b). Bone marrow colony stimulating activity in human sera: Results of two independent surveys in Buffalo and Melbourne. *British Journal of Haematology* **15:** 147–159.

Foster, R. J., and Mirand, E. A. (1970). Bone marrow colony stimulating factor following ureteral ligation in germ-free mice. *Proceedings of the Society for Experimental Biology and Medicine* **133:** 1223–1227.

Foulke, R. S., Marshall, M. H., Trotta, P. P., and Von Hoff, D. D. (1990). *In vitro* assessment of the effects of granulocyte-macrophage colony-stimulating factor on primary human tumors and derived lines. *Cancer Research* **50:** 6264–6267.

Francis, G. E., Berney, J. J., Chipping, T. M., and Hoffbrand, A. V. (1979). Stimulation of human haemopoietic cells by colony stimulating factor: Sensitivity of leukaemic cells. *British Journal of Haematology* **41:** 545–562.

Frendl, G. (1992). Interleukin 3: From colony-stimulating factor to pluripotent immunoregulatory cytokine. *International Journal of Immunopharmacology* **14:** 421–430.

Frisch, J., Ganser, A., Hoelzer, D., Brugger, W., Kanz, L., Mertelsmann, R., and Schulz, G. (1992). Interleukin-3 and granulocyte-macrophage colony-stimulating factor in combination: Clinical implication. *Medical and Pediatric Oncology, Supplement* **2:** 34–37.

Fujisawa, M., Kobayashi, Y., Okabe, T., Takaku, F., Komatsu, Y., and Itoh, S. (1986). Recombinant human granulocyte colony stimulating factor induces granulocytosis *in vivo*. *Japanese Journal of Cancer Research* **77:** 866–869.

Fukunaga, R., Ishizaka-Ikeda, E., and Nagata, S. (1990a). Purification and characterization of the receptor for murine granulocyte colony-stimulating factor. *Journal of Biological Chemistry* **265:** 14008–14015.

Fukunaga, R., Ishizaka-Ikeda, E., and Nagata, S. (1993). Growth and differentiation signals mediated by different regions in the cytoplasmic domain of granulocyte-stimulating factor receptor. *Cell* **74:** 1079–1087.

Fukunaga, R., Ishizaka-Ikeda, E., Pan, C. X., Seto, Y., and Nagata, S. (1991). Functional domains of the granulocyte colony-stimulating factor receptor. *EMBO Journal* **10:** 2855–2865.

Fukunaga, R., Ishizaka-Ikeda, E., Seto, Y., and Nagata, S. (1990b). Expression cloning of a receptor for murine granulocyte colony-stimulating factor. *Cell* **61:** 341–350.

Fukunaga, R., Seto, Y., Mizushima, S., and Nagata, S. (1990c). Three different mRNAs encoding human granulocyte colony-stimulating factor receptor. *Proceedings of the National Academy of Sciences, U.S.A.* **87:** 8702–8706.

Fung, M.-C., Hapel, A. J., Ymer, S., Cohen, D. R., Johnson, R. M., Campbell, H. D., and Young, I. G. (1984). Molecular cloning of cDNA for murine interleukin-3. *Nature (London)* **307:** 233–237.

Gabrilove, J. L., Jakubowski, A., Fain, K., Grous, J., Scher, H., Sternberg, C., Yagoda, A., Clarkson, B., Bonilla, M. A., Oettgen, H. F., Alton, K., Boone, T., Altrock, B., Welte, K., and Souza, L. (1988). Phase I study of granulocyte colony-stimulating factor in patients with transitional cell carcinoma of the urothelium. *Journal of Clinical Investigation* **82:** 1454–1461.

Gabrilove, J. L., Wong, G., Bollenbacher, E., White, K., Kojima, S., and Wilson, E. L. (1993). Basic fibroblast growth factor counteracts the suppressive effect of transforming growth factor-$\beta$1 on human myeloid progenitor cells. *Blood* **81:** 909–915.

Ganser, A., Lindemann, A., Seipelt, G., Ottmann, O. G., Herrmann, F., Eder, M., Frisch, J., Schulz, G., Mertelsmann, R., and Hoelzer, D. (1990a). Effects of recombinant human interleukin-3 in patients with normal hematopoiesis and in patients with bone marrow failure. *Blood* **76:** 666–676.

Ganser, A., Seipelt, G., Lindemann, A., Ottmann, O. G., Falk, S., Eder, M., Herrmann, F., Becher, R., Höffken, K., Buchner. T., Klausmann, M., Frisch, J., Schulz, G., Mertelsmann, R., and Hoelzer, D. (1990b). Effects of recombinant human interleukin-3 in patients with myelodysplastic syndromes. *Blood* **76:** 455–462.

Ganser, A., Völkers, B., Greher, J., Ottmann, O. G., Walther, F., Becher. R., Bergmann, L., Schulz, G., and Hoelzer, D. (1989). Recombinant human granulocyte-macrophage colony-stimulating factor in patients with myelodysplastic syndromes: A phase I/II trial. *Blood* **73:** 31–37.

Gasson, J. C. (1991). Molecular physiology of granulocyte-macrophage colony-stimulating factor. *Blood* **77:** 1131–1145.

Gasson, J. C., Kaufman, S. E., Weisbart, R. H., Tomonaga, M., and Golde, D. W. (1986). High-affinity binding of granulocyte-macrophage colony-stimulating factor to normal and leukemic human myeloid cells. *Proceedings of the National Academy of Sciences, U.S.A.* **83:** 669–673.

Gasson, J. C., Weisbart, R. H., Kauffman, S. E., Clark, S. C., Hewick, R. M., and Wong, G. G. (1984). Purified human granulocyte-macrophage colony-stimulating factor: Direct action on neutrophils. *Science (Washington)* **226:** 1339–1342.

Gearing, A., Metcalf, D., Moore, J. C., and Nicola, N. A. (1989a). Elevated levels of GM-CSF and IL-1 in the serum, peritoneal and pleural cavities of GM-CSF transgenic mice. *Immunology* **67:** 216–220.

Gearing, D. P., King, J. A., Gough, N. M., and Nicola, N. A. (1989b). Expression cloning of a receptor for human granulocyte-macrophage colony-stimulating factor. *EMBO Journal* **8:** 3667–3676.

Gerhartz, H. H., Engelhard, M., Meusers, P., Brittinger, G., Wilmanns, W., Schlimok, G., Mueller, P., Huhn, D., Musch, R., Siegert, W., Gerhartz, D., Hartlapp, J. H., Thiel, E., Huber, C., Peschl, C., Spann, W., Emmerich, B., Schadek, C., Westerhausen, M., Pees, H.-W., Radtke, H., Engert, A., Terhardt, E., Schick, H., Binder, T., Fuchs, R., Hasford, J., Brandmaier, R., Stern, A. C., Jones, T. C., Ehrlich, H. J., Stein, H., Parwaresch, M., Tiemann, M., and Lennert, K. (1993). Randomized, double-blind, placebo-controlled, phase III study of recombinant human granulocyte-macrophage colony-stimulating factor as adjunct to induction treatment of high-grade malignant non-Hodgkin's lymphomas. *Blood* **82:** 2329–2339.

Gerhartz, H. H., Visani, G., Delmer, A., Zwierzina, H., and Ribeiro, M. (1989). Low-dose Ara-C plus granulocyte-macrophage colony-stimulating factor for the treatment of myelodysplastic syndromes. *Bone Marrow Transplantation* **5:** 36–37.

Gianni, A. M., Bregni, M., Siena, S., Stern, A. C., Gandola, L., and Bonadonna, G. (1990). Recombinant human granulocyte-macrophage colony-stimulating factor reduces hematologic toxicity and widens clinical applicability of high-dose cyclophosphamide treatment in breast cancer and non-Hodgkin's lymphoma. *Journal of Clinical Oncology* **8:** 768–778.

Gianni, A. M., Siena, S., Bregni, M., Tarella, C., Stern, A. C., Pileri, A., and Bonadonna, G. (1989). Granulocyte-macrophage colony-stimulating factor to harvest circulating haemopoietic stem cells for autotransplantation. *Lancet* **2:** 580–585.

Gisselbrecht, S., Fichelson, S., Sola, B., Bordereaux, D., Hampe, A., Andre, C., Galibert, F., and Tambourin, P. (1987). Frequent c-fms activation by proviral insertion in mouse myeloblastic leukaemias. *Nature (London)* **329:** 259–261.

Giulian, D., and Ingeman, J. E. (1988). Colony-stimulating factors as promoters of ameboid microglia. *Journal of Neuroscience* **8:** 4707–4717.

Gliniak, B. C., Park, L. S., and Rohrschneider, L. R. (1992). A GM-colony-stimulating factor (CSF) activated ribonuclease system transregulates M-CSF receptor expression in the murine FDC-P1/MAC myeloid cell line. *Molecular Biology of the Cell* **3:** 535–544.

Gliniak, B. C., and Rohrschneider, L. R. (1990). Expression of M-CSF receptor is controlled post-transcriptionally by the dominant actions of GM-CSF or Multi-CSF. *Cell* **63:** 1073–1083.

Glocker, M. O., Arbogast, B., Schreurs, J., and Deinzer, M. L. (1993). Assignment of the inter- and intramolecular disulfide linkages in recombinant human macrophage colony stimulating factor using fast atom bombardment mass spectrometry. *Biochemistry* **32:** 482–488.

Golde, D. W., and Cline, M. (1975). Endotoxin-induced release of colony-stimulating activity in man. *Proceedings of the Society for Experimental Biology and Medicine* **149:** 845–848.

Goodall, G. J., Bagley, C. J., Vadas, M. A., and Lopez, A. F. (1993). A model for the interaction of the GM-CSF, IL-3, and IL-5 receptors with their ligands. *Growth Factors* **8:** 87–97.

Gordon, M. Y., Riley, G. P., Watt, S. M., and Greaves, M. F. (1987). Compartmentalization of a haematopoietic growth facor (GM-CSF) by glycosaminoglycans in the bone marrow microenvironment. *Nature (London)* **326:** 403–405.

Gordon-Smith, E. C., Yandle, A., Milne, A., Speck, B., Marmont, A., Willemze, R., and Kolb, H. (1991). Randomised placebo-controlled study of RH-GM-CSF following ALG in the treatment of aplastic anemia. *Bone Marrow Transplantation* **7:** (suppl. 2), 78–80.

Gorman, D. M., Itoh, N., Jenkins, N. A., Gilbert, D. J., Copeland, N. G., and Miyajima, A. (1992). Chromosomal localization and organization of the murine genes encoding the beta subunits (AIC2A and AIC2B) of the interleukin 3, granulocyte/macrophage colony-stimulating factor, and interleukin 5 receptors. *Journal of Biological Chemistry* **267:** 15842–15848.

Gorman, D. M., Itoh, N., Kitamura, T., Schreurs, J., Yonehara, S., Yahara, I., Arai, K., and Miyajima, A. (1990). Cloning and expression of a gene encoding an interleukin 3 receptor-like protein: Identification of another member of the cytokine receptor gene family. *Proceedings of the National Academy of Sciences, U.S.A.* **87:** 5459–5463.

Gottschalk, L. R., Giannola, D. M., and Emerson, S. G. (1993). Molecular regulation of the human IL-3 gene: Inducible T cell-restricted expression requires intact AP-1 and Elf-1 nuclear protein binding sites. *Journal of Experimental Medicine* **178:** 1681–1692.

Gough, N. M., Gearing, D. P., Nicola, N. A., Baker, E., Pritchard, M., Callen, D. F., and Sutherland, G. R. (1990). Localization of the human GM-CSF receptor gene to the X-Y pseudoautosomal region. *Nature (London)* **345:** 734–736.

Gough, N. M., Gough, J., Metcalf, D., Kelso, A., Grail, D., Nicola, N. A., Burgess, A. W., and Dunn, A. R. (1984). Molecular cloning of cDNA encoding a murine haematopoietic growth regular, granulocyte-macrophage colony stimulating factor. *Nature (London)* **309:** 763–767.

Gough, N. M., Grail, D., Gearing, D. P., and Metcalf, D. (1987). Mutagenesis of murine granulocyte/macrophage-colony-stimulating factor reveals critical residues near the N terminus. *European Journal of Biochemistry* **169:** 353–358.

Gough, N. M., and Kelso, A. (1989). GM-CSF expression is preferential to Multi-CSF (IL-3) expression in murine T lymphocyte clones. *Growth Factors* **1:** 287–298.

Grant, S. M., and Heel, R. C. (1992). Recombinant granulocyte-macrophage colony-stimulating factor (rGM-CSF): A review of its pharmacological properties and prospective role in the management of myelosuppression. *Drugs* **43:** 516–560.

Grau, G. E., Kindler, V., Piguet, P. F., Lambert, P.-H., and Vassalli, P. (1988). Prevention of experimental cerebral malaria by anticytokine antibodies: Interleukin 3 and granulocyte macrophage colony-stimulating factor are intermediates in increased tumor necrosis factor production and macrophage accumulation. *Journal of Experimental Medicine* **168:** 1499–1504.

Green, J. A., Trillet, V. N., and Manegold, C. (1991). r-met-HuG-CSF (G-CSF) with CDE chemotherapy in small cell lung cancer: Interim results from a randomized placebo controlled trial. *Proceedings of the American Society of Clinical Oncology* **10:** 243.

Griffin, J. D., and Löwenberg, B. (1986). Clonogenic cells in acute myeloblastic leukemia. *Blood* **68:** 1185–1195.

Groopman, J. E., Mitsuyasu, R. T., DeLeo, M. J., Oette, D. H., and Golde, D. W. (1987). Effects of recombinant human granulocyte-macrophage colony-stimulating factor on myelopoiesis in the acquired immunodeficiency syndrome. *New England Journal of Medicine* **317:** 593–598.

Grossberg, H. S., and Bonnem, E. M. (1989). GM-CSF with ganciclovir for the treatment of CMV retinitis in AIDS. *New England Journal of Medicine* **320:** 1560.

Gualtieri, R. J., Liang, C-M., Shadduck, R. K., Waheed, A., and Banks, J. (1987). Identification of the hematopoietic growth factors elaborated by bone marrow stromal cells using antibody neutralization analysis. *Experimental Hematology* **15:** 883–889.

Guilbert, L. J., and Stanley, E. R. (1986). The interaction of $^{125}$I-colony-stimulating factor-1 with bone marrow-derived macrophages. *Journal of Biological Chemistry* **261:** 4024–4032.

Guilbert, L. J., Tynan, P. W., and Stanley, E. R. (1986). Uptake and destruction of $^{125}$I-CSF-1 by peritoneal exudate macrophages. *Journal of Cellular Biochemistry* **31:** 203–216.

Halenbeck, R., Kawasaki, E., Wrin, J., and Koths, K. (1989). Renaturation and purification of biologically active recombinant human macrophage colony-stimulating factor expressed in *E. coli. Biotechnology* **7:** 710–715.

Hall, B. M. (1969). The effects of whole-body irradiation on serum colony stimulating factor and *in vitro* colony forming cells in the bone marrow. *British Journal of Haematology* **17:** 553–561.

Hallek, M., Lepisto, E. M., Slattery, K. E., Griffin, J. D., and Ernst, T. J. (1992). Interferon-gamma increases the expression of the gene encoding the beta subunit of the granulocyte-macrophage colony-stimulating factor receptor. *Blood* **80:** 1736–1742.

Hamilton, B. J., Nagy, E., Malter, J. S., Arrick, B. A., and Rigby, W. F. (1993). Association of heterogeneous nuclear ribonucleoprotein A1 and C proteins with reiterated AUUUA sequences. *Journal of Biological Chemistry* **268:** 8881–8887.

Hamilton, J. A., Vairo, G., and Lingelbach, S. R. (1988). Activation and proliferation signals in murine macrophages: Stimulation of gluclose uptake by hemopoietic growth factors and other agents. *Journal of Cellular Physiology* **134:** 405–412.

Hammer, S. M., Gillis, J. M., Pinkston, P., and Rose, R. M. (1990). Effect of zidovudine and granulocyte-macrophage colony-stimulating factor on human immunodeficiency virus replication in alveolar macrophages. *Blood* **75:** 1215–1219.

Hammond, W. P., Boone, T. C., Donahue, R. E., Souza, L. M., and Dale, D. C. (1990). A comparison of treatment of canine cyclic hematopoiesis with recombinant human granulocyte-macrophage colony-stimulating factor (GM-CSF), G-CSF, interleukin-3, and canine G-CSF. *Blood* **76:** 523–532.

Hammond, W. P., Chatta, G. S., Andrews, R. G., and Dale, D. C. (1992). Abnormal responsiveness of granulocyte-committed progenitor cells in cyclic neutropenia. *Blood* **79:** 2536–2539.

Hammond, W. P., Csiba, E., Canin, A., Hockman, H., Souza, L. M., Layton, J. E., and Dale, D. C. (1991). Chronic neutropenia: A new canine model induced by human granulocyte colony-stimulating factor. *Journal of Clinical Investigation* **87:** 704–710.

Hammond, W. P., Price, T. H., Souza, L. M., and Dale, D. C. (1989). Treatment of cyclic neutropenia with granulocyte colony-stimulating factor. *New England Journal of Medicine* **320:** 1306–1311.

Hanazono, Y., Chiba, S., Sasaki, K., Mano, H., Miyajima, A., Arai, K., Yazaki, Y., and Hirai, H. (1993). c-fps/fes protein-tyrosine kinase is implicated in a signaling pathway triggered by granulocyte-macrophage colony-stimulating factor and interleukin-3. *EMBO Journal* **12:** 1641–1646.

Hanazono, Y., Hosoi, T., Kuwaki, T., Matsuki, S., Miyazona, K., Miyagawa, K., and Takaku, F. (1990). Structural analysis of the receptors for granulocyte colony-stimulating factor on neutrophils. *Experimental Hematology* **18:** 1097–1103.

Hannum, C., Culpepper, J., Campbell, D., McClanahan, T., Zurawski, S., Bazan, J. F., Kastelein, R., Hudak, S., Wagner, J., Mattson, J., Luh, J., Duda, G., Martina, N., Peterson, D., Menon, S., Shanafelt, A., Muench, M., Kelner, G., Namikawa, R., Rennick, D., Roncarolo, M.-G., Zlotnik, A., Rosnet, O., Dubreuil, P., Birnbaum, D., and Lee, F. (1994). Ligand for FLT3/FLK2 receptor tyrosine kinase regulates growth of haematopoietic stem cells and is encoded by variant RNAs. *Nature (London)* **368:** 643–648.

Hapel, A. J., Fung, M.-C., Mak, N.-K., Morris, C., Metcalf, D., and Nicola, N. A. (1992). Bone marrow cells from A/J mice do not proliferate in interleukin-3 but express normal numbers of interleukin-3 receptors. *British Journal of Haematology* **82:** 488–493.

Hara, H., Kitamura, Y., Kawata, T., Kanamura, A., and Nagai, K. (1974). Synergism between lymph node and bone marrow cells for production of granulocytes. II. Enhanced colony-stimulating activity of sera of mice with graft-versus-host reaction. *Experimental Hematology* **2:** 43–49.

Hara, H., and Miyajima, A. (1992). Two distinct functional high affinity receptors for mouse interleukin-3 (IL-3). *EMBO Journal* **11:** 1875–1884.

Haran-Ghera, N., Peled, A., Krautghamer, R., and Resnitzky, P. (1992). Initiation and promotion in radiation-induced myeloid leukemia. *Leukemia* **6:** 689–695.

Hariharan, I. K., Adams, J. M., and Cory, S. (1988). *bcr-abl* oncogene renders myeloid cell line factor independent: Potential autocrine mechanism in chronic myeloid leukemia. *Oncogene Research* **3:** 387–399.

Harrington, M. A., Edenberg, H. J., Saxman, S., Pedigo, L. M., Daub, R., and Broxmeyer, H. E. (1991). Cloning and characterization of the murine promoter for the colony-stimulating factor-1-encoding gene. *Gene* **102:** 165–170.

Harrison, D. E. (1980). Competitive repopulation: A new assay for long-term stem cell functional capacity. *Blood* **55:** 77–81.

Haskill, S., Johnson, C., Eierman, D., Becker, S., and Warren, K. (1988). Adherence induces selective mRNA expression of monocyte mediators and proto-oncogenes. *Journal of Immunology* **140:** 1690–1694.

Havemann, K., Klausmann, M., Wolf, M., Fischer, J. R., Drings, P., and Oster, W. (1991). Effect of rhGM-CSF on haematopoietic reconstitution after chemotherapy in small-cell lung cancer. *Journal of Cancer Research in Clinical Oncology* **117:** (suppl. 4), S203–S207.

Hawley, R. G., Fong, A. Z. C., Burns, B. F., and Hawley, T. S. (1992). Transplantable myeloproliferative diseases induced in mice by an interleukin 6 retrovirus. *Journal of Experimental Medicine* **176:** 1149–1163.

Hayashida, K., Kitamura, T., Gorman, D. M., Arai, K., Yokota, T., and Miyajima, A. (1990). Molecular cloning of a second subunit of the receptor for human granulocyte-macrophage colony-stimulating factor (GM-CSF): Reconstitution of a high-affinity GM-CSF receptor. *Proceedings of the National Academy of Sciences, U.S.A.* **87:** 9655–9659.

Heard, J. M., Roussel, M. F., Rettenmier, C. W., and Sherr, C. J. (1987). Multilineage hematopoietic disorders induced by transplantation of bone marrow cells expressing the v-fms oncogene. *Cell* **51:** 663–673.

Hebert, J. C., O'Reilly, M., and Gamelli, R. L. (1990). Protective effect of recombinant human granulocyte colony-stimulating factor against pneumonococcal infections in splenectomized mice. *Archives of Surgery* **125:** 1075–1078.

Heimfield, S., Hudak, S., Weissman, I., and Rennick, D. (1991). The *in vitro* response of phenotypically defined mouse stem cells and myeloerythroid progenitors to single or multiple growth factors. *Proceedings of the National Academy of Sciences, U.S.A.* **88:** 9902–9906.

Herrmann, F., Schulz, G., Wieser, M., Kolbe, K., Nicolay, U., Noack, M., Lindemann, A., and Mertelsmann, R. (1990). Effect of granulocyte-macrophage colony-stimulating factor on neutropenia and related morbidity induced by myelotoxic chemotherapy. *American Journal of Medicine* **88:** 619–624.

Heyworth, C. M., Dexter, T. M., Kan, O., and Whetton, A. D. (1990). The role of hemopoietic growth factors in self-renewal and differentiation of IL-3-dependent multipotential stem cells. *Growth Factors* **2:** 197–211.

Hill, C. P., Osslund, T. D., and Eisenberg, D. (1993). The structure of granulocyte-colony-stimulating factor and its relationship to other growth factors. *Proceedings of the National Academy of Sciences, U.S.A.* **90:** 5167–5171.

Hilton, D. J., Nicola, N. A., Gough, N. M., and Metcalf, D. (1988). Resolution and purification of three distinct factors produced by Krebs ascites cells which have differentiation-inducing activity on murine myeloid leukemic cell lines. *Journal of Biological Chemistry* **263:** 9238–9243.

Hirano, T., Yasukawa, K., Harada, H., Taga, T., Watanabe, Y., Matsuda, T., Kashiwamura, S., Nakajima, K., Koyama, K., Iwamatsu, A., Tsunasawa, S., Sakiyama, F., Matsui, H., Takahara, Y., Taniguchi, T., and Kishimoto, T. (1986). Complementary DNA for a novel human interleukin (BSF-2) that induces B lymphocytes to produce immunoglobulin. *Nature (London)* **324:** 73–76.

Hodgson, G. S., and Bradley, T. R. (1979). Properties of haematopoietic stem cells surviving 5-fluorouracil treatment: Evidence for a pre-CFU-S cell? *Nature (London)* **281:** 381–382.

Hofstetter, W., Wetterwald, A., Cecchini, M. C., Felix, R., Fleisch, H., and Mueller, C. (1992). Detection of transcripts for the receptor for macrophage colony-stimulating factor, c-fms, in murine osteoclasts. *Proceedings of the National Academy of Sciences, U.S.A.* **89:** 9637–9641.

Hollingshead, L. M., and Goa, K. L. (1991). Recombinant granulocyte colony-stimulating factor (rG-CSF): A review of its pharmacological properties and prospective role in neutropenic conditions. *Drugs* **42:** 300–330.

Horiguchi, J., Sariban, E., and Kufe, D. (1988). Transcriptional and post-transcriptional regulation of CSF-1 gene expression in human monocytes. *Molecular and Cellular Biology* **8:** 3951–3954.

Horiguchi, J., Warren, M. K., Ralph, P., and Kufe, D. (1986). Expression of the macrophage specific colony-stimulating factor (CSF-1) during monocytic differentiation. *Biochemical and Biophysical Research Communications* **141:** 924–930.

Horowitz, M. C., Coleman, D. L., Flood, P. M., Kupper, T. S., and Jilka, R. L. (1989). Parathyroid hormone and lipopolysaccharide induce murine osteoblast-like cells to secrete a cytokine indistinguishable from granulocyte-macrophage colony-stimulating factor. *Journal of Clinical Investigation* **83:** 149–157.

Huebner, K. Isobe, M., Croce, C. M., Golde, D. W., Kaufman, S. E., and Gasson, J. C. (1985). The human gene encoding GM-CSF is at 5q21–q32, the chromosome region deleted in the 5q- anomaly. *Science (Washington)* **230:** 1282–1285.

Hultner, L., Staber, F. G., Mergenthaler, H.-G., and Dormer, P. (1982). Production of murine granulocyte-macrophage colony-stimulating factors (GM-CSF) by bone marrow-derived and non-hemopoietic cells *in vivo*. *Experimental Hematology* **10:** 798–808.

Hume, D. A., Pavli, P., Donahue, R. E., and Fidler, I. J. (1988). The effect of human recombinant macrophage colony-stimulating factor (CSF-1) on the murine mononuclear phagocyte system *in vivo*. *Journal of Immunology* **141:** 3405–3409.

Ichikawa, Y. (1969). Differentiation of a cell line of myeloid leukemia. *Journal of Cellular Physiology* **74:** 223–234.

Ichikawa, Y. (1970). Further studies on the differentiation of a cell line of myeloid leukemia. *Journal of Cellular Physiology* **76:** 175–184.

Ichikawa, Y., Pluznik, D. H., and Sachs, L. (1966). *In vitro* control of the development of macrophage and granulocyte colonies. *Proceedings of the National Academy of Sciences, U.S.A.* **56:** 488–495.

Ihle, J. N., Keller, J., Henderson, L., Klein, F., and Palaszynski, E. (1982). Procedures for the purification of interleukin 3 to homogeneity. *Journal of Immunology* **129:** 2431–2436.

Ihle, J. N., Keller, J., Oroszlan, S., Henderson, L. E., Copeland, T. D., Fitch, F., Prystowsky, M. B., Goldwasser, E., Schrader, J. W., Palaszynski, E., Dy, M., and Lebel, B. (1983). Biologic properties of homogeneous interleukin 3. I. Demonstration of WEHI-3 growth factor activity, mast cell growth factor activity, p cell-stimulating factor activity, colony-stimulating factor activity, and histamine-producing cell-stimulating factor activity. *Journal of Immunology* **131:** 282–287.

Ihle, J. N., Silver, J., and Kozak, C. A. (1987). Genetic mapping of the mouse interleukin 3 gene to chromosome 11. *Journal of Immunology* **138:** 3051–3054.

Ihle, J. N. Witthuhn, B., Tang, B., Yi, T., and Quelle, F. W. (1994). Cytokine receptors and signal transduction. In *Baillière's Clinical Haematology*, Vol. 7, 17–48.

Ikebuchi, K., Wong, G. G., Clark, S. C., Ihle, J. N., Hirai, Y., and Ogawa, M. (1987). Interleukin-6 enhancement of interleukin-3-dependent proliferation of multipotential hemopoietic progenitors. *Proceedings of the National Academy of Sciences, U.S.A.* **84:** 9035–9039.

Inaba, K., Inaba, M., Romani, N., Aya, H., Deguchi, M., Ikehara, S., Muramatsu, S., and Steinman, R. M. (1992a). Generation of large numbers of dendritic cells from mouse bone marrow cultures supplemented with granulocyte/macrophage colony-stimulating factor. *Journal of Experimental Medicine* **176:** 1693–1702.

Inaba, T., Yamada, N., Gotoda, T., Shimano, H., Shimada, M., Momomura, K., Kadowaki, T., Motoyoshi, K., Tsukada, T., Morisaki, N., Saito, Y., Yoshida, S., Takaku, F., and Yazaki, Y. (1992b). Expression of M-CSF receptor encoded by c-fms on smooth muscle cells derived from arteriosclerotic lesion. *Journal of Biological Chemistry* **267:** 5693–5699.

Inazawa, J., Fukunaga, R., Seto, Y., Nakagawa, H., Misawa, S., Abe, T., and Nagata, S. (1991). Assignment of the human granulocyte colony-stimulating factor gene (CSF3R) to chromosome 1 at region p35–p34.3. *Genomics* **10:** 1075–1078.

Isfort, R. J., and Ihle, J. N. (1990). Multiple hematopoietic growth factors signal through tyrosine phosphorylation. *Growth Factors* **2:** 213–220.

Ishibashi, T., Kimura, H., Shikama, Y., Uchida, T., Kariyone, S., Hirano, T., Kishimoto, T., Takatsuki, F., and Akiyama, Y. (1989a). Interleukin-6 is a potent thrombopoietic factor *in vivo* in mice. *Blood* **74:** 1241–1244.

Ishibashi, T., Kimura, H., Uchida, T., Kariyone, S., Friese, P., and Burstein, S. A. (1989b). Human interleukin 6 is a direct promoter of maturation of megakaryocytes *in vitro*. *Proceedings of the National Academy of Sciences, U.S.A.* **86:** 5953–5957.

Ishibashi, T., Miller, S. L., and Burstein, S. A. (1987). Type β transforming growth factor is a potent inhibitor of murine megakaryocytopoiesis *in vitro*. *Blood* **69:** 1737–1741.

Itoh, N., Yonehara, S., Schreurs, J., Gorman, D. M., Maruyama, K., Ishii, A., Yahara, I., Arai, K., and Miyajima, A. (1990). Cloning of an interleukin-3 receptor gene: A member of a distinct receptor gene family. *Science (Washington)* **247:** 324–327.

Jacobsen, S. E., Ruscetti, F. W., Dubois, C. M., Wine, J., and Keller, J. R. (1992). Induction of colony-stimulating factor receptor expression on hematopoietic progenitor cells: Proposed mechanism for growth factor synergism. *Blood* **80:** 678–687.

Jacobsen, S. E. W., Veiby, O. P., and Smeland, E. B. (1993). Cytotoxic lymphocyte maturation factor (interleukin-12) is a synergistic growth factor for hemotapoietic stem cells. *Journal of Experimental Medicine* **178:** 413–418.

Janowska-Wieczorek, A., Belch, A. R., Jacobs, A., Bowen, D., Padua, R.-A., Paietta, E., and Stanley, E. R. (1991). Increased circulating colony-stimulating factor-1 in patients with preleukemia, leukemia, and lymphoid malignancies. *Blood* **77:** 1796–1803.

Johnson, G. R., and Burgess, A. W. (1978). Molecular and biological properties of a macrophage colony-stimulating factor from mouse yolk sacs. *Journal of Cellular Biology* **77:** 35–47.

Johnson, G. R., Gonda, T. J., Metcalf, D., Hariharan, I. K., and Cory, S. (1989). A lethal myeloproliferative syndrome in mice transplanted with bone marrow cells infected with a retrovirus expressing granulocyte-macrophage colony-stimulating factor. *EMBO Journal* **8:** 441–448.

Johnson, G. R., and Metcalf, D. (1979). The commitment of multipotential hemopoietic stem cells: Studies *in vivo* and *in vitro*. In Le Douarin (ed.), *Cell Lineage, Stem Cells and Cell Determination, INSERM Symposium No. 10,* pp. 199–213. Amsterdam: Elsevier/North-Holland Biomedical Press.

Johnson, G. R., and Metcalf, D. (1980). Detection of a new type of mouse eosinophil colony by Luxol-Fast-Blue staining. *Experimental Hematology* **8:** 549–561.

Jubinsky, P. T., and Stanley, E. R. (1985). Purification of hemopoietin-1: A multilineage hemopoietic growth factor. *Proceedings of the National Academy of Sciences, U.S.A.* **82:** 2764–2768.

Kanakura, Y., Cannistra, S. A., Brown, C. B., Nakamura, M., Seelig, G. F., Prosise, W. W., Hawkins, J. C., Kaushansky, K., and Griffin, J. D. (1991). Identification of functionally distinct domains of human granulocyte-macrophage colony-stimulating factor using monoclonal antibodies. *Blood* **77:** 1033–1043.

Kanakura, Y., Druker. B., Cannistra, S. A., Furukawa, Y., Torimoto, Y., and Griffin, J. D. (1990). Signal transduction of the human granulocyte-macrophage colony-stimulating factor and interleukin-3 receptors involves tyrosine phosphorylation of a common set of cytoplasmic proteins. *Blood* **76:** 706–715.

Kanda, N., Fukushige, S., Murotsu, T., Yoshida, M. C., Tsuchiya, M., Asano, S., Kaziro, Y., and Nagata, S. (1987). Human gene coding for granulocyte-colony stimulating factor is assigned to the q21–q22 region of chromosome 17. *Somatic Cell Molecular Genetics* **13:** 679–684.

Kannourakis, G., and Johnson, G. R. (1990). Proliferative properties of unfractionated, purified, and single cell human progenitor populations stimulated by recombinant human interleukin-3. *Blood* **75:** 370–377.

Kastelein, R. A., and Shanafelt, A. B. (1993). GM-CSF receptor: Interactions and activation. *Oncogene* **8:** 231–236.

Kaushansky, K. (1989). Control of granulocyte-macrophage colony-stimulating factor production in normal endothelial cells by positive and negative regulatory elements. *Journal of Immunology* **143:** 2525–2529.

Kaushansky, K., Lin, N., and Adamson, J. W. (1988). Interleukin 1 stimulates fibroblasts to synthesize granulocyte-macrophage and granulocyte colony-stimulating factors: Mechanism for the hematopoietic response to inflammation. *Journal of Clinical Investigation* **81:** 92–97.

Kaushansky, K., Lok, S., Holly, R. D., Broudy, V. C., Lin, N., Bailey, M. C., Forstrom, J. W., Buddle, M. M., Oort, P. J., Hagen, F. S., Roth, G. R., Papayannopolou, T., and Foster, D. C. (1994). Murine thrombopoietin: The ligand for c-mpl expands megakaryocyte progenitors, induces their differentiation and stimulates platelet production. *Nature (London)* **369:** 568–571.

Kaushansky, K., Shoemaker, S. G., Alfaro, S., and Brown, C. (1989). Hematopoietic activity of granulocyte/macrophage colony-stimulating factor is dependent upon two distinct regions of the molecule: Functional analysis based upon the activities of interspecies hybrid growth factors. *Proceedings of the National Academy of Sciences, U.S.A.* **86:** 1213–1217.

Kaushansky, K., Shoemaker, S. G., Broudy, V. C., Lin, N. L., Matous, J. V., Alderman, E. M., Aghajanian, J. D., Szklut, P. J., Van Dyke, R. E., Pearce, M. K., and Abrams, J. S. (1992). Structure-function relationships of interleukin-3: An analysis based on the function and binding characteristics of a series of interspecies chimera of gibbon and murine interleukin-3. *Journal of Clinical Investigation* **90:** 1879–1888.

Kawakami, M., Tsutsumi, H., Kumakawa, T., Abe, H., Hirai, M., Kurosawa, S., Mori, M., and Fukushima, M. (1990). Levels of serum granulocyte colony-stimulating factor in patients with infections. *Blood* **76:** 1962–1964.

Kawano, Y., Takaue, Y., Motoyoshi, K., Minakuchi, J., Kawashima, S., Saito, S., Hirao, A., Sato, J., Shimizu, T., and Kuroda, Y. (1993a). Measurement of serum levels of macrophage colony-stimulating factor (M-CSF) patients with uremia. *Experimental Hematology* **21:** 220–223.

Kawano, Y., Takaue, Y., Saito, S., Sato, J., Shimizu, T., Suzue, T., Hirao, A., Okamoto, Y., Abe, T., Watanabe, T., Kurodo, Y., Kimura, F., Motoyoshi, K., and Asano, S. (1993b). Granulocyte colony-stimulating factor (CSF), macrophage-CSF, granulocyte-macrophage CSF, interleukin-3, and interleukin-6 levels in sera from children undergoing blood stem cell autografts. *Blood* **81:** 856–860.

Kawasaki, E. S., Ladner, M. B., Wang, A. M., Van Arsdell, J., Warren, M. K., Coyne, M. Y., Schweickart, V. L., Lee, M.-T., Wilson, K. J., Boosman, A., Stanley, E. R., Ralph, P., and Mark, D. F. (1985). Molecular cloning of complementary DNA encoding human macrophage-specific colony-stimulating factor (CSF-1). *Science (Washington)* **230:** 291–296.

Kay, A. B., Ying, S., Varney, V., Gaga, M., Durham, S. R., Moqbel, R., Wardlaw, A. J., and Hamid, Q. (1991). Messenger RNA expression of the cytokine gene cluster, interleukin 3 (IL-3), IL-4, IL-5, and granulocyte/macrophage colony-stimulating factor, in allergen-induced late-phase cutaneous reactions in atopic subjects. *Journal of Experimental Medicine* **173:** 775–778.

Kayashima, S., Tsuru, S., Shinomiya, N., Katsura, N., Motoyoshi, K., Rokutanda, M., and Nagata, N. (1991). Effects of macrophage colony stimulating factor on reduction of viable bacteria and survival of mice during Listeria monocytogenes infection: Characteristics of monocyte subpopulations. *Infection and Immunity* **59:** 4677–4680.

Kelleher, C. A., Wong, G. G., Clark, S. C., Schendel, P. F., Minden, M. D., and McCulloch, E. A. (1988). Binding of iodinated recombinant human GM-CSF to the blast cells of acute myeloblastic leukemia. *Leukemia* **2:** 211–215.

Keller, J. R., Jacobsen, S. E., Sill, K. T., Ellingsworth, L. R., and Ruscetti, F. W. (1991). Stimulation of granulopoiesis by transforming growth factor beta: Synergy with granulocyte/macrophage colony stimulating factor. *Proceedings of the National Academy of Sciences, U.S.A.* **88:** 7190–7194.

Kelso, A., and Gough, N. M. (1988). Coexpression of granulocyte-macrophage colony-stimulating factor, $\gamma$-interferon, and interleukins 3 and 4 is random in murine alloreactive T-lymphocyte clones. *Proceedings of the National Academy of Sciences, U.S.A.* **85:** 9189–9193.

Kelso, A., and Metcalf, D. (1990). T lymphocyte-derived colony-stimulating factors. *Advances in Immunology* **48:** 69–105.

Kerrigan, D. P., Castillo, A., Foucar, K., Townsend, K., and Neidhart, J. (1989). Peripheral blood morphologic changes after high-dose antineoplastic chemotherapy and recombinant human granulocyte colony-stimulating factor administration. *American Journal of Clinical Pathology* **92:** 280–285.

Kimura, S., Matsuda, J., Ikematsu, S., Miyazono, K., Ito, A., Nakahata, T., Minamitani, M., Shimada, K., Shiokawa, K., and Takaku, F. (1990). Efficacy of recombinant human granulocyte colony-stimulating factor in neutropenia in patients with AIDS. *AIDS* **4:** 1251–1255.

Kinashi, T., Inaba, K., Tsubata, T., Tashiro, K., Palacios, R., and Honjo, T. (1988). Differentiation of an interleukin 3-dependent precursor B-cell clone into immunoglobulin-producing cells *in vitro*. *Proceedings of the National Academy of Sciences, U.S.A.* **85:** 4473–4477.

Kincade, P. W., Lee, G., Fernandes, G., Moore, M. A. S., Williams, N., and Good, R. A. (1979). Abnormalities in clonable B lymphocytes and myeloid progenitors in autoimmune NZB mice. *Proceedings of the National Academy of Sciences, U.S.A.* **76:** 3464–3468.

Kindler, V., Thorens, B., De Kossodo, S., Allet, B., Eliason, J. F., Thatcher, D., Farber, N., and Vassali, P. (1986). Stimulation of haemopoiesis *in vivo* by recombinant bacterial murine interleukin-3. *Proceedings of the National Academy of Sciences, U.S.A.* **83:** 1001–1005.

Kishimoto, T., Akira, S., and Taga, T. (1992). Interleukin-6 and its receptor: A paradigm for cytokines. *Science (Washington)* **258:** 593–597.

Kita, H., Ohnishi, T., Okubo, Y., Weiler, D., Abrams, J. S., and Gleich, G. J. (1991). Granulocyte/macrophage colony-stimulating factor and interleukin 3 release from human peripheral blood eosinophils and neutrophils. *Journal of Experimental Medicine* **174:** 745–748.

Kitamura, T., Hayashida, K., Sakamaki, K., Yokota, T., Arai, K., and Miyajima, A. (1991a). Reconstitution of functional receptors for human granulocyte/macrophage colony-stimulating factor (GM-CSF): Evidence that the protein encoded by the AIC2B cDNA is a subunit of the murine GM-CSF receptor. *Proceedings of the National Academy of Sciences, U.S.A.* **88:** 5082–5086.

Kitamura, T., Sato, N., Arai, K., and Miyajima, A. (1991b). Expression of the human IL-3 receptor cDNA reveals a shared beta subunit for the human IL-3 and GM-CSF receptors. *Cell* **66:** 1165–1174.

Kittler, E. L., McGrath, H., Temeles, D., Crittenden, R. B., Kister, V. K., and Quesenberry, P. J. (1992). Biologic significance of constitutive and subliminal growth factor production by bone marrow stroma. *Blood* **79:** 3168–3178.

Klingemann, H.-G., Eaves, A. C., Barnett, M. J., Reece, D. E., Shepherd, J. D., Belch, A. R., Brandwein, J. M., Langleben, A., Koch, P. A., and Phillips, G. L. (1990). Recombinant GM-CSF in patients with poor graft function after bone marrow transplantation. *Clinical and Investigative Medicine* **13:** 77–81.

Knepper, T. P., Arbogast, B., Schreurs, J., and Deinzer, M. L. (1992). Determination of the glycosylation patterns, disulfide linkages, and protein heterogeneities of baculovirus-expressed mouse interleukin-3 by mass spectrometry. *Biochemistry* **31:** 11651–11659.

Kobayashi, M., Yumiba, C., Kawaguchi, Y., Tanaka, Y., Ueda, K., Komazawa, Y., and Okada, K. (1990). Abnormal responses of myeloid progenitor cells to recombinant human colony-stimulating factors in congenital neutropenia. *Blood* **75:** 2143–2149.

Kobayashi, Y., Okabe, T., Ozawa, K., Chiba, S., Hino, M., Miyazono, K., Urabe, A., and Takaku, F. (1989). Treatment of myelodysplastic syndromes with recombinant human granulocyte colony-stimulating factor: A preliminary report. *American Journal of Medicine* **86:** 178–182.

Kodama, H., Yamasaki, A., Nose, M., Niida, S., Ohgame, Y., Abe, M., Kumegawa, M., and Suda, T. (1991). Congenital osteoclast deficiency in osteopetrotic (op/op) mice is cured by injections of macrophage colony-stimulating factor. *Journal of Experimental Medicine* **173:** 269–272.

Koeffler, H. P., Gasson, J., Ranyard, J., Souza, L., Shepard, M., and Munker, R. (1987). Recombinant human TNF$\alpha$ stimulates production of granulocyte colony-stimulating factor. *Blood* **70:** 55–59.

Koeffler, H. P., Gasson, J., and Tobler, A. (1988). Transcriptional and post-transcriptional modulation of myeloid colony-stimulating factor expression by tumor necrosis factor and other agents. *Molecular and Cellular Biology* **8:** 3432–3438.

Kongsuwan, K., Allen, J., and Adams, J. M. (1989). Expression of Hox-2.4 homeobox gene directed by proviral insertion in a myeloid leukemia. *Nucleic Acids Research* **17:** 1881–1892.

Koyanagi, Y., O'Brien, W. A., Zhao, J. Q., Golde, D. W., Gasson, J. C., and Chen, I. S. Y. (1988). Cytokines alter production of HIV-1 from primary mononuclear phagocytes. *Science (Washington)* **241:** 1673–1675.

Kraulis, P. J. (1991). MOLSCRIPT: A program to produce both detailed and schematic plots of protein structures. *Journal of Applied Crystallography* **24:** 946–950.

Kremer, E., Baker, E., D'Andrea, R. J., Slim, R., Phillips, H., Moretti, P. A., Lopez, A. F., Petit, C., Vadas, M. A., Sutherland, G. R., and Goodall, G. J. (1993). A cytokine receptor gene cluster in the X-Y pseudoautosomal region? *Blood* **82:** 22–28.

Kuga, T., Komatsu, Y., Yamasaki, M., Sekine, S., Miyaji, H., Nishi, T., Sato, M., Yokoo, Y., Asano, M., Okabe, M., Morimoto, M., and Itoh, S. (1989). Mutagenesis of human granulocyte colony stimulating factor. *Biochemical and Biophysical Research Communications* **159:** 103–111.

Ladner, M. B., Martin, G. A., Noble, J. A., Nikoloff, D. M., Tal, R., Kawasaki, E. S., and White, T. J. (1987). Human CSF-1: Gene structure and alternative splicing of mRNA precursors. *EMBO Journal* **6:** 2693–2698.

Ladner, M. B., Martin, G. A., Noble, J. A., Wittmen, V. P., Warren, M. K., McGrogan, M., and Stanley, E. R. (1988). cDNA cloning and expression of murine macrophage colony-stimulating factor from L929 cells. *Proceedings of the National Academy of Sciences, U.S.A.* **85:** 6706–6710.

Laker, C., Stocking, C., Bergholz, U., Hess, N., DeLamarter, J. F., and Ostertag, W. (1987). Autocrine stimulation after transfer of the granulocyte/macrophage colony-stimulating factor gene and autonomous growth are distinct but interdependent steps in the oncogenic pathway. *Proceedings of the National Academy of Sciences, U.S.A.* **84:** 8458–8462.

Landau, T., and Sachs, L. (1971). Characterization of the inducer required for the development of macrophage and granulocyte colonies. *Proceedings of the National Academy of Sciences, U.S.A.* **68:** 2540–2544.

Lang, R. A., Cuthbertson, R. A., and Dunn, A. R. (1992). TNF$\alpha$, IL-1$\alpha$ and bFGF are implicated in the complex disease of GM-CSF transgenic mice. *Growth Factors* **6:** 131–138.

Lang, R. A., Metcalf, D., Cuthbertson, R. A., Lyons, I., Stanley, E., Kelso, A., Kannourakis, G., Williamson, D. J., Klintworth, G. K., Gonda, T. J., and Dunn, A. R. (1987). Transgenic mice expressing a hemopoietic growth factor gene (GM-CSF) develop accumulations of macrophages, blindness and a fatal syndrome of tissue damage. *Cell* **51:** 675–686.

Lang, R. A., Metcalf, D., Gough, N. M., Dunn, A. R., and Gonda, T. J. (1985). Expression of a hemopoietic growth factor cDNA in a factor-dependent cell line results in autonomous growth and tumorigenicity. *Cell* **43:** 531–542.

Lanotte, M., Metcalf, D., and Dexter, T. M. (1982). Production of monocyte/macrophage colony-stimulating factor by preadipocyte cell lines derived from murine marrow stroma. *Journal of Cellular Physiology* **112:** 123–127.

Lapidot, T., Sirarad, C., Vormoor, J., Murdoch, B., Hoang, T., Caceres-Cortes, J., Minden, M., Paterson, B., Caligiuri, M. A., and Dick, J. E. (1994). A cell initiating human acute myeloid leukaemia after transplantation into SCID mice. *Nature (London)* **367:** 645–648.

Larner, A. C., David, M., Feldman, G. M., Igarashi, K., Hackett, R. H., Webb, D. S., Sweitzer, S. M., Petricoin, E. F., III, and Finbloom, D. S. (1993). Tyrosine phosphorylation of DNA binding proteins by multiple cytokines. *Science (Washington)* **261:** 1730–1733.

Larsen, A., Davis, T., Curtis, B. M., Gimpel, S., Sims, J. E., Cosman, D., Park, L., Sorensen, E., March, C. J., and Smith, C. A. (1990). Expression cloning of a human granulocyte colony-stimulating factor receptor: A structural mosaic of hematopoietin receptor, immunoglobulin, and fibronectin domains. *Journal of Experimental Medicine* **172:** 1559–1570.

Layton, J. E., Hockman, H., Sheridan, W. B., and Morstyn, G. (1989). Evidence for a novel *in vivo* control mechanism of granulopoiesis: Mature cell-related control of a regulatory growth factor. *Blood* **74:** 1303–1307.

Layton, J. E., Morstyn, G., Fabri, L., Reid, G. E., Burgess, A. W., Simpson, R. J., and Nice, E. C. (1991). Identification of a functional domain of human granulocyte colony-stimulating factor using neutralizing monoclonal antibodies. *Journal of Biological Chemistry* **266:** 23815–23823.

Le Beau, M., Lemons, R. S., Carrino, J. J., Pettenati, M. J., Souza, L. M., Diaz, M. O., and Rowley, J. D. (1987). Chromosomal localization of the human G-CSF gene to 17q11 proximal to the breakpoint of the t(15;17) in acute promyelocytic leukemia. *Leukemia* **1:** 795–799.

Le Beau, M. M., Westbrook, C. A., Diaz, M. O., Larson, R. A., Rowley, J. D., Gasson, J. C., Golde, D. W., and Sherr, C. J. (1986). Evidence for the involvement of GM-CSF and FMS in the deletion (5q) in myeloid disorders. *Science (Washington)* **231:** 984–987.

Lee, F., Yokota, T., Otsuka, T., Gemmell, L., Larson, N., Luh, J., Arai, K., and Rennick, D. (1985). Isolation of cDNA for a human granulocyte-macrophage colony-stimulating factor by functional expression in mammalian cells. *Proceedings of the National Academy of Sciences, U.S.A.* **82:** 4360–4364.

Lee, M. Y., Eyre, D. R., and Osborne, W. R. A. (1991). Isolation of a murine osteoclast colony-stimulating factor. *Proceedings of the National Academy of Sciences, U.S.A.* **88:** 8500–8504.

Leutz, A., Damm, K., Sterneck, E., Kowenz, E., Ness, S., Frank, R., Gausepohl, H., Pan, Y. C., Smart, J., Hayman, M., and Graf, T. (1989). Molecular cloning of the chicken myelomonocytic growth factor (cMGF) reveals relationship to interleukin 6 and granulocyte colony stimulating factor. *EMBO Journal* **8:** 175–181.

Li, C. L., and Johnson, G. R. (1992). Rhodamine 123 reveals heterogeneity within murine Lin$^-$, Sca-1$^+$ hemopoietic stem cells. *Journal of Experimental Medicine* **175:** 1443–1447.

Li, W., and Stanley, E. R. (1991). Role of dimerization and modification of the CSF-1 receptor in its activation and internalization during the CSF-1 response. *EMBO Journal* **10:** 277–288.

Lieschke, G. J., Maher, D., Cebon, J., O'Connor, M., Green, M., Sheridan, W., Boyd, A., Rallings, M., Bonnem, E., Metcalf, D., Burgess, A. W., McGrath, K., Fox, R. M., and Morstyn, G. (1989). Effects of bacterially-synthesized recombinant human granulocyte-macrophage colony-stimulating factor in patients with advanced malignancy. *Annals of Internal Medicine* **110:** 357–364.

Lieschke, G. J., Maher, D., O'Connor, M., Green, M., Sheridan, W., Rallings, M., Bonnem, E., Burgess, A. W., McGrath, K., Fox, R. M., and Morstyn, G. (1990). Phase I study of intravenously administered bacterially synthesized granulocyte-macrophage colony-stimulating factor and comparison with subcutaneous administration. *Cancer Research* **50:** 606–614.

Lieschke, G. J., Stanley, E., Grail, D., Hodgson, G., Sinickas, V., Gall, J. A. M., Sinclair, R., and Dunn, A. R. (1994). Mice lacking both macrophage- and granulocyte-macrophage colony-stimulating factor have macrophages and co-existent osteopetrosis and severe lung disease. *Blood* **84:** 27–35.

Lin, H. S., and Stewart, L. (1974). Peritoneal exudate cells. I. Growth requirements of cells capable of forming colonies in soft agar. *Journal of Cellular Physiology* **83:** 369–378.

Lindemann, A., Herrmann, F., Oster, W., Haffner, G., Meyenburg, W., Souza, L. M., and Mertelsmann, R. (1989). Hematologic effects of recombinant human granulocyte colony-stimulating factor in patients with malignancy. *Blood* **74:** 2644–2651.

Link, H., Boogaerts, M., Carella, A., Ferrant, A., Gadner, H., Gorin, N. C., Harabacz, I., Harrousseau, F., Hervé, P., Kolb, H. J., Kreiger, O., Labar, B., Linkesch, W., Mandelli, F., Maraninchi, D., Nicolay, U., Niederweiser, D., Reiffers, J., Rizzoli, V., Siegert, W., Slavin, S., Vernant, J. P., and de Witte, T. (1990). Recombinant human granulocyte-macrophage colony-stimulating factor (rhGM-CSF) after autologous bone marrow transplantation for acute lymphoblastic leukemia and non-Hodgkin's lymphoma: A randomized double blind multicenter trial in Europe. *Blood* **76:** (Suppl. 1), 152a.

Linnekin, D., and Farrar, W. L. (1990). Signal transduction of human interleukin 3 and granulocyte-macrophage colony-stimulating factor through serine and tyrosine phosphorylation. *Biochemical Journal* **271:** 317–324.

Lock, P., Metcalf, D., and Nicola, N. A. (1994). Histidine-367 of the human common β chain of the receptor is critical for high-affinity binding of human granulocyte-macrophage colony-stimulating factor. *Proceedings of the National Academy of Sciences, U.S.A.* **91:** 252–256.

Logothetis, C. J., Dexeus, F. H., Sella, A., Amato, R. J., Kilbourn, R. G., Finn, L., and Gutterman, J. U. (1990). Escalated therapy for refractory urothelial tumors: Methotrexate-vinblastine-doxorubicin-cisplatin plus unglycosylated recombinant human granulocyte-macrophage colony-stimulating factor. *Journal of the National Cancer Institute* **82:** 667–672.

Lok, S., Kaushansky, K., Holly, R. D., Kuijper. J. L., Lofton-Day, C. E., Oort, P. J., Grant, F. J., Heipel, M. D., Burkhead, S. K., Kramer, J. M., Bell, L. A., Sprecher, C. A., Blumberg, H., Johnson, R., Prunkard, D., Ching, A. F. T., Bailey, M. C., Forstrom, J. W., Buddle, M. M., Osborn, S. G., Evans, S. J., Sheppard, P. O., Presnell, S. R., O'Hara, P. J., Hagen, F. S., Roth, G. R., and Foster, D. C. (1994). Murine thrombopoietin: Expression cloning cDNA sequence and stimulation of platelet production *in vivo*. *Nature (London)* **369:** 565–568.

Lokker, N. A., Strittmatter, U., Steiner, C., Fagg, B., Graff, P., Kocher, H. P., and Zenke, G. (1991). Mapping the epitopes of neutralizing anti-human IL-3 monoclonal antibodies: Implications for structure-activity relationship. *Journal of Immunology* **146:** 893–898.

Lopez, A. F., Eglinton, J. M., Gillis, D., Park, L. S., Clark, S., and Vadas, M. A. (1989). Reciprocal inhibition of binding between interleukin 3 and granulocyte-macrophage colony-stimulating factor to human eosinophils. *Proceedings of the National Academy of Sciences, U.S.A.* **86:** 7022–7026.

Lopez, A. F., Lyons, A. B., Eglinton, J. M., Park, L. S., To, L. B., Clark, S. C., and Vadas, M. A. (1990). Specific binding of human interleukin-3 and granulocyte-macrophage colony-stimulating factor to human basophils. *Journal of Allergy and Clinical Immunology* **85:** 99–102.

Lopez, A. F., Shannon, M. F., Barry, S., Phillips, J. A., Cambareri, B., Dottore, M., Simmons, P., and Vadas, M. A. (1992a). A human interleukin 3 analog with increased biological and binding activities. *Proceedings of the National Academy of Sciences, U.S.A.* **89:** 11842–11846.

Lopez, A. F., Shannon, M. F., Hercus, T., Nicola, N. A., Cambareri, B., Dottore, M., Layton, M. J., Eglinton, L., and Vadas, M. A. (1992b). Residue 21 of human granulocyte-macrophage colony-stimulating factor is critical for biological activity and for high but not low affinity binding. *EMBO Journal* **11:** 909–916.

Lopez, A. F., Vadas, M. A., Woodcock, J. M., Milton, S. E., Lewis, A., Elliott, M. J., Gillis, D., Ireland, R., Olwell, E., and Park, L. S. (1991). Interleukin-5, interleukin-3, and granulocyte-macrophage colony-stimulating factor cross-compete for binding to cell surface receptors on human eosinophils. *Journal of Biological Chemistry* **266:** 24741–24747.

Lopez, A. F., Williamson, D. J., Gamble, J. R., Begley, C. G., Harlan, J. M., Kebanoff, S. J., Waltersdorph, A., Wong, G., Clark, S. C., and Vadas, M. A. (1986). Recombinant human granulocyte-macrophage colony-stimulating factor stimulates *in vitro* mature human neutrophil and eosinophil function, surface receptor expression, and survival. *Journal of Clinical Investigation* **78:** 1220–1228.

Lord, B. I., Bronchud, M. H., Owens, S., Chang, J., Howell, A., Souza, L., and Dexter, T. M. (1989). The kinetics of human granulopoiesis following treatment with granulocyte colony-stimulating factor *in vivo*. *Proceedings of the National Academy of Sciences, U.S.A.* **86:** 9499–9503.

Lord, B. I., Molineux, G., Pojda, Z., Souza, L. M., Mermod, J.-J., and Dexter, T. M. (1991). Myeloid cell kinetics in mice treated with recombinant interleukin-3, granulocyte colony-stimulating (CSF), or granulocyte-macrophage CSF *in vivo*. *Blood* **77:** 2154–2159.

Lord, B. I., and Wright, E. G. (1984). Spatial organisation of CFU-S proliferation regulators in the mouse femur. *Leukemia Research* **8:** 1073–1083.

Lorimore, S. A., Eckmann, L., Pragnell, I. B., and Wright, E. G. (1990). Synergistic interactions allow colony formation *in vitro* by murine haemopoietic stem cells. *Leukemia Research* **14:** 481–489.

Lotem, J., Shabo, Y., and Sachs, L. (1989). Clonal variation in susceptibility to differentiation by different protein inducers in the myeloid leukemia cell line M1. *Leukemia* **3:** 804–807.

Lothrop, C., Jr., Warren, D. J., Souza, L. M., Jones, J. B., and Moore, M. A. S. (1988). Correction of cyclic hematopoiesis with recombinant human granulocyte colony stimulating factor. *Blood* **72:** 1324–1328.

Lovejoy, B., Cascio, D., and Eisenberg, D. (1993). Crystal structure of canine and bovine granulocyte-colony stimulating factor (G-CSF). *Journal of Molecular Biology* **234:** 640–653.

Löwenberg, B., and Touw, I. P. (1993). Hematopoietic growth factors and their receptors in acute leukemia. *Blood* **81:** 281–292.

Löwenberg, B., van Putten, W. L., Touw, I. P., Delwel, R., and Santini, V. (1993). Autonomous proliferation of leukemic cells *in vitro* as a determinant of prognosis in adult acute myeloid leukemia. *New England Journal of Medicine* **328:** 614–619.

Lu, H. S., Boone, T. C., Souza, L. M., and Lai, P. H. (1989). Disulfide and secondary structures of recombinant human granulocyte colony stimulating factor. *Archives of Biochemistry and Biophysics* **268:** 81–92.

Lu, H. S., Clogston, C. L., Wypych, J., Fausset, P. R., Lauren, S., Mendiaz, E. A., Zsebo, K. M., and Langley, K. E. (1991). Amino acid sequence and posttranslational modification of stem cell factor isolated from buffalo rat liver cell-conditioned medium. *Journal of Biological Chemistry* **266:** 8102–8107.

Lu, L., Walker, D., Graham, C. D., Waheed, A., Shadduck, R. K., and Broxmeyer, H. E. (1988). Enhancement of release from MHC class II antigen-positive monocytes of hematopoietic colony stimulating factors CSF-1 and G-CSF by recombinant human tumor necrosis factor-alpha: Synergism with recombinant human interferon-gamma. *Blood* **72:** 34–41.

Luger, T. A., Wirth, U., and Kock, A. (1985). Epidermal cells synthesize a cytokine with interleukin-3-like properties. *Journal of Immunology* **134:** 915–919.

Lyman, S. D., James, L., Vanden Bos, T., de Vries, P., Brasel, K., Gliniak, B., Hollingsworth, L. T., Picha, K. S., McKenna, H. J., Splett, R. R., Fletcher, F. A., Maraskovsky, E., Farrah, T., Foxworthe, D., Williams, D. E., and Beckmann, M. P. (1993). Molecular cloning of a ligand for the flt3/flk-2 tyrosine kinase receptor: A proliferative factor for primitive hemopoietic cells. *Cell* **75:** 1157–1167.

Maekawa, T., and Metcalf, D. (1989). Clonal suppression of HL60 and U937 cells by recombinant leukemia inhibitory factor in combination with GM-CSF or G-CSF. *Leukemia* **3:** 270–276.

Maekawa, T., Metcalf, D., and Gearing, D. P. (1990). Enhanced suppression of human myeloid leukemic cell lines by combinations of IL-6, LIF, GM-CSF and G-CSF. *International Journal of Cancer* **45:** 353–358.

Malik, S., and Balkwill, F. (1991). Epithelial ovarian cancer: A cytokine propelled disease? *British Journal of Cancer* **64:** 617–620.

Malter, J. S., McCrory, W. A., Wilson, M., and Gillis, P. (1990). Adenosine-uridine binding factor requires metals for binding to granulocyte-macrophage colony-stimulating factor mRNA. *Enzyme* **44:** 203–213.

Manos, M. M. (1988). Expression and processing of a recombinant human macrophage colony-stimulating factor in mouse cells. *Molecular and Cellular Biology* **8:** 5035–5039.

Mathey-Prevot, B., Andrews, N. C., Murphy, H. S., Kreissman, S. G., and Nathan, D. G. (1990). Positive and negative elements regulate human interleukin 3 expression. *Proceedings of the National Academy of Sciences, U.S.A.* **87:** 5046–5050.

Matsumoto, M., Matsubara, S., Matsuno, T., Tamura, M., Hattori, K., Nomura, H., Ono, M., and Yokota, T. (1987). Protective effect of human granulocyte colony-stimulating factor on microbial infection in neutropenic mice. *Infection and Immunity* **55:** 2715–2720.

Mayani, H., Dragowska, W., and Lansdorp, P. M. (1993). Lineage commitment in human hemopoiesis involves asymmetric cell division of multipotent progenitors and does not appear to be influenced by cytokines. *Journal of Cellular Physiology* **157:** 579–586.

Mayer, P., Valent, P., Schmidt, G., Liehl, E., and Bettelheim, P. (1989). The *in vivo* effects of recombinant human interleukin-3: Demonstration of basophil differentiation factor, histamine-producing activity, and priming of GM-CSF-responsive progenitors in non-human primates. *Blood* **74:** 613–621.

Mazur, E. M., Cohen, J. L., Wong, G. G., and Clark, S. C. (1987). Modest stimulatory effect of recombinant human GM-CSF on colony growth from peripheral blood human megakaryocyte progenitor cells. *Experimental Hematology* **15:** 1128–1133.

McArthur, G. A., Rohrschneider, L. R., and Johnson, G. R. (1994). Induced expression of *c-fms* in normal hematopoietic cells shows evidence for both conservation and lineage restriction of signal transduction in response to macrophage colony-stimulating factor. *Blood* **83:** 972–981.

McNiece, I. K., Langley, K., and Zsebo, K. M. (1991). Recombinant human stem cell factor synergises with GM-CSF, G-CSF, IL3 and Epo to stimulate human progenitor cells of myeloid and erythroid lineages. *Experimental Hematology* **19:** 226–231.

McNiece, I. K., Stewart, F. M., Deacon, D. M., and Quesenberry, P. J. (1988). Synergistic interactions between hematopoietic growth factors as detected by *in vitro* mouse bone marrow colony formation. *Experimental Hematology* **16:** 383–388.

Medlock, E. S., Kaplan, D. L., Cecchini, M., Ulich, T. R., del Castillo, J., and Andresen, J. (1993). Granulocyte colony-stimulating factor crosses the placenta and stimulates fetal rat granulopoiesis. *Blood* **81:** 916–922.

Meeker, T. C., Hardy, D., Willman, C., Hogan, T., and Abrams, J. (1990). Activation of the interleukin-3 gene by chromosome translocation in acute lymphocytic leukemia with eosinophilia. *Blood* **76:** 285–289.

Mempel, K., Pietsch, T., Menzel, T., Zeidler, C., and Welte, K. (1991). Increased serum levels of granulocyte colony-stimulating factor in patients with severe congenital neutropenia. *Blood* **77:** 1919–1922.

Meropol, N. J., Altmann, S. W., Shanafelt, A. B., Kastelein, R. A., Johnson, G. D., and Prystowsky, M. B. (1992). Requirement of hydrophilic amino-terminal residues for granulocyte-macrophage colony-stimulating factor bioactivity and receptor binding. *Journal of Biological Chemistry* **267:** 14266–14269.

Metcalf, D. (1968). Potentiation of bone marrow colony growth *in vitro* by the addition of lymphoid or bone marrow cells. *Journal of Cellular Physiology* **72:** 9–19.

Metcalf, D. (1969). The effect of bleeding on the number of *in vitro* colony-forming cells in the bone marrow. *British Journal of Haematology* **16:** 397–407.

Metcalf, D. (1970). Studies on colony formation *in vitro* by mouse bone marrow cells. II. Action of colony stimulating factor. *Journal of Cellular Physiology* **76:** 89–99.

Metcalf, D. (1971). Acute antigen-induced elevation of serum colony stimulating factor (CSF) levels. *Immunology* **21:** 427–436.

Metcalf, D. (1972). Effects of thymidine suiciding on colony formation *in vitro* by mouse hematopoietic cells. *Proceedings of the Society for Experimental Biology and Medicine* **139:** 511–514.

Metcalf, D. (1974a). Stimulation by human urine or plasma of granulopoiesis by human marrow cells in agar. *Experimental Hematology* **2:** 157–173.

Metcalf, D. (1974b). Depressed responses of the granulocyte-macrophage system to bacterial antigens following preimmunization. *Immunology* **26:** 1115–1125.

Metcalf, D. (1977). *In-vitro* cloning techniques for hemopoietic cells: Clinical applications. *Annals of Internal Medicine* **87:** 483–488.

Metcalf, D. (1979). Clonal analysis of the action of GM-CSF on the proliferation and differentiation of myelomonocytic leukemic cells. *International Journal of Cancer* **24:** 616–623.

Metcalf, D. (1980). Clonal analysis of proliferation and differentiation of paired daughter cells: Action of granulocyte-macrophage colony-stimulating factor on granulocyte-macrophage precursors. *Proceedings of the National Academy of Sciences, U.S.A.* **77:** 5327–5330.

Metcalf, D. (1982a). Regulator-induced suppression of myelomonocytic leukemic cells: Clonal analysis of early cellular events. *International Journal of Cancer* **30:** 203–210.

Metcalf, D. (1982b). Regulatory control of the proliferation and differentiation of normal and leukemia cells. *National Cancer Institute Monograph* **60:** 123–131.

Metcalf, D. (1984). *The Hemopoietic Colony Stimulating Factors.* Amsterdam: Elsevier.

Metcalf, D. (1985). Multi-CSF-dependent colony formation by cells of a murine hemopoietic cell line: Specificity and action of Multi-CSF. *Blood* **65:** 357–362.

Metcalf, D. (1988a). *The Molecular Control of Blood Cells.* Cambridge, MA: Harvard University Press.

Metcalf, D. (1988b). Mechanisms contributing to the sex difference in levels of granulocyte-macrophage colony-stimulating factor in the urine of GM-CSF mice. *Experimental Hematology* **16:** 794–800.

Metcalf, D. (1989). Actions and interactions of G-CSF, LIF and IL-6 on normal and leukemic murine cells. *Leukemia* **3:** 349–355.

Metcalf, D. (1991a). The Florey Lecture – The colony-stimulating factors: discovery to clinical use. *Philosophical Transactions of the Royal Society, London, Series B* **333:** 147–173.

Metcalf, D. (1991b). Lineage commitment of hemopoietic progenitor cells in developing blast cell colonies: Influence of colony stimulating factors. *Proceedings of the National Academy of Sciences, U.S.A.* **88:** 11310–11314.

Metcalf, D. (1991c). Transgenic mice as models of hemopoiesis. *Cancer* **67:** 2695–2699.

Metcalf, D. (1992). Mechanisms responsible for size differences between hemopoietic colonies: An analysis using a CSF-dependent hemopoietic cell line. *International Journal of Cell Cloning* **10:** 116–125.

Metcalf, D. (1993a). The cellular basis for enhancement interactions between stem cell factor and the colony stimulating factors. *Stem Cells* **11:** (suppl. 2), 1–11.

Metcalf, D. (1993b). Hemopoietic regulators: Redundancy or subtlety? *Blood* **82:** 3515–3523.

Metcalf, D. (1994). Hemopoietic regulators and leukemia development: A personal retrospective. *Advances in Cancer Research* **63:** 41–91.

Metcalf, D., Begley, C. G., Johnson, G. R., Nicola, N. A., Lopez, A. F., and Williamson, D. J. (1986a). Effects of purified bacterially synthesized murine Multi-CSF (IL-3) on hematopoiesis in normal adult mice. *Blood* **68:** 46–57.

Metcalf, D., Begley, C. G., Johnson, G. R., Nicola, N. A., Vadas, M. A., Lopez, A. F., Williamson, D. J., Wong, G. G., Clark, S. C., and Wang, E. A. (1986b). Biologic properties *in vitro* of a recombinant human granulocyte-macrophage colony-stimulating factor. *Blood* **67:** 37–45.

Metcalf, D., Begley, C. G., Nicola, N. A., and Johnson, G. R. (1987a). Quantitative responsiveness of murine hemopoietic populations *in vitro* and *in vivo* to recombinant Multi-CSF (IL-3). *Experimental Hematology* **15:** 288–295.

Metcalf, D., Begley, C. G., Williamson, D., Nice, E. C., DeLamarter, J., Mermod, J.-J., Thatcher, D., and Schmidt, A. (1987b). Hemopoietic responses in mice injected with purified recombinant murine GM-CSF. *Experimental Hematology* **15:** 1–9.

Metcalf, D., and Burgess, A. W. (1982). Clonal analysis of progenitor cell commitment to granulocyte or macrophage production. *Journal of Cellular Physiology* **111:** 275–283.

Metcalf, D., Burgess, A. W., Johnson, G. R., Nicola, N. A., Nice, E. C., DeLamarter, J., Thatcher, D. R., and Mermod, J.-J. (1986c). *In vitro* actions on hemopoietic cells of recombinant murine GM-CSF purified after production in *Escherichia coli*: Comparison with purified native GM-CSF. *Journal of Cellular Physiology* **128:** 421–431.

Metcalf, D., Chan, S. H., Gunz, F. W., Vincent, P., and Ravich, R. B. M. (1971). Colony-stimulating factor and inhibitor levels in acute granulocytic leukemia. *Blood* **38:** 143–152.

Metcalf, D., Elliott, M. J., and Nicola, N. A. (1992a). The excess numbers of peritoneal macrophages in granulocyte-macrophage colony-stimulating factor transgenic mice are generated by local proliferation. *Journal of Experimental Medicine* **175:** 877–884.

Metcalf, D., and Foster, R. (1967). Behavior on transfer of serum stimulated bone marrow colonies. *Proceedings of the Society for Experimental Biology and Medicine* **126:** 758–762.

Metcalf, D., and Johnson, G. R. (1979). Interactions between purified GM-CSF, purified erythropoietin and spleen conditioned medium on hemopoietic colony formation *in vitro*. *Journal of Cellular Physiology* **99:** 159–174.

Metcalf, D., Johnson, G. R., and Burgess, A. W. (1980). Direct stimulation by purified GM-CSF of the proliferation of multipotential and erythroid precursor cells. *Blood* **55:** 138–147.

Metcalf, D., Johnson, G. R., and Mandel, T. E. (1979). Colony formation in agar by multipotential hemopoietic cells. *Journal of Cellular Physiology* **98:** 401–420.

Metcalf, D., and MacDonald, H. R. (1975). Heterogeneity of *in vitro* colony- and cluster-forming cells in the mouse marrow: Segregation by velocity sedimentation. *Journal of Cellular Physiology* **85:** 643–654.

Metcalf, D., MacDonald, H. R., Odartchenko, N., and Sordat, B. (1975). Growth of mouse megakaryocyte colonies *in vitro*. *Proceedings of the National Academy of Sciences, U.S.A.* **72:** 1744–1748.

Metcalf, D., and Merchav, S. (1982). Effects of GM-CSF deprivation on precursors of granulocytes and macrophages. *Journal of Cellular Physiology* **112:** 411–418.

Metcalf, D., and Moore, J. G. (1988). Divergent disease patterns in GM-CSF transgenic mice associated with differing transgene insertion sites. *Proceedings of the National Academy of Sciences, U.S.A.* **85:** 7767–7771.

Metcalf, D., and Moore, M. A. S. (1971). *Haemopoietic Cells.* Amsterdam: North-Holland.

Metcalf, D., Moore, M. A. S., and Warner, N. L. (1969). Colony formation *in vitro* by myelomonocytic leukemic cells. *Journal of the National Cancer Institute* **43:** 983–1001.

Metcalf, D., and Nicola, N. A. (1983). Proliferative effects of purified granulocyte colony-stimulating factor (G-CSF) on normal mouse hematopoietic cells. *Journal of Cellular Physiology* **116:** 198–206.

Metcalf, D., and Nicola, N. A. (1985a). Role of the colony stimulating factors in the emergence and suppression of myeloid leukemia populations. In G. Holm, S. Hammarstrom, and P. Perlmann (eds.), *Molecular Biology of Tumor Cells,* pp. 215–232. New York: Raven.

Metcalf, D., and Nicola, N. A. (1985b). Synthesis by mouse peritoneal cells of G-CSF, the differentiation inducer for myeloid leukemia cells: Stimulation by endotoxin, M-CSF and Multi-CSF. *Leukemia Research* **1:** 35–50.

Metcalf, D., and Nicola, N. A. (1988). Tissue localization and fate in mice of injected multipotential colony-stimulating factor. *Proceedings of the National Academy of Sciences, U.S.A.* **85:** 3160–3164.

Metcalf, D., and Nicola, N. A. (1991). Direct proliferative actions of stem cell factor on murine bone marrow cells *in vitro*: Effects of combination with colony-stimulating factors. *Proceedings of the National Academy of Sciences, U.S.A.* **88:** 6239–6243.

Metcalf, D., and Nicola, N. A. (1992). The clonal proliferation of normal mouse hemopoietic cells: Enhancement and suppression by CSF combinations. *Blood* **79:** 2861–2866.

Metcalf, D., Nicola, N. A., Gearing, D. P., and Gough, N. M. (1990). Low-affinity placenta-derived receptors for human granulocyte-macrophage colony-stimulating factor can deliver a proliferative signal to murine hemopoietic cells. *Proceedings of the National Academy of Sciences, U.S.A.* **87:** 4670–4674.

Metcalf, D., Nicola, N. A., Gough, N. M., Elliott, M., McArthur, G., and Li, M. (1992b). Synergistic suppression: Anomalous inhibition of the proliferation of factor-dependent hemopoietic cells by combinations of two colony stimulating factors. *Proceedings of the National Academy of Sciences, U.S.A.* **89:** 2819–2823.

Metcalf, D., and Rasko, J. E. J. (1993). Leukemic transformation of immortalized FDC-P1 cells engrafted in GM-CSF transgenic mice. *Leukemia* **7:** 878–886.

Metcalf, D., and Stanley, E. R. (1971). Haematological effects in mice of partially purified colony-stimulating factor (CSF) prepared from human urine. *British Journal of Haematology* **21:** 481–492.

Metcalf, D., and Stevens, S. (1972). Influence of age and antigenic stimulation on granulocyte and macrophage progenitor cells in the mouse spleen. *Cell and Tissue Kinetics* **5:** 433–446.

Metcalf, D., and Wahren, B. (1968). Bone marrow colony stimulating activity of sera in infectious mononucleosis. *British Medical Journal* **3:** 99–101.

Meunch, M. D., Schneider, J. G., and Moore, M. A. S. (1992). Interaction amongst colony stimulating factors, IL-1β, IL-6 and kit-ligand in the regulation of primitive murine hematopoietic cells. *Experimental Hematology* **20:** 339–349.

Micklem, H. S., Anderson, N., and Ross, E. (1975). Limited potential of circulating hemopoietic stem cells. *Nature (London)* **256:** 41–43.

Migliaccio, A. R., Bruno, M., and Migliaccio, G. (1987). Evidence for direct action of human biosynthetic (recombinant) GM-CSF on erythroid progenitors in serum-free culture. *Blood* **70:** 1867–1871.

Migliaccio, A. R., Migliaccio, G., Adamson, J. W., and Torok-Storb, B. (1992a). Production of granulocyte colony-stimulating factor and granulocyte/macrophage- colony-stimulating factor after interleukin-1 stimulation of marrow stromal cell cultures from normal or aplastic anemia donors. *Journal of Cellular Physiology* **152:** 199–206.

Migliaccio, G., Migliaccio, A. R., Druzin, M. L., Giardina, P.-J. V., Zsebo, K. M., and Adamson, J. W. (1992b). Long-term generation of colony-forming cells in liquid culture of $CD34^+$ cord blood cells in the presence of recombinant human stem cell factor. *Blood* **79:** 2620–2627.

Migliaccio, G., Migliaccio, A. R., Valinsky, J., Langley, K., Zsebo, K., Visser, J. W. M., and Adamson, J. W. (1991). Stem cell factor induces proliferation and differentiation of highly enriched murine hematopoietic cells. *Proceedings of the National Academy of Sciences, U.S.A.* **88:** 7420–7424.

Milatovich, A., Kitamura, T., Miyajima, A., and Francke, U. (1993). Gene for the alpha-subunit of the human interleukin-3 receptor (IL3A) localized to the X-Y pseudoautosomal region. *American Journal of Human Genetics* **53:** 1146–1153.

Miles, S. A., Mitsuyasu, R. T., Moreno, J., Baldwin, G., Alton, N. K., Souza, L., and Glaspy, J. A. (1991). Combined therapy with recombinant granulocyte colony-stimulating factor and erythropoietin decreases hematologic toxicity from zidovudine. *Blood* **77:** 2109–2117.

Miura, N., Okada, S., Zsebo, K. M., Miura, Y., and Suda, T. (1993). Rat stem cell factor and IL-6 preferentially support the proliferation of *c-kit*-positive murine hemopoietic cells rather than their differentiation. *Experimental Hematology* **21:** 143–149.

Miyake, T., Kung, C. K.-H., and Goldwasser, E. (1977). Purification of human erythropoietin. *Journal of Biological Chemistry* **252:** 5558–5564.

Miyatake, S., Otsuka, T., Yokota, T., Lee, F., and Arai, K. (1985). Structure of the chromosomal gene for granulocyte-macrophage colony stimulating factor: Comparison of the mouse and human genes. *EMBO Journal* **4:** 2561–2568.

Miyatake, S., Seiki, M., Yoshida, M., and Arai, K. I. (1988). T-cell activation signals and human T-cell leukemia virus type I-encoded p40(x) protein activate the mouse granulocyte-macrophage colony-stimulating factor gene through a common DNA element. *Molecular and Cellular Biology* **8:** 5581–5587.

Miyatake, S., Shlomai, J., Arai, K., and Arai, N. (1991). Characterization of the mouse granulocyte-macrophage colony-stimulating factor (GM-CSF) gene promoter: Nuclear factors that interact with an element shared by three lymphokine genes – those for GM-CSF, interleukin-4 (IL-4), and IL-5. *Molecular and Cellular Biology* **11:** 5894–5901.

Miyauchi, J., Kelleher, C. A., Wong, G. G., Yang, Y.-C., Clark, S. C., Minkin, S., Minden, M. D., and McCulloch, E. A. (1988a). The effects of combinations of the recombinant growth factors GM-CSF, G-CSF, IL-3 and CSF-1 on leukemic blast cells in suspension culture. *Leukemia* **2:** 382–387.

Miyauchi, J., Wang, C., Kelleher, C. H., Wong, G. G., Clark, S. C., Minden, M. D., and McCulloch, E. A. (1988b). The effects of recombinant CSF-1 on the blast cells of acute myeloblastic leukemia in suspension culture. *Journal of Cellular Physiology* **135:** 55–62.

Molineux, G., Pojda, Z., and Dexter, T. M. (1990a). A comparison of hematopoiesis in normal and splenectomized mice treated with granulocyte colony-stimulating factor. *Blood* **75:** 563–569.

Molineux, G., Pojda, Z., Hampson, I. N., Lord, B. I., and Dexter, T. M. (1990). Transplantation potential of peripheral blood stem cells induced by granulocyte colony-stimulating factor. *Blood* **76:** 2153–2158.

Moonen, P., Mermod, J.-J., Ernst, J. F., Hirschi, M., and DeLamarter, J. F. (1987). Increased biological activity of deglycosylated recombinant human granulocyte/macrophage colony-stimulating factor produced by yeast or animal cells. *Proceedings of the National Academy of Sciences, U.S.A.* **84:** 4428–4431.

Moore, M. A. S. (1988). Interleukin 3: An overview. *Lymphokines* **15:** 219–280.

Moore, M. A. S., and Metcalf, D. (1970). Ontogeny of the haemopoietic system: Yolk sac origin of *in vivo* and *in vitro* colony forming cells in the developing mouse embryo. *British Journal of Haematology* **18:** 279–296.

Moore, M. A. S., Spitzer, G., Metcalf, D., and Penington, D. G. (1974a). Monocyte production of colony stimulating factor in familial cyclic neutropenia. *British Journal of Haematology* **27:** 47–55.

Moore, M. A. S., Spitzer, G., Williams, N., Metcalf, D., and Buckley, J. (1974b). Agar culture studies in 127 cases of untreated acute leukemia: The prognostic value of reclassification of leukemia according to *in vitro* growth characteristics. *Blood* **44:** 1–18.

Moore, M. A. S., and Warren, D. J. (1987). Synergy of interleukin-1 and granulocyte colony-stimulating factor: *In vivo* stimulation of stem cell recovery and haemopoietic regeneration following 5-fluorouracil treatment of mice. *Proceedings of the National Academy of Sciences, U.S.A.* **84:** 7134–7138.

Moore, M. A. S., and Williams, N. (1972). Physical separation of colony stimulating cells from *in vitro* colony forming cells in hemopoietic tissue. *Journal of Cellular Physiology* **80:** 195–206.

Moore, M. A. S., and Williams, N. (1973). Functional morphologic and kinetic analyses of the granulocyte-macrophage progenitor cell. In W. A. Robinson (ed.), *Hemopoiesis in Culture.* DHEW Publication No. 74-205, pp. 17–27, Washington: DHEW.

Moore, M. A. S., Williams, N., and Metcalf, D. (1973a). *In vitro* colony formation by normal and leukemic human hematopoietic cells: Characterization of the colony-forming cells. *Journal of the National Cancer Institute* **50:** 603–623.

Moore, M. A. S., Williams, N., and Metcalf, D. (1973b). *In vitro* colony formation by normal and leukemic human hematopoietic cells: Interaction between colony-forming and colony-stimulating cells. *Journal of the National Cancer Institute* **50:** 591–602.

Morley, A., Quesenberry, P., Bealmer, P., Stohlman, F., and Wilson, R. (1972). Serum colony stimulating factor levels in irradiated germfree and conventional CFW mice. *Proceedings of the Society for Experimental Biology and Medicine* **140:** 478–480.

Morris, S. W., Valentine, M. B., Shapiro, D. N., Sublett, J. E., Deaven, L. L., Foust, J. T., Roberts, W. M., Cerretti, D. P., and Look, A. T. (1991). Reassignment of the human CSF1 gene to chromosome 1p13–p21. *Blood* **78:** 2013–2020.

Morstyn, G., Campbell, L., Souza, L. M., Alton, N. K., Keech, J., Green, M., Sheridan, W., Metcalf, D., and Fox, R. (1988). Effect of granulocyte colony-stimulating factor on neutropenia induced by cytotoxic chemotherapy. *Lancet* **i:** 667–672.

Morstyn, G., Lieschke, G. J., Cebon, J., Dührsen, U., Villeval, J.-L., Sheridan, W., McGrath, K., and Layton, J. E. (1989a). Early clinical trials with colony-stimulating factors. *Cancer Investigation* **7:** 443–456.

Morstyn, G. Lieschke, G. L., Sheridan, W., Layton, J., and Cebon, J. (1989b). Pharmacology of the colony-stimulating factors. *Trends in Pharmacological Science* **10:** 154–159.

Morstyn, G., Ramenghi, U., Lieschke, G. J., Bishop, J. F., Stuart-Harris, R., Kafford, R. F., Raghavan, D., Cebon, J., Layton, J. E., and Sheridan, W. (1990). The impact of granulocyte-colony stimulating factor and granulocyte macrophage-colony stimulating factor on cancer therapy. In J. G. Fortner and J. E. Rhoads (eds.), *Accomplishments in Cancer Research, 1989,* pp. 204–211. Philadelphia: Lippincott.

Mui, A. L., Kay, R. J., Humphries, R. K., and Krystal, G. (1992). Purification of the murine interleukin 3 receptor. *Journal of Biological Chemistry* **267:** 16523–16530.

Mumcuoglu, M., Naparstek, E., and Slavin, S. (1990). The use of recombinant cytokines for enhancing immunohematopoietic reconstitution following bone marrow transplantation. II. The influence of lymphokines on CFU-GM colonies from human untreated, ASTA-Z or campath-IM treated bone marrow. *Bone Marrow Transplantation* **5:** 153–158.

Munker, R., Gasson, J., Ogawa, M., and Koeffer, H. P. (1986). Recombinant human TNF induces production of granulocyte-macrophage colony-stimulating factor. *Nature (London)* **323:** 79–82.

Murohashi, I., Tohda, S., Suzuki, T., Nagata, K., Yamashita, Y., and Nara, N. (1989). Autocrine growth mechanisms of the progenitors of blast cells in acute myeloblastic leukemia. *Blood* **74:** 35–41.

Musashi, M., Yang, Y-C., Paul, S. R., Clark, S. C., Sudo, T., and Ogawa, M. (1991). Direct and synergistic effects of interleukin 11 on murine hemopoiesis in culture. *Proceedings of the National Academy of Sciences, U.S.A.* **88:** 765–769.

Nabel, G., Galli, S. J., Dvorak, A. M., Dvorak, H. F., and Cantor, H. (1981). Inducer T lymphocytes synthesize a factor that stimulates proliferation of cloned mast cells. *Nature (London)* **291:** 332–334.

Nagata, S. (1990). Granulocyte colony-stimulating factor. *Handbook of Experimental Pharmacology* **95:** 699–722.

Nagata, S., Tsuchiya, M., Asano, S., Kaziro, Y., Yamazaki, T., Yamamoto, O., Hirata, Y., Kubota, N., Oheda, M., Nomura, H., and Ono, M. (1986a). Molecular cloning and expression of cDNA for human granulocyte colony-stimulating factor. *Nature (London)* **319:** 415–418.

Nagata, S., Tsuchiya, M., Asano, S., Yamamoto, O., Hirata, Y., Kubota, N., Oheda, M., Nomura, H., and Yamazaki, T. (1986b). The chromosomal gene structure and two mRNAs for human granulocyte colony-stimulating factor. *EMBO Journal* **5:** 575–581.

Nagler, A., Ginzton, N., Negrin, R., Bang, D., Donlon, T., and Greenberg, P. (1990). Effects of recombinant human granulocyte colony stimulating factor and granulocyte-monocyte colony stimulating factor on *in vitro* hemopoiesis in the myelodysplastic syndromes. *Leukemia* **4:** 193–202.

Nakahata, T., Gross, A. J., and Ogawa, M. (1982). A stochastic model of self-renewal and commitment to differentiation of the primitive hemopoietic stem cells in culture. *Journal of Cellular Physiology* **113:** 455–458.

Nakamura, Y., Komatsu, N., and Nakauchi, H. (1992). A truncated erythropoietin receptor that fails to prevent programmed cell death of erythroid cells. *Science (Washington)* **257:** 1138–1141.

Negrin, R. S., Haeuber, D. H., Nagler, A., Kobayashi, Y., Sklar, J., Donlon, T., Vincent, M., and Greenberg, P. L. (1990). Maintenance treatment of patients with myelodysplastic syndromes using human granulocyte colony-stimulating factor. *Blood* **76:** 36–43.

Negrin, R. S., Haeuber, D. H., Nagler, A., Olds, L. C., Donlon, T., Souza, L. M., and Greenberg, P. L. (1989). Treatment of myelodysplastic syndromes with recombinant human granulocyte colony-stimulating factor: A phase I/II trial. *Annals of Internal Medicine* **110:** 976–984.

Negrin, R. S., Stein, R., Vardiman, J., Doherty, K., Cornwell, J., Krantz, S., and Greenberg, P. L. (1993). Treatment of the anemia of myelodysplastic syndromes using recombinant human granulocyte colony-stimulating factor in combination with erythropoietin. *Blood* **82:** 737–743.

Neidhart, J., Mangalik, A., Kohler, W., Stidley, C., Saiki, J., Duncan, P., Souza, L., and Downing, M. (1989). Granulocyte colony-stimulating factor stimulates recovery of granulocytes in patients receiving dose-intensive chemotherapy without bone marrow transplantation. *Journal of Clinical Oncology* **7:** 1685–1692.

Nelson, S., Daifuku, R., and Andresen, J. (1994). Use of filgrastim (r-metHuG-CSF) in infectious diseases. In G. Morstyn and T. M. Dexter (eds.), *Filgrastim (r-metHuG-CSF) in Clinical Practice,* pp. 253–266. New York: Dekker.

Nelson, S., Summer, W., Bagby, G., Nakamura, C., Stewart, L., Lipscomb, G., and Andresen, J. (1991). Granulocyte colony-stimulating factor enhances pulmonary host defenses in normal and ethanol-treated rats. *Journal of Infectious Diseases* **164:** 901–906.

Nemunaitis, J. (1993). Macrophage function activating cytokines: Potential clinical application. *Critical Reviews in Oncology-Hematology* **14:** 152–171.

Nemunaitis, J., Shannon-Dorey, K., Appelbaum, F. R., Meyers, J., Owens, A., Day, R., Ando, D., O'Neill, C., Buckner, D., and Singer, J. (1993).

Long-term follow-up of patients with invasive fungal disease who received adjunctive therapy with recombinant human macrophage colony-stimulating factor. *Blood* **82:** 1422–1427.

Nemunaitis, J., Singer, J. W., Buckner, C. D., Durnam, D., Epstein, C., Hill, R., Storb, R., Thomas, E. D., and Appelbaum, F. R. (1990). Use of recombinant human granulocyte-macrophage colony-stimulating factor in graft failure after bone marrow transplantation. *Blood* **76:** 245–253.

Nemunaitis, J., Singer, J. W., Buckner, C. D., Hill, R., Storb, R., Thomas, E. D., and Appelbaum, F. R. (1988). Use of recombinant human granulocyte-macrophage colony-stimulating factor in autologous marrow transplantation for lymphoid malignancies. *Blood* **72:** 834–836.

Neta, R., Oppenheim, J. J., and Douches, S. D. (1988). Interdependence of the radioprotective effects of human recombinant interleukin 1$\alpha$, tumor necrosis factor $\alpha$, granulocyte colony-stimulating factor and murine recombinant granulocyte-macrophage colony-stimulating factor. *Journal of Immunology* **140:** 108–111.

Nicholson, S. E., Oates, A. C., Harpur, A. G., Ziemiecki, A., Wilks, A. F., and Layton, J. E. (1994). Tyrosine kinase jak1 is associated with the granulocyte colony stimulating factor receptor and both become tyrosine phosphorylated after receptor activation. *Proceedings of the National Academy of Sciences, U.S.A.* **91:** 2985–2988.

Nicola, N. A. (1985). Granulocyte colony-stimulating factor. In G. D. Sabato (ed.), *Methods in Enzymology, 1985,* pp. 600–619. New York: Academic.

Nicola, N. A. (1987a). Why do hemopoietic growth factor receptors interact with each other? *Immunology Today* **8:** 134–140.

Nicola, N. A. (1987b). Kinetic aspects of the interactions of colony-stimulating factors with cellular receptors. In R. P. Gale and D. W. Golde (eds.), *Recent Advances in Leukemia and Lymphoma, 1987,* pp. 215–228. New York: Liss.

Nicola, N. A. (1991a). Structural and functional characteristics of receptors for colony-stimulating factors (CSFs). In P. J. Quesenberry, S. Asano, and K. Saito (eds.), *Hemopoietic Growth Factors, 1991,* pp. 101–120. Amsterdam: Excerpta Medica.

Nicola, N. A. (1991b). Receptors for colony-stimulating factors. *British Journal of Haematology* **77:** 133–138.

Nicola, N. A., Begley, C. G., and Metcalf, D. (1985). Identification of the human analogue of a regulator that induces differentiation in murine leukaemic cells. *Nature (London)* **314:** 625–628.

Nicola, N. A., Burgess, A. W., and Metcalf, D. (1979a). Similar molecular properties of granulocyte-macrophage colony-stimulating factors produced by different mouse organs *in vitro* and *in vivo. Journal of Biological Chemistry* **254:** 5290–5299.

Nicola, N. A., Burgess, A. W., Staber, F. G., Johnson, G. R., Metcalf, D., and Battye, F. L. (1980). Differential expression of lectin receptors during hemopoietic differentiation: Enrichment for granulocyte-macrophage progenitor cells. *Journal of Cellular Physiology* **103:** 217–237.

Nicola, N. A., and Cary, D. (1992). Affinity conversion of receptors for colony stimulating factors: Properties of solubilized receptors. *Growth Factors* **6:** 119–129.

Nicola, N. A., and Metcalf, D. (1981). Biochemical properties of differentiation factors for murine myelomonocytic leukemic cells in organ conditioned media. Separation from colony stimulating factors. *Journal of Cellular Physiology* **109:** 253-264.

Nicola, N. A., and Metcalf, D. (1984). Differentiation induction in leukemic cells by normal growth regulators: Molecular and binding properties of purified granulocyte colony-stimulating factor. In J. M. Bishop, J. D. Rowley, and M. Greaves (eds.), *Genes and Cancer, 1984,* pp. 591-610. New York: Liss.

Nicola, N. A., and Metcalf, D. (1985a). The colony-stimulating factors and myeloid leukaemia. *Cancer Surveys* **4:** 789-815.

Nicola, N. A., and Metcalf, D. (1985b). Binding of $^{125}$I-labeled granulocyte colony-stimulating factor to normal murine hemopoietic cells. *Journal of Cellular Physiology* **124:** 313-321.

Nicola, N. A., and Metcalf, D. (1986). Binding of iodinated multipotential colony-stimulating factor (interleukin-3) to murine bone marrow cells. *Journal of Cellular Physiology* **128:** 180-188.

Nicola, N. A., and Metcalf, D. (1988). Binding, internalization and degradation of $^{125}$I-multipotential colony-stimulating factor (interleukin-3) by FDC-P1 cells. *Growth Factors* **1:** 29-39.

Nicola, N. A., and Metcalf, D. (1991). Subunit promiscuity among hemopoietic growth factor receptors. *Cell* **67:** 1-4.

Nicola, N. A., Metcalf, D., Johnson, G. R., and Burgess, A. W. (1979b). Separation of functionally-distinct human granulocyte-macrophage colony-stimulating factors. *Blood* **54:** 614-627.

Nicola, N. A., Metcalf, D., Matsumoto, M., and Johnson, G. R. (1983). Purification of a factor inducing differentiation in murine myelomonocytic leukemia cells: Identification as granulocyte colony-stimulating factor. *Journal of Biological Chemistry* **258:** 9017-9023.

Nicola, N. A., and Peterson, L. (1986). Identification of distinct receptors for two hemopoietic growth factors (granulocyte colony-stimulating factor and multipotential colony-stimulating factor) by chemical cross-linking. *Journal of Biological Chemistry* **261:** 12384-12389.

Nicola, N. A., Peterson, L., Hilton, D. J., and Metcalf, D. (1988). Cellular processing of murine colony-stimulating factor (Multi-CSF, GM-CSF, G-CSF) receptors by normal hemopoietic cells and cell lines. *Growth Factors* **1:** 41-49.

Nicola, N. A., Vadas, M. A., and Lopez, A. F. (1986). Down-modulation of receptors for granulocyte colony-stimulating factor on human neutrophils by granulocyte-activating agents. *Journal of Cellular Physiology* **128:** 501-509.

Nicola, N. A., Wycherley, K., Boyd, A. W., Layton, J. E., Cary, D., and Metcalf, D. (1993). Neutralizing and non-neutralizing monoclonal antibodies to the human granulocyte-macrophage colony-stimulating factor receptor alpha-chain. *Blood* **82:** 1724-1731.

Niemeyer, C. M., Sieff, C. A., Mathey-Prevot, B., Wimperis, J. Z., Bierer, B. B., Clark, S. C., and Nathan, D. G. (1989). Expression of human interleukin-3 (multi-CSF) is restricted to human lymphocytes and T-cell tumor lines. *Blood* **73:** 945-951.

Nimer, S. D., Champlin, R. E., and Golde, D. W. (1988a). Serum cholesterol-lowering activity of granulocyte-macrophage colony-stimulating factor. *Journal of American Medical Association* **260:** 3297-3300.

Nimer, S., Fraser, J., Richards, J., Lynch, M., and Gasson, J. (1990). The repeated sequence CATT(A/T) is required for granulocyte-macrophage colony-stimulating factor promoter activity. *Molecular and Cellular Biology* **10:** 6084–6088.

Nimer, S. D., Gates, M. J., Koeffler, H. P., and Gasson, J. C. (1989). Multiple mechanisms control the expression of granulocyte-macrophage colony-stimulating factor by human fibroblasts. *Journal of Immunology* **143:** 2374–2377.

Nimer, S. D., Morita, E. A., Martis, M. J., Wachsman, W., and Gasson, J. C. (1988b). Characterization of the human granulocyte-macrophage colony-stimulating factor promoter region by genetic analysis: Correlation with DNase I footprinting. *Molecular and Cellular Biology* **8:** 1979–1984.

Nishida, J., Yoshida, M., Arai, K., and Yokota, T. (1991). Definition of a GC-rich motif as regulatory sequence of the human IL-3 gene: Coordinate regulation of the IL-3 gene by CLE2/GC box of the GM-CSF gene in T cell activation. *International Immunology* **3:** 245–254.

Nishizawa, M., and Nagata, S. (1990). Regulatory elements responsible for inducible expression of the granulocyte colony-stimulating factor gene in macrophages. *Molecular and Cellular Biology* **10:** 2002–2011.

Nishizawa, M., Tsuchiya, M., Watanabe-Fukunaga, R., and Nagata, S. (1990). Multiple elements in the promoter of granulocyte colony-stimulating factor gene regulate its constitutive expression in human carcinoma cells. *Journal of Biological Chemistry* **265:** 5897–5902.

Nomura, H., Imazeki, I., Oheda, M., Kubota, N., Tamura, M., Ono, M., Ueyama, Y., and Asano, S. (1986). Purification and characterization of human granulocyte colony-stimulating factor (G-CSF). *EMBO Journal* **5:** 871–876.

Nunez, G., London, L., Hockenberry, D., Alexander, M., McKearn, J. P., and Korshmeyer, H. (1990). Deregulated *bcl*-2 gene expression selectively prolongs survival of growth factor-deprived hemopoietic cell lines. *Journal of Immunology* **144:** 3602–3610.

Ogawa, M., Porter, P. N., and Nakahata, T. (1983). Renewal and commitment of differentiation of hemopoietic stem cells (an interpretative review). *Blood* **61:** 823–829.

Oheda, M., Hase, S., Ono, M., and Ikenaka, T. (1988). Structures of the sugar chains of recombinant human granulocyte-colony-stimulating factor produced by Chinese hamster ovary cells. *Journal of Biochemistry (Tokyo)* **103:** 544–546.

Oheda, M., Hasegawa, M., Hattori, K., Kuboniwa, H., Kojima, T., Orita, T., Tomonou, K., Yamazaki, T., and Ochi, N. (1990). O-linked sugar chain of human granulocyte colony-stimulating factor protects it against polymerization and denaturation allowing it to retain its biological activity. *Journal of Biological Chemistry* **265:** 11432–11435.

Ohno, R., Hiraoka, A., Tanimoto, M., Asou, N., Kuriyama, K., Kobayashi, T., Yoshida, M., Teshima, H., Saito, H., and Fujimoto, K. (1993). No increase of leukemia relapse in newly diagnosed patients with acute myeloid leukemia who received granulocyte colony-stimulating factor for life-threatening infection during remission induction and consolidation therapy. *Blood* **81:** 561–562.

Ohno, R., Tomonaga, M., Kobayashi, T., Kanamura, A., Shirakawa, S., Masaoka, T., Omine, M., Oh, H., Nomura, T., and Sakai, Y. (1990). Effect of granulocyte colony-stimulating factor after intensive induction therapy in relapsed or refractory acute leukemia. *New England Journal of Medicine* **323:** 871–877.

Ohta, M., Greenberger, J. S., Anklesaria, P., Bassols, A., and Massague, J. (1987). Two forms of transforming growth factor-beta distinguished by multipotential haematopoietic progenitor cells. *Nature (London)* **329:** 539–541.

Okabe, M., Asano, M., Kuga, T., Komatsu, Y., Yamasaki, M., Yokoo, Y., Itoh, S., Morimoto, M., and Oka, T. (1990). In vitro and in vivo hematopoietic effect of mutant human granulocyte colony-stimulating factor. *Blood* **75:** 1788–1793.

Okuda, K., Sanghera, J. S., Pelech, S. L., Kanakura, Y., Hallek, M., Griffin, J. D., and Druker, B. J. (1992). Granulocyte-macrophage colony-stimulating factor, interleukin-3, and Steel factor induce rapid tyrosine phosphorylation of p42 and p44 MAP kinase. *Blood* **79:** 2880–2887.

Omori, F., Okamura, S., Shimoda, K., Otsuka, T., Harada, M., and Niho, Y. (1992). Levels of human serum granulocyte colony-stimulating factor and granulocyte colony-stimulating factor under pathological conditions. *Biotherapy* **4:** 147–153.

Orchard, P. J., Dahl, N., Aukerman, S. L., Blazar, B. R., and Key, L., Jr. (1992). Circulating macrophage colony-stimulating factor is not reduced in malignant osteopetrosis. *Experimental Hematology* **20:** 103–105.

Oster, W., Lindemann, A., Ganser, A., Mertelsmann, R., and Herrmann, F. (1988). Constitutive expression of hematopoietic growth factor genes by acute myeloblastic leukemia cells. *Behring Institute Mitteilungen* **83:** 68–79.

Ottmann, O. G., Ganser, A., Seipelt, I. G., Eder, M., Schulz, G., and Hoelzer, D. (1990). Effects of recombinant human interleukin-3 on human hematopoietic progenitor and precursor cells *in vivo. Blood* **76:** 1494–1502.

Palacios, R., Henson, G., Steinmetz, M., and McKearn, J. P. (1984). Interleukin-3 supports growth of mouse pre-B-cell clones *in vitro. Nature (London)* **309:** 126–131.

Pampfer, S., Daiter, E., Barad, D., and Pollard, J. W. (1992). Expression of the colony-stimulating factor-1 receptor (c-fms proto-oncogene product) in the human uterus and placenta. *Biology of Reproduction* **46:** 48–57.

Pandit, J., Bohm, A., Jancarik, J., Halenbeck, R., Koths, K., and Kim, S. H. (1992). Three-dimensional structure of dimeric human recombinant macrophage colony-stimulating factor. *Science (Washington)* **258:** 1358–1362.

Paran, M., and Sachs, L. (1968). The continuous requirement for inducers for the development of macrophage and granulocyte colonies. *Journal of Cellular Physiology* **72:** 247–250.

Park, J. H., Kaushansky, K., and Levitt, L. (1993). Transcriptional regulation of interleukin 3 (IL3) in primary human T lymphocytes: Role of AP-1- and octamer-binding proteins in control of IL3 gene expression. *Journal of Biological Chemistry* **268:** 6299–6308.

Park, L. S., Friend, D., Gillis, S., and Urdal, D. L. (1986). Characterization of the cell surface receptor for human granulocyte/macrophage colony-stimulating factor. *Journal of Experimental Medicine* **164:** 251–262.

Park, L. S., Friend, D., Price, V., Anderson, D., Singer, J., Prickett, K. S., and Urdal, D. L. (1989). Heterogeneity in human interleukin-3 receptors: A subclass that binds human granulocyte/macrophage colony stimulating factor. *Journal of Biological Chemistry* **264:** 5420–5427.

Park, L. S., Martin, U., Sorenson, R., Luhr, S., Morrissey, P. J., Cosman, D., and Larsen, A. (1992). Cloning of the low-affinity murine granulocyte-macrophage colony-stimulating factor receptor and reconstitution of a high affinity receptor complex. *Proceedings of the National Academy of Sciences, U.S.A.* **89:** 4295–4299.

Parry, A. D., Minasian, E., and Leach, S. J. (1988). Conformational homologies among cytokines: Interleukins and colony stimulating factors. *Journal of Molecular Recognition* **1:** 107–110.

Parry, A. D., Minasian, E., and Leach, S. J. (1991). Cytokine conformations: Predictive studies. *Journal of Molecular Recognition* **4:** 63–75.

Peleraux, A., and Eliason, J. F. (1989). Proliferation of single hemopoietic progenitor cells in the absence of colony-stimulating factors and serum. *Experimental Hematology* **17:** 1032–1037.

Perkins, A., and Cory, S. (1993). Conditioned immortalization of mouse myelomonocytic, megakaryocytic and mast cell progenitors by the *Hox*2.4 homeobox gene. *EMBO Journal* **12:** 3835–3846.

Perkins, A. Kongsuwan, K., Visvader, J., Adams, J. M., and Cory, S. (1990). Homeobox gene expression plus autocrine growth factor production elicits myeloid leukemia. *Proceedings of the National Academy of Sciences, U.S.A.* **87:** 8398–8402.

Perno, C. F., Yarchoan, R., Cooney, D. A., Hartman, N. R., Webb, D. S. A., Hao, Z., Mitsuya, H., Johns, D. G., and Broder, S. (1989). Replication of human immunodeficiency virus in monocytes: Granulocyte/macrophage colony-stimulating factor (GM-CSF) potentiates viral production yet enhances the antiviral effect mediated by 3′-azido-2′3′-dideoxythymidine (AZT) and other dideoxynucleoside congeners of thymidine. *Journal of Experimental Medicine* **169:** 933–951.

Peters, W. P., Rosner, G., Ross, M., Vredenburgh, J., Meisenberg, B., Gilbert, C., and Kurtzberg, J. (1993). Comparative effects of granulocyte-macrophage colony-stimulating factor (GM-CSF) and granulocyte colony-stimulating factor (G-CSF) on priming peripheral blood progenitor cells for use with autologous bone marrow after high-dose chemotherapy. *Blood* **81:** 1709–1719.

Pettengell, R., Demuynck, H., Testa, N. G., and Dexter, T. M. (1992). The engraftment capacity of peripheral blood progenitor cells mobilized with chemotherapy +/− G-CSF. In P. Henon and C. Juttner (eds.), *Peripheral Blood Stem Cell Autografts. Proceedings of the Second International Symposium,* pp.59–61. Dayton, OH: Alphamed.

Plaut, M., Pierce, J. H., Watson, C. J., Hanley-Hyde, J., Nordan, R. P., and Paul, W. E. (1989). Mast cell lines produce lymphokines in response to cross-linkage of Fc$\epsilon$RI or to calcium ionophores. *Nature (London)* **339:** 64–67.

Ploemacher, R. E., van der Sluijs, J. P., van Beurden, A. J., Baert, M. R. M., and Chan, P. L. (1991). Use of limiting-dilution type long-term marrow cultures in frequency analysis of marrow-repopulating and spleen colony-forming hematopoietic stem cells in the mouse. *Blood* **78:** 2527–2533.

Ploemacher, R. E., van Soest, P. L., Boudewijn, A., and Neben, S. (1993). Interleukin-12 enhances interleukin-3 dependent multilineage hematopoietic colony formation stimulated by interleukin-11 or Steel factor. *Leukemia* **7:** 1374–1380.

Pluda, J. M., Yarchoan, R., Smith, P. D., McAtee, N., Shay, L. E., Oette, D., Maha, M., Wahl, S. M., Myers, C. E., and Broder, S. (1990). Subcutaneous recombinant granulocyte-macrophage colony-stimulating factor used as a single agent and in an alternating regimen with azidothymidine in leukopenic patients with severe human immunodeficiency virus infection. *Blood* **76:** 463–472.

Pluznik, D. H., Bickel, M., and Mergenhagen, S. E. (1989). B lymphocyte derived hematopoietic growth factors. *Immunological Investigations* **18:** 103–116.

Pluznik, D. H., Cunningham, R. E., and Noguchi, P. D. (1984). Colony-stimulating factor (CSF) controls proliferation of CSF-dependent cells by acting during the G1 phase of the cell cycle. *Proceedings of the National Academy of Sciences, U.S.A.* **81:** 7451–7455.

Pluznik, D. H., and Sachs, L. (1966). The induction of clones of normal "mast" cells by a substance in conditioned medium. *Experimental Cell Research* **43:** 553–563.

Pojda, Z., Molineux, G., and Dexter, T. M. (1990). Hemopoietic effects of short-term *in vivo* treatment of mice with various doses of rhG-CSF. *Experimental Hematology* **18:** 27–31.

Pollard, J. W., Bartocci, A., Arceci, R., Orlofsky, A., Ladner, M. B., and Stanley, E. R. (1987). Apparent role of the macrophage growth factor, CSF-1, in placental development. *Nature (London)* **330:** 484–486.

Pollard, J. W., Hunt, J. S., Wiktor-Jedrzejczak, W., and Stanley, E. R. (1991). A pregnancy defect in the osteopetrotic (op/op) mouse demonstrates the requirement for CSF-1 in female fertility. *Developmental Biology* **148:** 273–283.

Postmus, R. E., Gietema, J. A., Damsma, O., Biesma, B., Limburg, P. C., Vellenga, E., and de Vries, E. G. E. (1992). Effects of recombinant interleukin-3 in patients with relapsed small-cell lung cancer treated with chemotherapy: A dose-finding study. *Journal of Clinical Oncology* **10:** 1131–1140.

Powles, R., Smith, C., Milan, S., Treleaven, J., Millar, J., McElwain, T., Gordon-Smith, E., Milliken, S., and Tiley, C. (1990). Human recombinant GM-CSF in allogeneic bone marrow transplantation for leukaemia: Double-blind, placebo-controlled trial. *Lancet* **336:** 1417–1420.

Price, L. K., Choi, H. U., Rosenberg, L., and Stanley, E. R. (1992). The predominant form of secreted colony stimulating factor-1 is a proteoglycan. *Journal of Biological Chemistry* **267:** 2190–2199.

Quesenberry, P. J., and Gimbrone, M. A. (1980). Vascular endothelium as a regulator of granulopoiesis. Production of colony-stimulating activity by cultured human endothelial cells. *Blood* **56:** 1060–1067.

Quinn, T. P., Peters, K. G., de Vries, C., Ferrara, N., and Williams, L. T. (1993). Fetal liver kinase 1 is a receptor for vascular endothelial growth factor and is selectively expressed in vascular endothelium. *Proceedings of the National Academy of Sciences, U.S.A.* **90:** 7533–7537.

Raines, M. A., Liu, L., Quan, S. G., Joe, V., Di Persio, J. F., and Golde, D. W. (1991). Identification and molecular cloning of a soluble human granulocyte-macrophage colony-stimulating factor receptor. *Proceedings of the National Academy of Sciences, U.S.A.* **88:** 8203–8207.

Rambaldi, A., Young, D. C., and Griffin, J. D. (1987). Expression of the M-CSF (CSF-1) gene by human monocytes. *Blood* **69:** 1409–1413.

Rappold, G., Willson, T. A., Henke, A., and Gough, N. M. (1992). Arrangement and localization of the human GM-CSF receptor alpha chain gene CSF2RA within the X-Y pseudoautosomal region. *Genomics* **14:** 455–461.

Redman, B. C., Flaherty, L., Chan, T. H., Kraut, M., Martino, S., Simon, M., Valdivieso, M., and Groves, E. (1992). Phase I trial of recombinant macrophage colony-stimulating factor by rapid intravenous infusion in patients with cancer. *Journal of Immunotherapy* **12:** 50–54.

Reedijk, M., Liu, X., Van der Geer, P., Letwin, K., Waterfield, M. D., Hunter, T., and Pawson, T. (1992). Tyn 721 regulates specific binding of the CSF-1 receptor kinase insert to PI 3′-kinase SH2 domains: A model for SH2-mediated receptor-target interactions. *EMBO Journal* **11:** 1365–1372.

Rennick, D., Yang, G., Gemmell, L., and Lee, F. (1987a). Control of hemopoiesis by a bone marrow stomal cell clone: Lipopolysaccharide- and interleukin-1-inducible production of colony stimulating factors. *Blood* **69:** 682–691.

Rennick, D., Yang, G., Muller-Sieburg, C., Smith, C., Arai, N., Takabe, Y., and Gemmell, L. (1987b). Interleukin 4 (B-cell stimulatory factor-1) can enhance or antagonize the factor-dependent growth of hemopoietic progenitor cells. *Proceedings of the National Academy of Sciences, U.S.A.* **84:** 6889–6893.

Resnick, M., Roguel-Resnick, N., Bercovier, H., Levy, L., Toledo, J., and Zipori, D. (1990). Detection of interleukin-3 in the serum of mice infected with Mycobacterium lepraemurium. *Journal of Infectious Disease* **162:** 1202–1204.

Rettenmier, C. W., and Roussel, M. F. (1988). Differential processing of colony-stimulating factor 1 precursors encoded by two human cDNAs. *Molecular and Cellular Biology* **8:** 5026–5034.

Rettenmier, C. W., Roussel, M. F., Ashmun, R. A., Ralph, P., Price, K., and Sherr, C. J. (1987). Synthesis of membrane-bound colony-stimulating factor 1 (CSF-1) and downmodulation of CSF-1 receptors in NIH 3T3 cells transformed by cotransfection of the human CSF-1 and c-fms (CSF-1 receptor) genes. *Molecular and Cellular Biology* **7:** 2378–2387.

Rich, I. N. (1986). A role for the macrophage in normal hemopoiesis. I. Functional capacity of bone-marrow-derived macrophages to release hemopoietic growth factors. *Experimental Hematology* **14:** 738–745.

Richman, C. M., Weiner, R. S., and Yankee, R. A. (1976). Increase in circulating stem cells following chemotherapy in man. *Blood* **47:** 1031–1039.

Ridge, S. A., Worwood, M., Oscier, D., Jacobs, A., and Padua, R. A. (1990). Fms mutations in myelodysplastic, leukemic, and normal subjects. *Proceedings of the National Academy of Sciences, U.S.A.* **87:** 1377–1380.

Roberts, A. W., and Metcalf, D. (in press). Granulocyte colony stimulating factor induces selective elevations of progenitor cells in the peripheral blood of mice. *Experimental Hematology.*

Roberts, W. M., Look, A. T., Roussel, M. F., and Sherr, C. J. (1988). Tandem linkage of human CSF-1 receptor (c-fms) and PDGF receptor genes. *Cell* **55:** 655–661.

Roberts, W. M., Shapiro, L. H., Ashmun, R. A., and Look, A. T. (1992). Transcription of the human colony-stimulating factor-1 receptor gene is regulated by separate tissue-specific promoters. *Blood* **79:** 586–593.

Robinson, W. A., Metcalf, D., and Bradley, T. R. (1967). Stimulation by normal and leukaemic mouse sera of colony formation *in vitro* by mouse bone marrow cells. *Journal of Cellular and Comparative Physiology* **69:** 83–92.

Robinson, W. A., Stanley, E. R., and Metcalf, D. (1969). Stimulation of bone marrow colony growth *in vitro* by human urine. *Blood* **33:** 396–399.

Rothwell, V. M., and Rohrschneider, L. R. (1987). Murine c-fms cDNA: Cloning, sequence analysis and retroviral expression. *Oncogene Research* **1:** 311–324.

Roussel, M. F., Cleveland, J. L., Shurtleff, S. A., and Sherr, C. J. (1991). Myc rescue of a mutant CSF-1 receptor impaired in mitogenic signalling. *Nature (London)* **353:** 361–363.

Roussel, M. F., Downing, J. R., Rettenmier, C. W., and Sherr, C. J. (1988). A point mutation in the extracellular domain of the human CSF-1 receptor (c-fms proto-oncogene product) activates its transforming potential. *Cell* **55:** 979–988.

Roussel, M. F., and Sherr, C. J. (1989). Mouse NIH 3T3 cells expressing human colony-stimulating factor 1 (CSF-1) receptors overgrow in serum-free medium containing human CSF-1 as their only growth factor. *Proceedings of the National Academy of Sciences, U.S.A.* **86:** 7924–7927.

Roussel, M. F., and Sherr, C. J. (1993). Signal transduction by the macrophage colony-stimulating factor receptor. *Current Opinion in Hematology* **1:** 11–18.

Roussel, M. F., Shurtleff, S. A., Downing, J. R., and Sherr, C. J. (1990). A point mutation at tyrosine 809 in the human colony-stimulating factor 1 receptor impairs mitogenesis without abrogating tyrosine kinase activity, association with phosphatidylinositol 3-kinase, or induction of c-fos and jun B genes. *Proceedings of the National Academy of Sciences, U.S.A.* **87:** 6738–6742.

Rugo, H. S., O'Hanley, P., Bishop, A. G., Pearce, M. K., Abrams, J. S., Howard, M., and O'Garra, A. (1992). Local cytokine production in a murine model of *Escherichia coli* pyelonephritis. *Journal of Clinical Investigation* **89:** 1032–1039.

Ryan, G. R., Milton, S. E., Lopez, A. F., Bardy, P. G., Vadas, M. A., and Shannon, M. F. (1991). Human interleukin-3 mRNA accumulation is controlled at both the transcriptional and posttranscriptional level. *Blood* **77:** 1195–1202.

Sachs, L. (1987). The Wellcome Foundation Lecture, 1986. The molecular regulators of normal and leukaemic blood cells. *Proceedings of the Royal Society of London Biological Sciences* **231:** 289–312.

Sachs, L. (1990). The proteins that control haemopoiesis and leukaemia. In G. Bock and J. Marsh (eds.), *Molecular Control of Haemopoiesis* (Ciba Foundation Symposium) **148:** 5–19. Chichester: Wiley.

Saito, M., Saito, S., Nakagawa, T., Ichijo, M., and Motoyoshi, K. (1992a). Origin of macrophage colony-stimulating factor (M-CSF) and granulocyte colony-stimulating factor (G-CSF) in amniotic fluid. *Asia Oceania Journal of Obstetrics and Gynecology* **18:** 355–361.

Saito, S., Motoyoshi, K., Ichijo, M., Saito, M., and Takaku, F. (1992b). High serum human macrophage colony-stimulating factor level during pregnancy. *International Journal of Hematology* **55:** 219–225.

Sakamaki, K., Miyajima, I., Kitamura, T., and Miyajima, A. (1992). Critical cytoplasmic domains of the common beta subunit of the human GM-CSF, Il-3 and IL-5 receptors for growth signal transduction and tyrosine phosphorylation. *EMBO Journal* **11:** 3541–3549.

Sallerfors, B., and Olofsson, T. (1991). Granulocyte-macrophage colony-stimulating factor (GM-CSF) and granulocyte colony-stimulating factor (G-CSF) in serum during induction treatment of acute leukaemia. *British Journal of Haematology* **78:** 343–351.

Sallerfors, B., Olofsson, T., and Lenhoff, S. (1991). Granulocyte-macrophage colony stimulating factor (GM-CSF) and granulocyte colony-stimulating factor (G-CSF) in serum in bone marrow transplanted patients. *Bone Marrow Transplantation* **8:** 191–195.

Salmon, S. E., and Lui, R. (1989). Effects of granulocyte-macrophage colony-stimulating factor on the *in vitro* growth of human solid tumors. *Journal of Clinical Oncology* **7:** 1346–1350.

Sanda, M. G., Yang, J. C., Topalian, S. L., Groves, E. S., Childs, A., Belfort, R., Jr., de Smet, M. D., Schwartzentruber, D. J., White, D. E., Lotze, M. T., and Rosenberg, S. A. (1992). Intravenous administration of recombinant human macrophage colony-stimulating factor to patients with metastatic cancer: A Phase I study. *Journal of Clinical Oncology* **10:** 1643–1649.

Sanderson, C. J. (1992). Interleukin-5, eosinophils and disease. *Blood* **79:** 3101–3109.

Sandoval, C., Adams-Graves, P., Parganas, E., Wang, W., and Ihle, J. N. (1993). The cytoplasmic portion of the G-CSF receptor is normal in patients with Kostmann syndrome. *Blood* **82:** (suppl. 1), 185a.

Sato, N., Sakamaki, K., Terada, N., Arai, K., and Miyajima, A. (1993). Signal transduction by the high-affinity GM-CSF receptor: Two distinct cytoplasmic regions of the common beta subunit responsible for different signaling. *EMBO Journal* **12:** 4181–4189.

Sawada, K., Krantz, S. B., Dai, C.-H., Sato, N., Ieko, M., Sakurama, S., Yasukouchi, T., and Nakagawa, S. (1991). Transitional change of colony stimulating factor requirements for erythroid progenitors. *Journal of Cellular Physiology* **149:** 1–8.

Saxena, S. K., Crouse, D. A., and Sharp, J. G. (1993). Effect of systemic interleukin-3 administration on epithelial cell proliferation in mouse intestine. *Life Sciences (England)* **53:** 473–477.

Scarffe, J. H. (1991). Emerging clinical uses for GM-CSF. *European Journal of Cancer* **27:** 1493–1504.

Schaub, R. G., Bree, M. P., Hayes, L. L., Rudd, M. A., Rabbani, L., Loscalzo, J., and Clinton, S. K. (1994). Recombinant human macrophage colony-stimulating factor reduces plasma cholesterol and carrageenin granuloma foam cell formation in Watanabe heritable hyperlipidemic rabbits. *Arteriosclerosis and Thrombosis* **14:** 70–76.

Schlessinger, J., and Ullrich, A. (1992). Growth factor signalling by receptor tyrosine kinases. *Neuron* **9:** 383–391.

Schmidt, G. M., Snieciski, D. S., Snyder, D. S., O'Donnell, M. R., Parker, P. M., Stein, A., Smith, E., Stepan, D. E., Molina, A., Taguchi, J., Margolin, K. A., Somlo, G., and Forman, S. J. (1992). G-CSF primed peripheral blood stem cell autografts in patients with advanced lymphoid malignancies. *Proceedings of the American Society of Clinical Oncology* **11:** 317.

Schreurs, J., Arai, K., and Miyajima, A. (1990). Evidence for a low-affinity interleukin-3 receptor. *Growth Factors* **2:** 221–233.

Schrimsher, J. L., Rose, K., Simona, M. G., and Wingfield, P. (1987). Characterization of human and mouse granulocyte-macrophage-colony-stimulating factors derived from *Escherichia coli. Biochemical Journal* **247:** 195–199.

Schumacher, A., and Nordheim, A. (1992). Progress towards a molecular understanding of cyclosporin A-mediated immunosuppression. *Clinical Investigator* **70:** 773–779.

Seelentag, W. K., Mermod, J.-J., Montesano, R., and Vassalli, P. (1987). Additive effects of interleukin 1 and tumour necrosis factor-alpha on the accumulation of the three granulocyte and macrophage colony-stimulating factor mRNAs in human endothelial cells. *EMBO Journal* **6:** 2261–2265.

Seelig, G. F., Prosise, W. W., and Scheffler, J. E. (1994). A role for the carboxyl terminus of human granulocyte-macrophage colony-stimulating factor in the binding of ligand to the $\alpha$-structure of the high affinity receptor. *Journal of Biological Chemistry* **269:** 5548–5553.

Seto, Y., Fukunaga, R., and Nagata, S. (1992). Chromosomal gene organization of the human granulocyte colony-stimulating factor receptor. *Journal of Immunology* **148:** 259–266.

Shabo, Y., Lotem, J., Rubinstein, M., Revel, M., Clark, S. C., Wolf, S. F., Kamen, R., and Sachs, L. (1988). The myeloid blood cell differentiation-inducing protein MGI-2A is interleukin 6. *Blood* **72:** 2070–2073.

Shadduck, R. K., and Nanna, N. G. (1971). Granulocyte colony stimulating factor. III. Effects of alkylating agent-induced granulocytopenia. *Proceedings of the Society for Experimental Biology and Medicine* **137:** 1479–1482.

Shanafelt, A. B., Johnson, K. E., and Kastelein, R. A. (1991a). Identification of critical amino acid residues in human and mouse granulocyte-macrophage colony-stimulating factor and their involvement in species specificity. *Journal of Biological Chemistry* **266:** 13804–13810.

Shanafelt, A. B., and Kastelein, R. A. (1989). Identification of critical regions in mouse granulocyte-macrophage colony-stimulating factor by scanning-deletion analysis. *Proceedings of the National Academy of Sciences, U.S.A.* **86:** 4872–4876.

Shanafelt, A. B., and Kastelein, R. A. (1992). High affinity ligand binding is not essential for granulocyte-macrophage colony-stimulating factor receptor activation. *Journal of Biological Chemistry* **267:** 25466–25472.

Shanafelt, A. B., Miyajima, A., Kitamura, T., and Kastelein, R. A. (1991b). The amino-terminal helix of GM-CSF and IL-5 governs high affinity binding to their receptors. *EMBO Journal* **10:** 4105–4112.

Shannon, M. F., Coles, L. S., Fielke, R. K., Goodall, G. J., Lagnado, C. A., and Vadas, M. A. (1992). Three essential promoter elements mediate tumour necrosis factor and interleukin-1 activation of the granulocyte-colony stimulating factor gene. *Growth Factors* **7:** 181–193.

Shannon, M. F., Gamble, J. R., and Vadas, M. A. (1988). Nuclear proteins interacting with the promoter region of the human granulocyte/macrophage colony-stimulating factor gene. *Proceedings of the National Academy of Sciences, U.S.A.* **85:** 674–678.

Shannon, M. F., Pell, L. M., Lenardo, M. J., Kuczek, E. S., Occhiodoro, F. S., Dunn, S. M., and Vadas, M. A. (1990). A novel tumor necrosis factor-responsive transcription factor which recognizes a regulatory element in hemopoietic growth factor genes. *Molecular and Cellular Biology* **10:** 2950–2959.

Shaw, G., and Kamen, R. (1986). A conserved AU sequence from the 3′ untranslated region of GM-CSF mRNA mediates selective mRNA degradation. *Cell* **46:** 659–667.

Shen, Y., Baker, E., Callen, D. F., Sutherland, G. R., Willson, T. A., Rakar, S., and Gough, N. M. (1992). Localization of the human GM-CSF receptor beta chain gene (CSF2RB) to chromosome 22q12.2 → q13.1. *Cytogenetics and Cell Genetics* **61:** 175–177.

Sheridan, J. W., and Metcalf, D. (1972). Studies on the bone marrow colony stimulating factor (CSF): Relation of tissue CSF to serum CSF. *Journal of Cellular Physiology* **80:** 129–140.

Sheridan, J. W., and Metcalf, D. (1973a). A low molecular weight factor in lung-conditioned medium stimulating granulocyte and monocyte colony formation in vitro. *Journal of Cellular Physiology* **81:** 11–24.

Sheridan, J. W., and Metcalf, D. (1973b). The bone marrow colony stimulating factor (CSF): Relation of serum CSF to urine CSF. *Proceedings of the Society for Experimental Biology and Medicine* **144:** 785–788.

Sheridan, J. W., and Stanley, E. R. (1971). Tissue sources of bone marrow colony stimulating factor. *Journal of Cellular Physiology* **78:** 451–460.

Sheridan, W. P., Begley, C. G., Juttner, C. A., Szer, J., To, L. B., Maher, D., McGrath, K. M., Morstyn, G., and Fox, R. M. (1992). Effect of peripheral-blood progenitor cells mobilized by Filgrastim (G-CSF) on platelet recovery after high-dose chemotherapy. *Lancet* **339:** 640–644.

Sheridan, W. P., Morstyn, G., Wold, M., Dodds, A., Lusk, J., Maher, D., Layton, J. E., Green, M. D., Souza, L., and Fox, R. M. (1989). Granulocyte colony-stimulating factor and neutrophil recovery after high-dose chemotherapy and autologous bone marrow transplantation. *Lancet* **ii:** 891–895.

Sherr, C. J. (1990). Colony-stimulating factor-1 receptor. *Blood* **75:** 1–12.

Sherr, C. J. (1993). Mammalian G1 cyclins. *Cell* **73:** 1059–1065.

Sherr, C. J., Rettenmier, C. W., Sacca, R., Roussel, M. F., Look, A. T., and Stanley, E. R. (1985). The c-fms proto-oncogene product is related to the receptor for the mononuclear phagocyte growth factor, CSF-1. *Cell* **41:** 665–676.

Shikita, M., Tsuneoka, K., Harigawa, S., and Tsurufuji, S. (1981). A granulocyte-macrophage colony-stimulating factor (GM-CSA) produced by carrageenin-induced inflammatory cells of mice. *Journal of Cellular Physiology* **109:** 161–169.

Shimoda, K., Okamura, S., Mizuno, Y., Harada, N., Kubota, A., Yamada, M., Hara, T., Aoki, T., Akeda, H., and Ueda, K. (1993). Human macrophage colony-stimulating factor levels in cerebrospinal fluid. *Cytokine* **5:** 250–254.

Shoemaker, S. G., Hromas, R., and Kaushansky, K. (1990). Transcriptional regulation of interleukin 3 gene expression in T lymphocytes. *Proceedings of the National Academy of Sciences, U.S.A.* **87:** 9650–9654.

Sieff, C. A., Tsai, S., and Faller, D. V. (1987). Interleukin-1 induces cultured human endothelial cell production of granulocyte-macrophage colony stimulating factor. *Journal of Clinical Investigation* **79:** 48–51.

Silvennoinen, O., Schindler, C., Schlessinger, J., and Levy, D. E. (1993a). Ras-independent growth factor signaling by transcription factor tyrosine phosphorylation. *Science (Washington)* **261:** 1736–1739.

Silvennoinen, O., Witthuhn, B. A., Quelle, F. W., Cleveland, J. L., Yi, T., and Ihle, J. N. (1993b). Structure of the murine Jak2 protein-tyrosine kinase and its role in interleukin 3 signal transduction. *Proceedings of the National Academy of Sciences, U.S.A.* **90:** 8429–8433.

Silver, G. M., Gamelli, R. L., and O'Reilly, M. (1989). The beneficial effect of granulocyte colony-stimulating factor (G-CSF) in combination with gentamicin on survival after *Pseudomonas* burn wound infection. *Surgery* **106:** 452–455.

Simmers, R. N., Webber, L. M., Shannon, M. F., Garson, O. M., Wong, G., Vadas, M. A., and Sutherland, G. R. (1987). Localization of the G-CSF gene on chromosome 17 proximal to the breakpoint in the t(15;17) in acute promyelocytic leukemia. *Blood* **70:** 330–332.

Singer, J. W., Fialkow, P. J., Dow, L. W., Ernst, C., and Steinmann, L. (1979). Unicellular or multicellular origin of human granulocyte-macrophage colonies *in vitro. Blood* **54:** 1395–1399.

Singer, J. W., James, M. C., and Thomas, E. D. (1977). Serum colony stimulating factor. A marker for graft-versus-host disease in humans. In S. J. Baum and G. D. Ledney (eds.), *Experimental Hematology Today,* pp. 221–231. New York: Springer.

Smith, M. R., De Gudicibus, S. J., and Stacey, D. W. (1986). Requirement for c-ras proteins during viral oncogene transformation. *Nature (London)* **320:** 540–543.

Smith, S. L., Bender, J. G., Maples, P. B., Unverzagt, K., Schilling, M., Lum, L., Williams, S., and Van Epps, D. E. (1993). Expansion of neutrophil precursors and progenitors in suspension cultures of CD34$^+$ cells enriched from human bone marrow. *Experimental Hematology* **21:** 870–877.

Socinski, M. A., Cannistra, S. A., Elias, A., Antman, K. H., Schnipper, L., and Griffin, J. D. (1988a). Granulocyte-macrophage colony-stimulating factor expands the circulating haemopoietic progenitor cell compartment in man. *Lancet* **i:** 1194–1198.

Socinski, M. A., Cannistra, S. W., Sullivan, R., Elias, A., Antman, K., Schnipper, L., and Griffin, J. D. (1988b). Granulocyte-macrophage colony-stimulating factor induces the expression of the CD11b surface adhesion molecule on human granulocytes *in vivo. Blood* **72:** 691–697.

Sola, B., Simon, D., Mattei, M. G., Fichelson, S., Bordereaux, D., Tambourin, P. E., Guenet, J. L., and Gisselbrecht, S. (1988). Fim-1, Fim-2/c-fms, and Fim-3, three common integration sites of Friend murine leukemia virus in myeloblastic leukemias, map to mouse chromosomes 13, 18 and 3, respectively. *Journal of Virology* **62:** 3973–3978.

Sorensen, P., Farber, N. M., and Krystal, G. (1986). Identification of the interleukin-3 receptor using an iodinatable, cleavable, photoreactive crosslinking agent. *Journal of Biological Chemistry* **261:** 9094–9097.

Sorensen, P., Mui, A. L., and Krystal, G. (1989). Interleukin-3 stimulates the tyrosine phosphorylation of the 140-kilodalton interleukin-3 receptor. *Journal of Biological Chemistry* **264:** 19253–19258.

Souza, L. M., Boone, T. C., Gabrilove, J., Lai, P. H., Zsebo, K. M., Murdock, D. C., Chazin, V. R., Bruszewski, J., Lu, H., Chen, K. K., Barendt, J., Platzer, E., Moore, M. A. S., Mertelsmann, R., and Welte, K. (1986). Recombinant human granulocyte colony-stimulating factor: Effects on normal and leukemic myeloid cells. *Science (Washington)* **232:** 61–65.

Spangrude, G. J., Heimfeld, S., and Weissman, I. L. (1988). Purification and characterization of mouse hematopoietic stem cells. *Science (Washington)* **241:** 58–62.

Sparrow, L. G., Metcalf, D., Hunkapiller, M. W., Hood, L. E., and Burgess, A. W. (1985). Purification and partial amino acid sequence of asialo murine granulocyte-macrophage colony stimulating factor. *Proceedings of the National Academy of Sciences, U.S.A.* **82:** 292–296.

Spertini, O., Kansas, G. S., Munro, J. M., Griffin, J. D., and Tedder, T. F. (1991). Regulation of leukocyte migration by activation of the leukocyte adhesion molecule-1 (LAM-1) selectin. *Nature (London)* **349:** 691–694.

Spitzer, G., Dunphy, F. R., Velasquez, W. S., Petruska, P. J., and Adkins, D. R. (1994). Filgrastim (r-met HuG-CSF) in bone marrow and peripheral blood cell transplantation. In G. Morstyn and T. M. Dexter (eds.), *Filgrastim (r-met HuG-CSF) in Clinical Practice,* pp. 173–195. New York: Dekker.

Sprang, S. R., and Bazan, J. F. (1993). Cytokine structural taxonomy and mechanisms of receptor engagement. *Current Opinion in Structural Biology* **3:** 815–827.

Stahl, N., and Yancopoulos, G. D. (1993). The alphas, betas, and kinases of cytokine receptor complexes. *Cell* **74:** 587–590.

Stanley, E., Lieschke, G. J., Grail, D., Metcalf, D., Hodgson, G., Gall, J. A. M., Maher, D. W., Cebon, J., Sinickas, V., and Dunn, A. R. (1994). Granulocyte-macrophage colony-stimulating factor-deficient mice show no major perturbation of hematopoiesis but develop a characteristic pulmonary pathology. *Proceedings of the National Academy of Sciences, U.S.A.* **91:** 5592–5596.

Stanley, E., Metcalf, D., Sobieszczuk, P., Gough, N. M., and Dunn, A. R. (1985). The structure and expression of the murine gene encoding granulocyte-macrophage colony stimulating factor: Evidence for utilisation of alternative promoters. *EMBO Journal* **4:** 2569–2573.

Stanley, E. R., Bartocci, A., Patinkin, D., Rosendaal, K., and Bradley, T. R. (1986). Regulation of very primitive, multipotent, hemopoietic cells by hemopoietin-1. *Cell* **45:** 667–674.

Stanley, E. R., Bradley, T. R., and Sumner, M. A. (1971). Properties of the mouse embryo conditioned medium factor(s) stimulating colony formation by mouse bone marrow cells grown *in vitro. Journal of Cellular Physiology* **78:** 301–317.

Stanley, E. R., and Guilbert, L. J. (1981). Methods for the purification assay, characterization and target cell binding of a colony stimulating factor (CSF-1). *Journal of Immunological Methods* **42:** 253–284.

Stanley, E. R., Hansen, G., Woodcock, J., and Metcalf, D. (1975). Colony stimulating factor and the regulation of granulopoiesis and macrophage production. *Federation Proceedings* **34:** 2272–2278.

Stanley, E. R., and Heard, P. M. (1977). Factors regulating macrophage production and growth: Purification and some properties of the colony stimulating factor from medium conditioned by mouse L cells. *Journal of Biological Chemistry* **252:** 4305–4312.

Stanley, E. R., and Metcalf, D. (1969). Partial purification of some properties of the factor in normal and leukaemic human urine stimulating mouse bone marrow colony growth *in vitro. Australian Journal of Experimental Biology and Medical Science* **47:** 467–483.

Stanley, E. R., Metcalf, D., Maritz, J. S., and Yeo, G. F. (1972). Standardized bioassay for bone marrow colony stimulating factor in human urine: Levels in normal man. *Journal of Laboratory Clinical Medicine* **79:** 657–668.

Stein, J., Borzillo, G. V., and Rettenmier, C. W. (1990). Direct stimulation of cells expressing receptors for macrophage colony-stimulating factor (CSF-1) by a plasma membrane-bound precursor of human CSF-1. *Blood* **76:** 1308–1314.

Stephenson, J. R., Axelrad, A. A., McLeod, D. L., and Shreeve, M. M. (1971). Induction of colonies of hemoglobin-synthesizing cells by erythropoietin *in vitro. Proceedings of the National Academy of Sciences, U.S.A.* **68:** 1542–1546.

Steward, W. P., Scarffe, J. H., Austin, R., Bonnem, E., Thatcher, N., Morgenstern, G., and Crowther, D. (1989). Recombinant human granulocyte macrophage colony stimulating factor (rhGM-CSF) given as daily short infusions – a phase I dose-toxicity study. *British Journal of Cancer* **59:** 142–145.

Steward, W. P., Scarffe, J. H., Dirix, L. Y., Chang, J., Radford, J. A., Bonnem, E., and Crowther, D. (1990). Granulocyte-macrophage colony stimulating factor (GM-CSF) after high-dose melphalan in patients with advanced colon cancer. *British Journal of Cancer* **61:** 749–754.

Strife, A., Lambek, C., Wisniewski, D., Gulati, S., Gasson, J. C., Golde, D. W., Welte, K., Gabrilove, J. L., and Clarkson, B. (1987). Activities of four purified growth factors on highly enriched human hematopoietic progenitor cells. *Blood* **69:** 1508–1523.

Stoudemire, J. B., and Garnick, M. B. (1991). Effects of recombinant human macrophage colony-stimulating factor on plasma cholesterol levels. *Blood* **77:** 750–755.

Suda, J., Suda, T., and Ogawa, M. (1984). Analysis of differentiation of mouse hemopoietic stem cells in culture by sequential replating of paired progenitors. *Blood* **64:** 393–399.

Suda, T., Suda, J., Kajigaya, S., Nagata, S., Asano, S., Saito, M., and Miura, Y. (1987). Effects of recombinant murine granulocyte colony-stimulating factor on granulocyte-macrophage and blast colony formation. *Experimental Hematology* **15:** 958–965.

Sullivan, G. W., Carper, H. T., and Mandell, G. L. (1993). The effect of three human recombinant hematopoietic growth factors (granulocyte-macrophage colony-stimulating factor, granulocyte colony-stimulating factor, and interleukin-3) on phagocyte oxidative activity. *Blood* **81:** 1863–1870.

Suzu, S., Ohtsuki, T., Makishima, M., Yanai, N., Kawashima, T., Nagata, N., and Motoyoshi, K. (1992a). Biological activity of a proteoglycan form of macrophage colony-stimulating factor and its binding to type V collagen. *Journal of Biological Chemistry* **267:** 16812–16815.

Suzu, S., Ohtsuki, T., Yanai, N., Takatsu, Z., Kawashima, T., Takaku, F., Nagata, N., and Motoyoshi, K. (1992b). Identification of a high molecular weight macrophage colony-stimulating factor as a glycosaminoglycan-containing species. *Journal of Biological Chemistry* **267:** 4345–4348.

Suzumura, A., Sawada, M., Yamamoto, H., and Marunouchi, T. (1990). Effects of colony stimulating factors on isolated microglia *in vitro. Journal of Neuroimmunology* **30:** 111–120.

Taga, T., Hibi, M., Hirata, Y., Yamasaki, K., Yasukawa, K., Matsuda, T., Hirano, T., and Kishimoto, T. (1989). Interleukin-6 triggers the association of its receptor with a possible signal transducer, gp130. *Cell* **58:** 573–581.

Takahashi, K., Naito, M., Morioka, Y., and Schultz, D. (1993). Immunophenotypic and ultrastructural differentiation and maturation of nonlymphoid dendritic cells in osteopetrotic (op) mice with the total absence of macrophage colony stimulating factor activity. *Advances in Experimental Medicine and Biology* **329:** 293–297.

Takahashi, S., Asano, S., Masaoka, T., Takaku, F., Niitsu, Y., Shibuya, A., Saito, H., Sekine, I., Sanpi, K., Hanada, R., Ohto, M., Ito, T., Ohira, M., Mugishima, H., Kodama, F., Seki, S., Shirakawa, S., and Konishi, S. (1991). Clinical evaluation of recombinant human granulocyte colony-stimulating factor (rhuG-CSF) in autologous bone marrow transplantation. *Rinsho-Ketsueki* **32:** 221–226.

Talmadge, J. F., Tribble, H., Pennington, R., Bowersox, O., Schneider, M. A., Castelli, P., Black, P. C., and Abe, F. (1989). Protective, restorative and therapeutic properties of recombinant colony stimulating factors. *Blood* **73:** 2093–2103.

Tamura, M., Hattori, K., Nomura, H., Oheda, M., Kubota, N., Imazeki, I., Ono, M., Ueymama, Y., Nagata, S., Shirafuji, N., and Asano, S. (1987). Induction of neutrophilic granulocytosis in mice by administration of purified human native granulocyte colony-stimulating factor (G-CSF). *Biochemical and Biophysical Research Communications* **142:** 454–460.

Tamura, M., Hattori, K., Ono, M., Hata, S., Hayata, I., Asano, S., Bessho, M., and Hirashima, K. (1989). Effects of recombinant human granulocyte colony-stimulating factor (rG-CSF) on murine myeloid leukemia: Stimulation of proliferation of leukemia cells *in vitro* and inhibition of leukemia *in vivo*. *Leukemia* **3:** 853–858.

Tanaka, S., Takahashi, N., Udagawa, N., Tamura, T., Akatsu, T., Stanley, E. R., Kurokawa, T., and Suda, T. (1993). Macrophage colony-stimulating factor is indispensable for both proliferation and differentiation of osteoclast progenitors. *Journal of Clinical Investigation* **91:** 257–263.

Tanikawa, S., Nose, M., Aoki, Y., Tsuneoka, K., Shikita, M., and Nara, N. (1990). Effects of recombinant human granulocyte colony-stimulating factor on the hematologic recovery and survival of irradiated mice. *Blood* **76:** 445–449.

Tao, M.-H., and Levy, R. (1993). Idiotype/granulocyte-macrophage colony-stimulating factor fusion protein as a vaccine for B-cell lymphoma. *Nature (London)* **362:** 755–758.

Tavernier, J., Devos, R., Cornelis, S., Tuypens, T., Van der Heyden, J., Fiers, W., and Plaetinck, G. (1991). A human high affinity interleukin-5 receptor (IL5R) is composed of an IL5-specific alpha chain and a beta chain shared with the receptor for GM-CSF. *Cell* **66:** 1175–1184.

Taylor, G. R., Reedijk, M., Rothwell, V., Rohrschneider, L., and Pauson, T. (1989a). The unique insert of cellular and viral fms protein tyrosine kinase domain is dispensable for enzymatic and transforming activities. *EMBO Journal* **8:** 2029–2037.

Taylor, K. M., Jagannath, S., Spitzer, G., Spinolo, J. A., Tucker, S. L., Fogel, B., Cabanillas, F. F., Hagemeister, F. B., and Souza, L. M. (1989b). Recombinant human granulocyte colony-stimulating factor hastens granulocyte recovery after high-dose chemotherapy and autologous bone marrow transplantation in Hodgkin's disease. *Journal of Clinical Oncology* **7:** 1791–1799.

Tazi, A., Nioche, S., Chastre, J., Smiejan, J. M., and Hance, A. J. (1991). Spontaneous release of granulocyte colony-stimulating factor (G-CSF) by alveolar macrophages in the course of bacterial pneumonia and sarcoidosis: Endotoxin-dependent and exotoxin-independent G-CSF release by cells recovered by bronchoalveolar lavage. *American Journal of Respiratory Cell and Molecular Biology* **4:** 140–147.

Teshima, T., Shibuya, T., Harada, M., Akashi, K., Taniguchi, S., Okamura, T., and Niho, Y. (1990). Granulocyte-macrophage colony-stimulating factor suppresses induction of neutrophil alkaline phosphatase synthesis by granulocyte colony-stimulating factor. *Experimental Hematology* **18:** 316–321.

Thomas, S., Clark, S. C., Rappeport, J. M., Nathan, D. G., and Emerson, S. G. (1990). Deficient T-cell granulocyte-macrophage colony stimulating factor production in allogeneic bone marrow transplant recipients. *Transplantation* **49:** 703–708.

Thorens, B., Mermod, J.-J., and Vassalli, P. (1987). Phagocytosis and inflammatory stimuli induce GM-CSF mRNA in macrophages through post-transcriptional regulation. *Cell* **48:** 671–679.

Till, J. E., and McCulloch, E. A. (1961). A direct measurement of the radiation sensitivity of normal mouse bone marrow cells. *Radiation Research* **14:** 213–222.

Tobal, K., Pagliuca, A., Bhatt, B., Bailey, N., Layton, D. M., and Mufti, G. S. (1990). Mutation of the human fms gene (M-CSF receptor) in myelodysplastic syndromes and acute myeloid leukemia. *Leukemia* **4:** 486–489.

Toda, H., Murata, A., Matsuura, N., Uda, K., Oka, Y., Tanaka, N., and Mori, T. (1993). Therapeutic efficacy of granulocyte colony stimulating factor against rat cecal ligation and puncture model. *Stem Cells* **11:** 228–234.

Todokoro, K., Yamamoto, A., Amanuma, H., and Ikawa, Y. (1985). Isolation and characterization of a genomic DDD mouse interleukin-3 gene. *Gene* **39:** 103–107.

Toksoz, D., Zsebo, K. M., Smith, K. A., Hu, S., Brankow, D., Suggs, S. V., Martin, F. H., and Williams, D. A. (1992). Support of human hematopoiesis in long-term bone marrow cultures by murine stromal cells selectively expressing the membrane-bound and secreted forms of the human homolog of the Steel gene product, stem cell factor. *Proceedings of the National Academy of Sciences, U.S.A.* **89:** 7350–7354.

Tokumitsu, H., Masuda, E. S., Tsuboi, A., Arai, K., and Arai, N. (1993). Purification of the 120 kDa component of the human nuclear factor of activated T cells (NF-AT): Reconstitution of binding activity to the cis-acting element of the GM-CSF and IL-2 promoter with AP-1. *Biochemical and Biophysical Research Communications* **196:** 737–744.

Tran, H. T. T., Metcalf, D., and Cheers, C. (1990). Anti-bacterial activity of peritoneal cells from transgenic mice producing high levels of GM-CSF. *Immunology* **71:** 377–382.

Trentin, J. J. (1989). Hemopoietic microenvironments. In M. Tavassoli (ed.), *Handbook of the Hemopoietic Microenvironment,* pp. 1–86. Clifton, NJ: Humana.

Trillet-Lenoir, V., Arpin, D., and Brune, J. (1993a). Optimal delivery of dose in cancer chemotherapy with the support of haematopoietic growth factors. *European Journal of Cancer* **29A:** (suppl. 5), S14–S16.

Trillet-Lenoir, V., Green, J., Manegold, C., Von Pawel, J., Gatzemeier, U., Lebeau, B., Depierre, A., Johnson, P., Decoster, G., Tomita, D., and Ewen, C. (1993b). Recombinant granulocyte colony stimulating factor reduces the infectious complications of cytotoxic chemotherapy. *European Journal of Cancer* **29A:** 313–324.

Troutt, A. B., and Kelso, A. (1992). Enumeration of lymphokine mRNA-containing cells *in vivo* in a murine graft-versus-host reaction using the PCR. *Proceedings of the National Academy of Sciences, U.S.A.* **89:** 5276–5280.

Troutt, A. B., and Lee, F. (1989). Tissue distribution of murine hemopoietic growth factor mRNA production. *Journal of Cellular Physiology* **138:** 38–44.

Trudgett, A., McNeill, T. A., and Killen, M. (1973). Granulocyte-macrophage precursor cell and colony-stimulating factor responses of mice infected with Salmonella typhimurium. *Infection and Immunity* **8:** 450–455.

Tsuchiya, M., Asano, S., Kaziro, Y., and Nagata, S. (1986). Isolation and characterization of the cDNA for murine granulocyte colony-stimulating factor. *Proceedings of the National Academy of Sciences, U.S.A.* **83:** 7633–7637.

Tsuchiya, M., Kaziro, Y., and Nagata, S. (1987). The chromosomal gene structure for murine granulocyte colony-stimulating factor. *European Journal of Biochemistry* **165:** 7–12.

Tsujimoto, Y., Finger, L. R., Yunis, J., Nowell, P. C., and Croce, C. M. (1984). Cloning of the chromosome breakpoint of neoplastic B cells with the t(14; 18) chromosome translocation. *Science (Washington)* **226:** 1097–1099.

Tushinski, R. J., Oliver, I. T., Guilbert, L. J., Tynan, P. W., Warner, J. N., and Stanley, E. R. (1982). Survival of mononuclear phagocytes depends on a lineage-specific growth factor that the differentiated cells selectively destroy. *Cell* **28:** 71–81.

Twentyman, P. R., and Wright, K. A. (1991). Failure of GM-CSF to influence the growth of small cell and non-small cell lung cancer cell lines *in vitro*. *European Journal of Cancer* **27:** 6–8.

Urdal, D. L., Mochizuki, D., Conlon, P. J., March, C. J., Remerowski, M. L., Eisenman, J., Ramthun, C., and Gillis, S. (1984). Lymphokine purification by reversed-phase high-performance liquid chromatography. *Journal of Chromatography* **296:** 171–179.

Uzumaki, H., Okabe, T., Sasaki, N., Hagiwara, K., Takaku, F., and Itoh, S. (1988). Characterization of receptor for granulocyte colony-stimulating factor on human circulating neutrophils. *Biochemical and Biophysical Research Communications* **156:** 1026–1032.

Uzumaki, H., Okabe, T., Sasaki, N., Hagiwara, K., Takaku, F., Tobita, M., Yasukawa, K., Ito, S., and Umezawa, Y. (1989). Identification and characterization of receptors for granulocyte colony-stimulating factor on human placenta and trophoblastic cells. *Proceedings of the National Academy of Sciences, U.S.A.* **86:** 9323–9326.

Vadhan-Raj, S., Buescher, S., Broxmeyer, H. E., Le Maistre, A., Lepe-Zuniga, J. L., Ventura, G., Jeha, S., Horwitz, L. J., Trujillo, J. M., Gillis, S., and Hittelman, W. N. (1988). Stimulation of myelopoiesis in patients with aplastic anemia by recombinant human granulocyte-macrophage colony-stimulating factor. *New England Journal of Medicine* **319:** 1628–1634.

Vadhan-Raj, S., Jena, S. S., Buescher, S., LeMaistre, A., Yee, G., Lu, L., Lloreta, J., Hoots, W. K., Hittelman, W. N., Gutterman, J. U., and Broxmeyer, H. E. (1990). Stimulation of myelopoiesis in a patient with congenital neutropenia: Biology and nature of response to recombinant human granulocyte-macrophage colony-stimulating factor. *Blood* **75:** 858–864.

Vadhan-Raj, S., Keating, M., LeMaistre, A., Hittleman, W. N., McCredie, K., Trujillo, J. M., Broxmeyer, H. E., Henney, C., and Gutterman, J. U. (1987). Effects of recombinant human granulocyte-macrophage colony-stimulating factor in patients with myelodysplastic syndrome. *New England Journal of Medicine* **317:** 1545–1552.

Vairo, G., and Hamilton, J. A. (1988). Activation and proliferation signals in murine macrophages: Stimulation of $Na^+$, $K^+$-ATPase activity by hemopoietic growth factors and other agents. *Journal of Cellular Physiology* **134:** 13–24.

Valtieri, M., Tweardy, D. J., Caracciolo, D., Johnson, K., Mavilio, F., Altmann, S., Santoli, D., and Rovera, G. (1987). Cytokine-dependent granulocytic differentiation: Regulation of proliferative and differentiative responses in a murine progenitor cell line. *Journal of Immunology* **138:** 3829–3835.

Van Daalen Wetters, T., Hawkins, S. A., Roussel, M. F., and Sherr, C. J. (1992). Random mutagenesis of CSF-1 receptor (FMS) reveals multiple sites for activating mutations within the extracellular domain. *EMBO Journal* **11:** 551–557.

Van de Pol, C. J., and Garnick, M. B. (1991). Clinical applications of recombinant macrophage-colony stimulating factor (rhM-CSF). *Biotechnology Therapeutics* **2:** 231–239.

Van den Berghe, H., Vermaelen, K., Mecucci, C., Barbieri, D., and Tricot, G. (1985). The 5q- anomaly. *Cancer Genetics and Cytogenetics* **17:** 189–255.

Van der Geer, P., and Hunter, T. (1993). Mutation of Tyr 697, a GRB-2 binding site, and Tyr 721, a PI-3[1]-kinase binding site, abrogates signal transduction by the murine CSF-1 receptor expressed in Rat-2 fibroblasts. *EMBO Journal* **12:** 5161–5172.

Vaux, D. L., Cory, S., and Adams, J. M. (1988). *bcl*-2 gene promotes haemopoietic cell survival and cooperates with *c-myc* to immortalise pre-B cells. *Nature (London)* **335:** 440–442.

Vellenga, E., Rambaldi, A., Ernst, T. J., Ostapovicz, D., and Griffin, J. D. (1988). Independent regulation of M-CSF and G-CSF gene expression in human monocytes. *Blood* **71:** 1529–1532.

Verhoef, G. E. G., De Schouwer, P., Ceuppens, J. L., Van Damme, J., Goossens, W., and Boogaerts, M. A. (1992). Measurement of serum cytokine levels in patients with myelodysplastic syndromes. *Leukemia* **6:** 1268–1272.

Villeval, J.-L., Dührsen, U., Morstyn, G., and Metcalf, D. (1990). Effect of recombinant human granulocyte-macrophage colony-stimulating factor on progenitor cells in patients with advanced malignancies. *British Journal of Haematology* **74:** 36–44.

Visvader, J., and Verma, I. M. (1989). Differential transcription of exon 1 of the human c-fms gene in placental trophoblasts and monocytes. *Molecular and Cellular Biology* **9:** 1336–1341.

von Melchner, H., and Hoffken, K. (1985). Commitment to differentiation of human promyelocytic leukemia cells (HL60): An all-or-none event preceded by reversible losses of self-renewal potential. *Journal of Cellular Physiology* **125:** 573–581.

Wakiyama, H., Tsuru, S., Hata, N., Shinomiya, M., Shinomiya, N., Noritake, M., Umezawa, Y., and Rokutanda, M. (1993). Therapeutic effect of granulocyte colony-stimulating factor and cephem antibiotics against experimental infections in neutropenic mice induced by cyclophosphamide. *Clinical and Experimental Immunology* **92:** 218–224.

Walker, F., and Burgess, A. W. (1985). Specific binding of radioiodinated granulocyte-macrophage colony-stimulating factor to hemopoietic cells. *EMBO Journal* **4:** 933–939.

Walker, F., and Burgess, A. W. (1987). Internalisation and recycling of the granulocyte-macrophage colony-stimulating factor (GM-CSF) receptor on a murine myelomonocytic leukemia. *Journal of Cellular Physiology* **130:** 255–261.

Walker, F., Nicola, N. A., Metcalf, D., and Burgess, A. W. (1985). Hierarchical down-modulation of hemopoietic growth factor receptors. *Cell* **43:** 269–276.

Walter, M. R., Cook, W. J., Ealick, S. E., Nagabhushan, T. L., Trotta, P. P., and Bugg, C. E. (1992). Three-dimensional structure of recombinant human granulocyte- macrophage colony-stimulating factor. *Journal of Molecular Biology* **224:** 1075–1085.

Wang, H. M., Ogorochi, T., Arai, K., and Miyajima, A. (1992). Structure of mouse interleukin-3 (IL-3) binding protein (AIC2A): Amino acid residues critical for IL-3 binding. *Journal of Biological Chemistry* **267:** 979–983.

Wang, Z. E., Myles, G. M., Brandt, C. S., Lioubin, M. N., and Rohrschneider, L. (1993). Identification of the ligand-binding regions in the macrophage colony-stimulating factor receptor extracellular domain. *Molecular and Cellular Biology* **13:** 5348–5359.

Watari, S., Asano, S., Shirafuji, N., Kodo, H., Ozawa, K., Takaku, F., and Kamachi, S. (1989). Serum granulocyte colony-stimulating factor levels in healthy volunteers and patients with various disorders as estimated by enzyme immunoassay. *Blood* **73:** 117–122.

Weber, B., Horiguchi, J., Leubbers, R., Sherman, M., and Kufe, D. (1989). Posttranscriptional stabilization of c-fms mRNA by a labile protein during human monocytic differentiation. *Molecular and Cellular Biology* **9:** 769–775.

Welham, M. J., Duronio, V., Sanghera, J. S., Pelech, S. L., and Schrader, J. W. (1992). Multiple hemopoietic growth factors stimulate activation of mitogen-activated protein kinase family members. *Journal of Immunology* **149:** 1683–1693.

Welte, K., Bonilla, M. A., Gabrilove, J. L., Gillio, A. P., Potter, G. K., Moore, M. A. S., O'Reilly, R. J., Boone, T. C., and Souza, L. M. (1987). Recombinant human granulocyte-colony stimulating factor: *In vitro* and *in vivo* effects on myelopoiesis. *Blood Cells* **13:** 17–30.

Welte, K. E., Platzer, E., Lu, L., Gabrilove, J. L., Levi, E., Mertelsmann, R., and Moore, M. A. S. (1985). Purification and biochemical characterization of human pluripotent hematopoietic colony-stimulating factor. *Proceedings of the National Academy of Sciences, U.S.A.* **82:** 1526–1530.

Welte, K., Zeidler, C., Reiter, A., Müller, W., Odenwald, E., Souza, L., and Riehm, H. (1990). Differential effects of granulocyte-macrophage colony-stimulating factor and granulocyte colony-stimulating factor in children with severe congenital neutropenia. *Blood* **75:** 1056–1063.

Wheeler, E. F., Askew, D., May, S., Ihle, J. N., and Sherr, C. J. (1987). The v-fms oncogene induces factor-independent growth and transformation of the interleukin-3-dependent myeloid cell line FDC-P1. *Molecular and Cellular Biology* **7:** 1673–1680.

Wheeler, E. F., Rettenmier, C. W., Look, A. T., and Sherr, C. J. (1986). The *v-fms* oncogene induces factor independence and tumorigenicity in CSF-1 dependent macrophage cell line. *Nature (London)* **324:** 377–380.

Whetton, A. D., and Dexter, T. M. (1983). Effect of haematopoietic cell growth factor on intracellular ATP levels. *Nature (London)* **303:** 629–631.

Wiktor-Jedrzejczak, W., Ratajczak, M. Z., Ptasznik, A., Sell, K. W., Ahmed-Ansari, A., and Ostertag, W. (1992). CSF-1 deficiency in the op/op mouse has differential effects on macrophage populations and differentiation stages. *Experimental Hematology* **20:** 1004–1010.

Wiktor-Jedrzejczak, W., Urbanowska, E., Aukerman, S. L., Pollard, J. W., Stanley, E. R., Ralph, P., Ansari, A. A., Sell, K. W., and Szperl, M. (1991). Correction by CSF-1 of defects in the osteopetrotic *op/op* mouse suggests local, developmental and humoral requirements for this growth factor. *Experimental Hematology* **19:** 1049–1054.

Willemze, R., van der Lely, N., Zwierzina, H., Suciu, S., Solbu, G., Gerhartz, H., Labar, B., Visani, G., Peetermans, M. E., Jacobs, A., Stryckmans, P.,

Fenaux, P., Haak, H. L., Ribeiro, M. M., Baumelou, E., Baccarani, M., Mandelli, F., Jaksic, B., Louwagie, A., Thyss, A., Hayat, M., de Cataldo, F., Stern, A. C., and Zittoun, R. (1993). A randomized Phase I/II multicenter study of recombinant human granulocyte-macrophage colony-stimulating factor (GM-CSF) therapy for patients with myelodysplastic syndromes and a relatively low risk of acute leukemia. *Annals of Hematology* **64:** 173-180.

Williams, D. E., Eisenman, J., Baird, A., Rauch, C., Van Ness, K., March, C. J., Park, L. S., Martin, U., Mochizuki, D. Y., Boswell, H. S., Burgess, G. S., Cosman, D., and Lyman, S. D. (1990a). Identification of a ligand for the c-kit proto-oncogene. *Cell* **63:** 167-174.

Williams, G. T., Smith, C. A., Spooncer, E., Dexter, T. M., and Taylor, D. R. (1990b). Haemopoietic colony stimulating factors promote cell survival by suppressing apoptosis. *Nature (London)* **343:** 76-79.

Williamson, D. J., Begley, C. G., Vadas, M. A., and Metcalf, D. (1988). The detection and initial characterization of colony-stimulating factors in synovial fluid. *Clinical and Experimental Immunology* **72:** 67-73.

Willman, C. L., Sever, C. E., Pallavicini, M. G., Harada, H., Tanaka, N., Slovak, M. L., Yamamoto, H., Harada, K., Meeker, T. C., List, A. F., and Taniguchi, T. (1993). Deletion of IRF-1, mapping to chromosome 5q31.1, in human leukemia and preleukemic myelodysplasia. *Science (Washington)* **259:** 968-971.

Wing, E. J., Magee, D. M., Whiteside, T. L., Kaplan, S. S., and Shadduck, R. K. (1989). Recombinant human granulocyte/macrophage colony-stimulating factor enhances monocyte cytotoxicity and secretion of tumor necrosis factor $\alpha$ and interferon in cancer patients. *Blood* **73:** 643-646.

Witmer-Pack, M. D., Hughes, D. A., Schuler, G., Lawson, L., McWilliam, A., Inaba, K., Steinman, R. M., and Gordon, S. (1993). Identification of macrophage and dendritic cells in the osteopetrotic (op/op) mouse. *Journal of Cellular Science* **104:** 1021-1029.

Wodnar-Filipowicz, A., Heusser, C. H., and Moroni, C. (1989). Production of the haemopoietic growth factors GM-CSF and interleukin-3 by mast cells in response to IgE receptor-mediated activation. *Nature (London)* **339:** 150-152.

Wong, G. G., Temple, P. A., Leary, A. C., Witek-Giannotti, J. S., Yang, Y-C., Ciarletta, A. B., Chung, M., Murtha, D., Kriz, R., Kaufman, R. J., Ferenz, C. R., Sibley, B. S., Turner, K. J., Hewick, R. M., Clark, S. C., Yanai, N., Yokota, H., Yamada, M., Saito, M., Motoyoshi, K., and Takaku, F. (1987). Human CSF-1: Molecular cloning and expression of 4kb encoding the human urinary protein. *Science (Washington)* **235:** 1504-1508.

Wong, G. G., Witek, J. S., Temple, P. A., Wilkens, K. M., Leary, A. G., Luxenberg, D. P., Jones, S. S., Brown, E. L., Kay, R. M., Orr, E. C., Shoemaker, C., Golde, D. W., Kaufmann, R. J., Hewick, R. M., Wang, E. A., and Clark, S. C. (1985). Human GM-CSF: Molecular cloning of the complementary DNA and purification of the natural and recombinant proteins. *Science (Washington)* **228:** 810-815.

Woolford, J., McAuliffe, A., and Rohrschneider, L. R. (1988). Activation of the feline c-fms proto-oncogene: Multiple alterations are required to generate a fully transformed phenotype. *Cell* **55:** 965-977.

Yamada, H., Iwase, S., Mohri, M., and Kufe, D. (1991). Involvement of a nuclear factor-kappa B-like protein in induction of the macrophage colony-stimulating factor gene by tumor necrosis factor. *Blood* **78:** 1988-1995.

Yamanishi, K., Randawa, Z. I., Brown, D., Masui, Y., Yasuda, S., Takahashi, M., and Adachi, M. (1993). Structural analysis of recombinant human carboxyl-terminal-truncated macrophage colony-stimulating factor. *Journal of Biochemistry (Tokyo)* **113:** 81–87.

Yang, Y.-C., Ciarletta, A. B., Temple, P. A., Chung, M. P., Kovacic, S., Witek-Giannotti, J. S., Leary, A. C., Kriz, R., Donahue, R. E., Wong, G. G., and Clark, S. C. (1986). Human IL-3 (Multi-CSF): Identification by expression cloning of a novel hematopoietic growth factor related to murine IL-3. *Cell* **47:** 3–10.

Yang, Y. C., Kovacic, S., Kriz, R., Wolf, S., Clark, S. C., Wellems, T. E., Nienhuis, A., and Epstein, N. (1988). The human genes for GM-CSF and IL3 are closely linked in tandem on chromosome 5. *Blood* **71:** 958–961.

Yasuda, H., Ajiki, Y., Shimozato, T., Kasahara, M., Kawada, H., Iwata, M., and Shimizu, K. (1990). Therapeutic efficacy of granulocyte colony-stimulating factor alone and in combination with antibiotics against *Pseudomonas aeruginosa* infections in mice. *Infection and Immunity* **58:** 2502–2509.

Ymer, S., Tucker, W. Q., Sanderson, C. J., Hapel, A. J., Campbell, H. D., and Young, I. G. (1985). Constitutive synthesis of interleukin-3 by leukaemia cell line WEHI-3B is due to retroviral insertion near the gene. *Nature (London)* **317:** 255–258.

Yokota, T., Lee, F., Rennick, D., Hall, C., Arai, N., Mosmann, T., Nabel, G., Cantor, H., and Arai, K. (1984). Isolation and characterisation of a mouse cDNA clone that expresses mast cell growth factor activity in monkey cells. *Proceedings of the National Academy of Sciences, U.S.A.* **81:** 1070–1074.

Yong, K., Salooja, N., Donahue, R. E., Hedge, U., and Linch, D. C. (1992). Human macrophage colony-stimulating factor levels are elevated in pregnancy and in immune thrombocytopenia. *Blood* **80:** 2897–2902.

Yonish-Rouach, E., Resnitzky, D., Lotem, J., Sachs, L., Kimchi, A., and Oren, M. (1991). Wild-type p53 induces apoptosis of myeloid leukaemic cells that is inhibited by interleukin-6. *Nature (London)* **352:** 345–347.

Yoshida, H., Hayashi, S., Kunisada, T., Ogawa, M., Nishkawa, S., Okamura, H., Sudo, T., Shultz, L. D., and Nishikawa, S. (1990). The murine mutation osteopetrosis is in the coding region of the macrophage colony stimulating factor gene. *Nature (London)* **345:** 442–444.

Yoshida, H., Hirashima, K., Asano, S., and Takaku, F. (1991). A phase II trial of recombinant human granulocyte colony-stimulating factor in the myelodysplastic syndromes. *British Journal of Haematology* **78:** 378–384.

Young, D. C., and Griffin, J. D. (1986). Autocrine secretion of GM-CSF in acute myeloblastic leukemia. *Blood* **68:** 1178–1181.

Young, D. C., Wagner, K., and Griffin, J. D. (1987). Constitutive expression of the granulocyte-macrophage colony-stimulating factor gene in acute myeloblastic leukemia. *Journal of Clinical Investigation* **79:** 100–106.

Yue, X., Favot, P., Dunn, T. L., Cassady, A. I., and Hume, D. A. (1993). Expression of mRNA encoding the macrophage colony-stimulating factor receptor (c-fms) is controlled by a constitutive promoter and tissue-specific transcription elongation. *Molecular and Cellular Biology* **13:** 3191–3201.

Yujiri, T., Shinohara, K., and Kurimoto, F. (1992). Fluctuations in serum cytokine levels in the patient with cyclic neutropenia. *American Journal of Hematology* **39:** 144–145.

Zenke, G., Lokker, N. A., Strittmatter, U., Fagg, B., Geisse, S., Huber, W. G., and Kocher, H. P. (1991). Purification and characterization of natural human interleukin-3. *Lymphokine and Cytokine Research* **10:** 329–335.

Zhu, N., Liggitt, D., Liu, Y., and Debs, R. (1993). Systemic gene expression after intravenous DNA delivery into adult mice. *Science (Washington)* **261:** 209–211.

Ziegler, I., Hultner, L., Egger, D., Kempkes, B., Mailhammer, R., Gillis, S., and Rodl, W. (1993). In a concerted action kit ligand and interleukin 3 control the synthesis of serotonin in murine bone marrow-derived mast cells: Up-regulation of GTP cyclohydrolase I and tryptophan 5-monooxygenase activity by the kit ligand. *Journal of Biological Chemistry* **268:** 12544–12551.

Ziltener, H. J., Clark-Lewis, I., Fazekas de St Groth, B., Hood, L. E., Kent, S. B., and Schrader, J. W. (1987). Antipeptide antibodies define the NH2-terminal structure of the pan-specific hemopoietin interleukin 3. *Journal of Immunology* **138:** 1105–1108.

Ziltener, H. J., Clark-Lewis, I., Fazekas de St Groth, B., Orban, P. C., Hood, L. E., Kent, S. B., and Schrader, J. W. (1988a). Monoclonal antipeptide antibodies recognize IL-3 and neutralize its bioactivity in vivo. *Journal of Immunology* **140:** 1182–1187.

Ziltener, H. J., Fazekas de St Groth, B., Leslie, K. B., and Schrader, J. W. (1988b). Multiple glycosylated forms of T cell-derived interleukin 3 (IL-3): Heterogeneity of IL-3 from physiological and nonphysiological sources. *Journal of Biological Chemistry* **263:** 14511–14517.

Zsebo, K. M., Wypych, J., McNiece, I. K., Lu, H. S., Smith, K. A., Kakare, S. B., Sachdev, R. K., Yuschenkoff, V. N., Birkett, N. C., Williams, L. R., Satyagal, V. N., Tung, W., Bosselman, R. A., Mendiaz, E. A., and Langley, K. E. (1990). Identification, purification and biological characterization of hematopoietic stem cell factor from Buffalo rat liver-conditioned medium. *Cell* **63:** 195–201.

Zucali, J. R., Dinarello, C. A., Oblon, D. J., Gross, M. A., Anderson, L., and Weiner, R. S. (1986). Interleukin-1 stimulates fibroblasts to produce granulocyte-macrophage colony-stimulating activity and prostaglandin E. *Journal of Clinical Investigation* **77:** 1857–1863.

# Index